Evidence-Based Critical Care: A Case-Based Approach

Evidence-Based Critical Care: A Case-Based Approach

Edited by Ronan Holland

AMERICAN
MEDICAL PUBLISHERS
www.americanmedicalpublishers.com

American Medical Publishers,
41 Flatbush Avenue,
1st Floor, New York,
NY 11217, USA

Visit us on the World Wide Web at:
www.americanmedicalpublishers.com

ISBN: 978-1-63927-101-6

Cataloging-in-Publication Data

Evidence-based critical care : a case-based approach / edited by Ronan Holland.
p. cm.
Includes bibliographical references and index.
ISBN 978-1-63927-101-6
1. Critical care medicine. 2. Emergency medicine. 3. Intensive care units.
4. Medical emergencies. I. Holland, Ronan.

RC86.7 .C75 2022

616.028--dc23

Table of Contents

Preface

The medical specialty that deals with the care of patients suffering from injuries or illnesses that require immediate medical attention is known as emergency medicine. It is also referred to as accident and emergency medicine. The field is concerned with immediate recognition, care, examination and stabilization of patients in the phase of acute injury and illness. Critical care, hyperbaric medicine, disaster medicine, sports medicine, ultrasonography and aerospace medicine are some of the sub-fields of this discipline. Critical care refers to the identification and management of patients that are at risk of or are recovering from life-threatening conditions. It involves the study of some crucial aspects like invasive monitoring techniques, life support, resuscitation and end-of-life care. Emergency medicine is an upcoming field of medicine that has undergone rapid development over the past few decades. The book studies, analyses and upholds the pillars of this discipline and its utmost significance in modern times. As this field is emerging at a rapid pace, the contents of this book will help the readers understand the modern concepts and applications of the subject.

This book is a comprehensive compilation of works of different researchers from varied parts of the world. It includes valuable experiences of the researchers with the sole objective of providing the readers (learners) with a proper knowledge of the concerned field. This book will be beneficial in evoking inspiration and enhancing the knowledge of the interested readers.

In the end, I would like to extend my heartiest thanks to the authors who worked with great determination on their chapters. I also appreciate the publisher's support in the course of the book. I would also like to deeply acknowledge my family who stood by me as a source of inspiration during the project.

Editor

1

Associations between bolus infusion of hydrocortisone, glycemic variability and insulin infusion rate variability in critically ill patients under moderate glycemic control

Roosmarijn T. M. van Hooijdonk[1*], Jan M. Binnekade[1], Lieuwe D. J. Bos[1,2], Janneke Horn[1], Nicole P. Juffermans[1,2], Ameen Abu-Hanna[3] and Marcus J. Schultz[1,2]

Abstract

Background: We retrospectively studied associations between bolus infusion of hydrocortisone and variability of the blood glucose level and changes in insulin rates in intensive care unit (ICU) patients.

Methods: 'Glycemic variability' and 'insulin infusion rate variability' were calculated from and expressed as the standard deviation (SD) of all blood glucose levels and insulin infusion rates during stay in the ICU, respectively. Glycemic and insulin infusion rate variability in patients who received bolus infusion of hydrocortisone were compared to those in patients who never received bolus infusion of hydrocortisone. Multivariate analysis was performed to correct for potential covariates including disease severity.

Results: We included 6409 patients over 6 years; of them 962 received bolus infusion of hydrocortisone. Compared to patients who never received bolus infusion of hydrocortisone, patients who received hydrocortisone had their blood glucose level measured more frequently, had higher glycemic variability; were more frequently treated with intravenous insulin and had higher insulin infusion rate variability. The association between hydrocortisone treatment and glycemic variability was independent of disease severity, but the effect of hydrocortisone treatment on blood glucose variability was less strong in the more severely ill patients. The association between hydrocortisone and insulin infusion rate variability was also independent of disease severity, and independent of glycemic variability.

Conclusions: Bolus infusion of hydrocortisone is independently associated with higher glycemic variability and higher insulin infusion rate variability in ICU patients. Studies are needed to see if continuous infusion of hydrocortisone prevents higher glycemic variability and higher insulin infusion rate variability.

Keywords: Hydrocortisone, Bolus infusion, Blood glucose control, Glycemic control, Blood glucose variability, Insulin, Insulin infusion rate variability

Background

Low-dose hydrocortisone treatment is an accepted therapy for patients with refractory shock [1]. Bolus infusion of hydrocortisone, however, could induce short episodes of hyperglycemia frequently requiring temporary adjustments of the insulin infusion rate in critically ill patients [2, 3]. While experienced intensive care unit (ICU) nurses usually are capable of preventing large swings in the blood glucose level [4], they could be less skilled in avoiding hydrocortisone-induced dysglycemia. Furthermore, preventing hydrocortisone-induced dysglycemia could largely increase nurse labor and costs associated with blood glucose monitoring, as temporary adjustments of insulin infusion rates could also increase the frequency of blood glucose measurements [3, 5].

*Correspondence: r.t.vanhooijdonk@amc.uva.nl
[1] Department of Intensive Care Medicine, Academic Medical Center, University of Amsterdam, Meibergdreef 9, 1105 AZ Amsterdam, The Netherlands
Full list of author information is available at the end of the article

Notably, glycemic variability is associated with increased mortality in critically ill patients [6].

It is unknown to what extent bolus infusion of hydrocortisone increases glycemic variability and adjustments in insulin infusion rates in patients under moderate glycemic control. Therefore, in a cohort of patients receiving blood glucose control aiming at blood glucose levels between 90 and 144 mg/dL, we tested the two following hypotheses: (a) bolus infusion of hydrocortisone is associated with glycemic variability, and (b) bolus infusion of hydrocortisone is associated with insulin infusion rate variability.

Methods

Study design

This was a retrospective cohort study performed in a 32-bed mixed medical-surgical ICU in a university hospital in the Netherlands (the Academic Medical Center, Amsterdam, The Netherlands). The Institutional Review Board approved the study protocol and waived the need for individual patient consent or ethical approval to collect and analyze data from registries that exclude patient-identifying information.

Study setting

The ICU was a closed-format unit with patients under the direct care of a team of board-certified ICU nurses and physicians. The nurse to patient ratio was 1:2. All beds were equipped with the MetaVision® patient data management system (iMDsoft, Tel Aviv, Israel) in which all blood glucose levels and insulin infusion rates were stored automatically.

Blood glucose control

The local guideline for moderate blood glucose control did not change during the period of data collection, and has been described before [7–9]. In short, experienced ICU nurses carefully titrated insulin aiming at a blood glucose level between 90 and 144 mg/dL. For this, continuous insulin infusion was started when the blood glucose level exceeded 144 mg/dL, and adjustments were made following a flow chart (see Additional file 1). Insulin infusion was stopped, and a bolus of 50 mL dextrose 20 % was given when the blood glucose level dropped <63 mg/dL. The flow chart provided recommendations regarding timing of follow-up blood glucose measurement, which could vary from 20 min to 4 h. Blood glucose levels were exclusively measured in blood samples obtained via an arterial catheter using a RapidLab 1265 blood gas analyzer (Siemens Healthcare Diagnostics, The Hague, The Netherlands) located in the ICU.

Indications for and protocol of hydrocortisone therapy

Indications for bolus infusions of hydrocortisone did not change during the period of data collection. ICU physicians prescribed bolus infusion of hydrocortisone in patients with refractory shock, defined as shock that was non-responsive to fluid resuscitation and poorly responsive to vasopressor therapy. Bolus infusion of hydrocortisone started at 100 mg every 8 h for 1 week, after which it was slowly tapered, according to international guidelines [10]. Bolus infusion of hydrocortisone was also initiated in patients with proven or suspected adrenal insufficiency, e.g., patients who received longstanding treatment with glucocorticosteroids before ICU admission.

Study population

The study cohort consisted of patients admitted to the ICU during a six-year period, lasting from January 2007 to December 2012. Patients <18 years old, readmitted patients and patients who were discharged alive within 24 h were excluded from the analysis. Furthermore, we excluded patients who had their blood glucose level measured fewer than three times during the entire stay in the ICU. Finally, patients who received treatment with glucocorticosteroids other than hydrocortisone, and patients who received continuous infusion instead of bolus infusion of hydrocortisone were excluded.

Data collected

Blood glucose levels, insulin infusion rates and boluses of hydrocortisone were extracted from the patient data management system. Demographic data were extracted from the National Intensive Care Evaluation (NICE) database, a validated database with high quality of data maintained by the NICE Foundation [11], including gender, age, length, weight, admission diagnosis, admission type, the Acute Physiology and Chronic Health Evaluation (APACHE) II score [12], ICU length of stay, hospital length of stay, ICU and hospital mortality.

Primary and secondary endpoints

The primary endpoint was glycemic variability. The secondary endpoints were the insulin infusion rate variability and the number of blood glucose measurements during stay in ICU. Glycemic variability was calculated from and expressed as the SD of all blood glucose levels per patient over the entire stay in ICU, as described before [6, 13] and as recommended in the consensus guidelines [14]. We chose to use the SD, as this is the most frequently used metric for glycemic variability. Insulin infusion rate variability was calculated from and expressed as the SD of insulin infusion rates per patient over the entire stay in ICU.

Power analysis

We did not perform a power calculation, as this was a retrospective observational exploratory analysis. We assumed to have sufficient numbers of patients when including the whole cohort over a period of 6 years.

Analysis plan

Demographic, blood glucose and insulin metrics were summarized and compared between patients who did and did not receive a bolus infusion of hydrocortisone during ICU admission. Data were compared using the Student's *t* test, the Mann–Whitney *U* test or the Chi-Square test. Statistical significance was considered to be at a *P* value <0.05. When appropriate, statistical uncertainty was expressed by the 95 % confidence levels.

We used univariate and multivariate linear regression analysis to test whether bolus infusion of hydrocortisone was independently associated with increased glycemic variability and insulin infusion rate variability. For this, glycemic variability was logarithmically transformed (using the natural logarithm) to obtain a more normal distribution. We categorized insulin infusion rate variability to 'no insulin infusion rate variability' (which included patients who never received insulin during the entire stay in ICU, and patients with fewer than three changes in the insulin infusion rate), and the three tertiles of the SD of the insulin infusion rate.

Thus, two separate multivariate models were developed, one model for glycemic variability and one model for insulin infusion rate variability. We first investigated if disease severity, expressed as the APACHE II score, was a significant interaction term with hydrocortisone. We stratified for the APACHE II scores into three groups [15, 16], when the *P* value of the interaction term was significant and the model fit improved (based on Akaike Information Criterion). The models included variables that were established as confounders [17]. A confounder was defined as a variable that is not on the casual path between hydrocortisone infusion and glycemic or insulin variability. Thus, for instance, we did not include vasopressor use as we considered it likely that vasopressor use is on the casual path. The following variables were tested for confounding: gender, BMI and type of admission (non-surgical, elective surgery, emergency surgery). All these variables met the theoretical criteria for confounding because they are (surrogate) causes or risk factors of outcome; and associated with the exposure (but not affected by it) [17].

Correlation between covariates was assessed to investigate collinearity. Pearson correlation coefficients were all under 0.5 showing no significant collinearity. The effect of covariates on the glucose variability was reported as the percentage of change in the glucose variability with the confidence interval. The effects of covariates on the insulin infusion rate variability were reported as odds ratios with the 95 % confidence interval. This odds ratios represent the odds of having a high insulin infusion rate variability (the highest tertile of the SD) compared to having no variability, or a small or moderate insulin infusion rate variability (the lowest and middle tertile of the SD), the odds of having moderate and high insulin infusion rate variability versus no or small insulin infusion rate variability, and the odds of having small, moderate and high insulin infusion variability rate versus having no variability. Finally, an ordinal regression was made to test if bolus infusion of hydrocortisone, independently of glycemic variability, was associated with insulin infusion rate variability.

In a post hoc analysis, we used the glycemic lability index (GLI) for glycemic variability, as this metric for glycemic variability takes into account the time interval between measurements [18]. The median GLI per day per patient was used in the analysis.

Diabetic status can be a potential confounder, but diabetic status was not captured, or captured incompletely, in the first 2 years of the cohort. We performed a second post hoc analysis, including only patients in whom diabetic status was reliably captured.

Analyses were performed using R (version: 3.1.1; R Foundation for Statistical Computing, Vienna, Austria).

Results

Patients

Of 11,946 patients 4638 met the exclusion criteria for the present analysis (Fig. 1). One hundred eighty patients had fewer than three blood glucose measurements available, necessary to calculate glycemic variability, and 718 patients received treatment with other glucocorticosteroids than hydrocortisone. Continuous infusion of hydrocortisone was never used. Table 1 shows demographic data of the remaining 6409 patients. Patients treated with hydrocortisone were older, more severely ill according to APACHE II scores, more often non-surgical patients and died more frequently.

Blood glucose metrics and insulin infusion metrics

Hypoglycemia and hyperglycemic measurements were more frequently found in patients treated with bolus infusions of hydrocortisone (Table 2). Glycemic variability was higher in patients who received hydrocortisone. The total number of blood glucose measurements during stay in ICU, and the median number of blood glucose measurements per day was higher in patients who received hydrocortisone.

Patients treated with bolus infusions of hydrocortisone were treated with insulin more frequently (Table 3). They

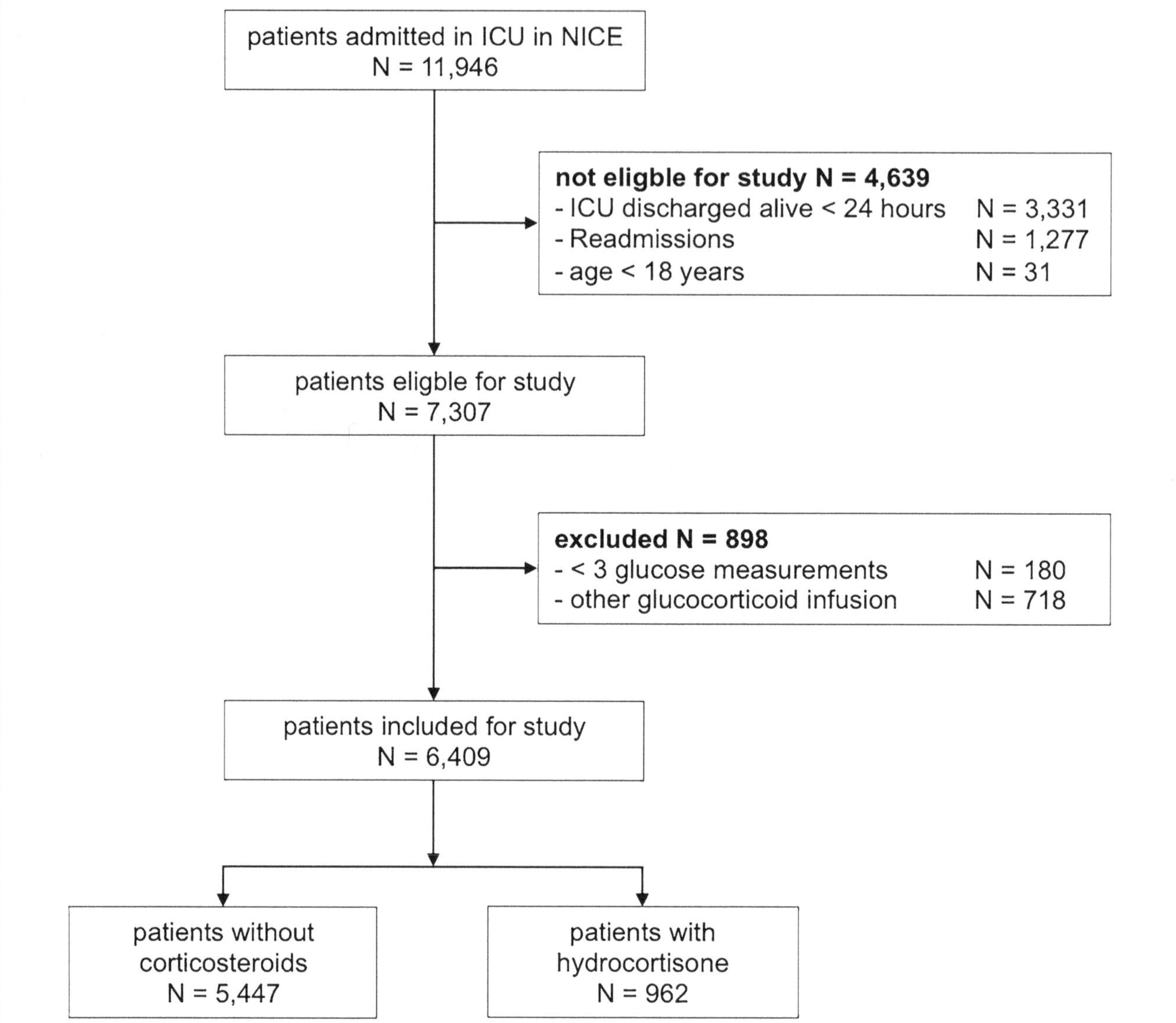

Fig. 1 CONSORT diagram of the study

received more boluses of insulin, and had more frequent adjustments in the insulin infusion rate. Consequently, they had higher insulin infusion rate variability.

Univariate and multivariate analyses

Tables 4 and 5 detail the results for the univariate and multivariate analyses. For all the three models, APACHE II score was a significant interaction term and therefore the analysis was stratified per APACHE II score category. In all three APACHE II score categories, bolus infusion of hydrocortisone was independently associated with higher glycemic variability expressed as the SD, though the effect was less strong in more severely ill patients.

Patients who received bolus infusion of hydrocortisone had higher odds of having higher insulin infusion rate variability, independently of confounders. The association between bolus infusion of hydrocortisone and insulin infusion rate variability remained statistically significant when glycemic variability was included as confounder.

Post hoc analyses

In the first post hoc analysis, bolus infusion of hydrocortisone was independently associated with higher GLI in the group of patients with APACHE II score between 15 and 24 (Additional file 1: Table S1). Entering GLI as confounder between bolus infusion of hydrocortisone and

Table 1 Patient characteristics

Characteristics	Patients who did not receive bolus infusion of hydrocortisone (N = 5447)	Patients who received bolus infusion of hydrocortisone (N = 962)	P value	Total cohort (N = 6409)
Age (years, median [IQR])	63 [51–73]	65 [55–74]	<0.001	63 [52–73]
Male gender [no (%)]	3431 (63.0)	571 (59.4)	0.035	4002 (62.4)
BMI (kg/m^2, median [IQR])	25 [23–28]	25 [23–29]	0.968	25 [23–28]
Admission diagnosis [no (%)]			<0.001	
Non-surgical	2159 (39.6)	542 (56.3)		2701 (42.1)
Emergency surgery	993 (18.2)	200 (20.8)		1193 (18.6)
Elective surgery	2295 (42.1)	220 (22.9)		2515 (39.2)
History of diabetes [no (%)]				
Diabetes	550 (14.7)	102 (16.5)	0.281	652 (15.0)
Non diabetes	3188 (85.3)	517 (83.5)		3705 (85.0)
Missing values	1709	343		2052
APACHE II scores (median [IQR])	18 [14–24}	24 [19–30]	<0.001	19 [14–25]
SAPS II score	40 [31–52]	55 [44–67]	<0.001	42 [32–54]
ICU LOS (days, median [IQR])	2 [1–4]	6 [3–12]	<0.001	3 [2–5]
Hospital LOS (days, median [IQR])	10 [6–20]	16 [8–36]	<0.001	11 [6–22]
ICU mortality [no (%)]	658 (12.1)	306 (31.8)	<0.001	961 (15.0)
Hospital mortality [no (%)]	944 (17.3)	391 (40.6)	<0.001	1335 (20.8)

APACHE acute physiology and chronic health evaluation, *BMI* body mass index, *ICU* intensive care unit, *IQR* interquartile range, *LOS* length of stay

Table 2 Blood glucose metrics

	Patients who did not receive bolus infusion of hydrocortisone (N = 5447)	Patients who received bolus infusion of hydrocortisone (N = 962)	P value	Total cohort (N = 6409)
Number of measurements (median [IQR])	20 [13–35]	53 [30–97]	<0.001	22 [13–42]
Median number of measurements per day (median [IQR])	6 [5–8]	7 [6–9]	<0.001	6 [5–8]
Median number of measurements per day with hydrocortisone (median [IQR])		8 [7–10]		
Median number of measurements per day without hydrocortisone (median [IQR])		6 [4–7]		
Mean blood glucose level (mg/dL, median [IQR])	136 [125–148]	136 [127–148]	0.043	136 [126–148]
Median blood glucose level (mg/dL, median [IQR])	132 [122–144]	132 [123–141]	0.588	132 [123–144]
Standard deviation of blood glucose level (mg/dL, median [IQR])	28 [20–39]	35 [26–47]	<0.001	29 [21–40]
Glycemic Lability Index (mg/dL^2/hour/day median [IQR])	942 [371–2236]	1322 [594–2883]	<0.001	994 [400–2369]
Maximum blood glucose level (mg/dL, median [IQR])	193 [166–234]	231 [193–285]	<0.001	198 [169–241]
Minimum blood glucose level (mg/dL, median [IQR])	90 [77–101]	70 [56–85]	<0.001	88 [74–99]
Mild hypoglycemia, <70 mg/dL (%)	826 (15.2)	451 (46.9)	<0.001	1277 (19.9)
Severe hypoglycemia, <40 mg/dL (%)	115 (2.1)	80 (8.3)	<0.001	195 (3.0)
Hyperglycemia, >180 mg/dL (%)	3438 (63.1)	824 (85.7)	<0.001	4262 (66.5)

IQR interquartile range, *IU* international units

Table 3 Insulin metrics

	Patients who did not receive bolus infusion of hydrocortisone (N = 5447)	Patients who received infusion of hydrocortisone (N = 962)	P value	Total cohort (N = 6409)
Patients receiving insulin infusion [no (%)]	3693 (67.8)	875 (91.0)	<0.001	4568 (71.3)
Patients receiving boluses of insulin infusion [no (%)]	490 (9.0)	248 (25.8)	<0.001	738 (11.5)
Number of insulin rate adjustments (median [IQR])	3 [0–8]	17 [6–35]	<0.001	4 [0–12]
Median number of insulin rates per day (median [IQR])	1 [0–2]	2 [1–3]	<0.001	1 [0–2]
Median number of insulin rates per day with hydrocortisone (median [IQR])		3 [1–4]		
Median number of insulin rates per day without hydrocortisone (median [IQR])		1 [0–2]		
Patients in insulin infusion rate variability category:				
No insulin infusion rate variability	2494 (45.8)	136 (14.1)		2630 (41.0)
Small insulin infusion rate variability	887 (16.3)	111 (11.5)		998 (15.6)
Moderate insulin infusion rate variability	1104 (20.3)	260 (27.0)		1364 (21.3)
High insulin infusion rate variability	962 (17.7)	455 (47.3)		1417 (22.1)
Standard deviation of insulin rate (IU/h, median [IQR])	0.6 [0–1.3]	1.6 [0.8–6.2]	<0.001	0.7 [0–1.6]

IQR interquartile range, *IU* international units

Table 4 Results of univariate and multivariate analysis with glycemic variability

Variable	Univariate		Multivariate	
	Percentage of change in glycemic variability [95 % CI]	P value	Percentage of change in glycemic variability [95 % CI]	P value
APACHE II score <15				
Bolus infusion of hydrocortisone	20 [5 – 36]	0.008	23 [8 – 40][a]	0.0018
APACHE II score 15–24				
Bolus infusion of hydrocortisone	22 [16 – 29]	<0.001	23 [16 – 30][b]	< 0.001
APACHE II score >24				
Bolus infusion of hydrocortisone	15 [8–21]	<0.001	14 [8–20][c]	< 0.001

APACHE acute physiology and chronic health evaluation, *BMI* body mass index, *CI* confidence interval

[a] Multivariate model includes the significant confounders Admission Type, and BMI

[b] Multivariate model includes the significant confounders Admission Type, gender and BMI

[c] Multivariate model includes the significant confounders Admission Type, and gender

insulin infusion rate variability did not affect the association (Additional file 1: Table S2).

In the second post hoc analysis, including only patients in whom diabetic status was reliably captured, the association between bolus infusion of hydrocortisone and glycemic and insulin variability remained statistically significant when diabetic status was included as confounder (Additional file 1: Tables S3, S4).

Discussion

The results of this retrospective analysis of blood glucose levels and insulin infusion rates in ICU patients under moderate glycemic control show that bolus infusion of hydrocortisone is associated with higher glycemic variability and insulin rate variability, more frequent BG measurements and a greater need for insulin boluses. These associations were independent of several factors,

Table 5 Results of univariate and multivariate analysis with insulin infusion rate variability

Variable	Univariate	Multivariate	Multivariate including glycemic variability
	Odds ratio [95 % CI]	Odds ratio [95 % CI]	Odds ratio [95 % CI]
APACHE II score <15			
Bolus infusion of hydrocortisone	3.8 [2.4–6.0]	4.2 [2.6–6.7][a]	4.1 [2.5–6.7]
APACHE II score 15–24			
Bolus infusion of hydrocortisone	4.0 [3.3–4.9]	4.0 [3.3–4.9]	3.6 [2.9–4.4]
APACHE II score >24			
Bolus infusion of hydrocortisone	3.1 [2.6–3.7]	3.1 [2.6–3.7]	3.1 [2.5–3.7]

APACHE acute physiology and chronic health evaluation, *BMI* body mass index, *CI* confidence interval

[a] Multivariate model includes the significant confounder BMI

including severity of disease and also diabetic status. One salient finding in the present analysis was that the associations between bolus infusions of hydrocortisone and glycemic variability and insulin infusion rate variability were less strong in patients who were more severely ill. It could be that the impact of severity of disease on variability of the blood glucose level and the insulin infusion rate is much stronger than the impact of bolus infusions of hydrocortisone. This could partly blur the associations, which we were interested in. Furthermore, when GLI was used to express glycemic variability, the independent association between bolus infusion and glycemic variability was significant only in patients with an APACHE II score between 15 and 24. The GLI takes into account the time interval and SD does not, which might explain the different results. Still, both measures do not capture all glucose excursions, as we were not continuously measuring the glucose level and thereby missing, by definition, blood glucose excursions between two glucose measurements.

We chose to develop a metric for insulin infusion rate variability, a new metric, based on the standard deviation similar to the one we used for glycemic variability. It should be noticed that insulin infusion rate variability may not reflect changes in insulin resistance or insulin sensitivity, but it could be a measure indicating changes in nursing workload. This was exactly the reason for developing this new metric, as most other metrics in the domain of blood glucose control do not consider workload by nurses. The number of measurements per day was considered before as measure indicating the nursing workload [3]. However, it is not only the blood glucose measurements which is time consuming, also the interpretation of the blood glucose measurement and the change in the insulin infusion pump takes time. In addition, trained nurses are necessary to perform the blood glucose control or when available decision support could be used.

The results are, at least in part, in line with those from several previous studies. First, in a randomized controlled study in cardiac surgery patients, peroperative treatment with dexamethasone was associated with elevated blood glucose levels for as long as 15 h after surgery, requiring more intensive treatment with insulin [19]. In addition, in a double-blind placebo-controlled randomized study, it was shown that treatment with methylprednisolone was associated with higher blood glucose levels and higher daily insulin doses in patients with COPD exacerbation needing mechanical ventilation [20]. Interestingly, a recent randomized study comparing bolus infusion with continuous infusion of hydrocortisone in septic shock patients showed no differences in the mean blood glucose level, but more hyperglycemic events and more frequent changes in the insulin infusion rate were found in patients receiving bolus infusion of hydrocortisone [3]. Higher glycemic variability was found in patients treated with hydrocortisone, although the difference with patients not treated with hydrocortisone remained statistically insignificant, probably due to the small sample size of fewer than 50 patients. Furthermore, the dosing regimen was different as they used a dose of 50 mg every 6 h opposed to our regimen of 100 mg hydrocortisone every 8 h. It is possible that the higher doses of hydrocortisone in the present study result in greater glucose variability and this might be the reason why we did find an independent association. Our investigation confirms the results of the randomized controlled trial [3] that bolus infusion of hydrocortisone indeed influences glycemic variability and insulin infusion dosing.

It was a practice to infuse a bolus of hydrocortisone every 8 h, and because of its relatively short half-life time of 90 min, we could have expected large swings in blood glucose levels and or insulin infusion rates with this treatment, depending on how the local guideline of glucose control allowed changes in the insulin infusion rate. We were specifically interested in associations between hydrocortisone therapy and glycemic variability, as glycemic variability is considered as one of the domains for quality of blood glucose control and associated with mortality [6, 21]. Previous studies investigating the effect of bolus hydrocortisone on the blood glucose levels in septic shock patients focused on hyperglycemia and not glycemic variability [2, 3, 22]. We are the first to show an independent association between bolus infusion of hydrocortisone and glycemic variability in a large cohort of critically ill patients, though the question remains whether prevention of bolus infusion of hydrocortisone-induced dysglycemia is beneficial. One randomized controlled trial comparing strict blood glucose control with conventional blood glucose control in patients receiving low-dose hydrocortisone for refractory shock did not find clinical benefit from prevention of bolus infusion of hydrocortisone-induced dysglycemia [22]. Notably, this trial did not report metrics of glycemic variability, making it impossible to see whether the intervention in that trial truly influenced glycemic variability. Future studies are necessary to determine whether it is possible to prevent hydrocortisone-induced glycemic variability, and if so whether this improves outcome. There could be a role for continuous glucose monitoring devices that are now slowly entering the market, but this certainly needs confirmation in future studies as well. Notably, a recent retrospective study showed that use of subcutaneous continuous glucose monitoring was not associated with lower glycemic variability in critically ill patients [23].

The results of the present study clearly show that action was required upon hydrocortisone-induced glycemic variability, as the total number of blood glucose level measurements were almost three times as many as in patients not receiving hydrocortisone treatment. Furthermore, adjustments of the insulin infusion rate occurred much more often. While we could not perform a cost analysis, it is clear that costs associated with blood glucose monitoring and adjustments of the insulin infusion rate in patients treated with hydrocortisone exceed those in patients not receiving hydrocortisone. Several studies show that continuous infusion of hydrocortisone is associated with a less steep rise of the blood glucose level than bolus infusion of hydrocortisone [2, 3]. This suggests that continuous infusion of hydrocortisone may need less frequent blood glucose measurements and adjustments of the insulin infusion rate. However, we should bear in mind that continuous infusion of hydrocortisone comes at a price: it may need an additional lumen of a central line or an extra peripheral venous access, but most important it mandates, often expensive, syringe pumps.

Strengths of this study include the large cohort of patients and blood glucose levels without any change in the local guidelines for blood glucose control or indication for bolus infusion of hydrocortisone. Furthermore, the target of the guideline for blood glucose control is a commonly used target in other hospitals, increasing generalizability of the results. Weaknesses of the present study include its retrospective design. Therefore, the data cannot support any causal relationship between steroid treatment and glycemic or insulin variability. In addition, patients receiving boluses of hydrocortisone in the study cohort were almost without exception suffering from septic shock, while most patients not receiving boluses of hydrocortisone were not. Thus, one could argue that differences in blood glucose variability between the two patient groups were simply reflecting differences induced by septic shock. Important in this context is that sepsis may be associated with increased glycemic variability [24]. Indeed, patients with septic shock have increased insulin resistance [25], as also suggested by the other metrics of blood glucose control in our study. However, while insulin resistance is suggested to be dependent on disease severity [25], this was not confirmed here as the effect of hydrocortisone treatment on blood glucose variability was independent of APACHE II scores. The finding that the associations were less strong in more severely ill patients may have been caused by already high blood glucose variability in these patients. Finally, results could have been different when glucocorticosteroids other than hydrocortisone would have been used because half-life times and glucocorticoid effects differ between various glucocorticosteroids agents.

There are several measures to calculate the glycemic variability. We used two measures and found that the association was only significant for both measures in the group of patients with APACHE II score between 15 and 24. It is possible the results will be different when using other measures for glycemic variability [6, 23].

One other major limitation of our analysis is that the frequency of the blood glucose level measurements affects the SD of the blood glucose level [13]. Nevertheless, in previous investigations, glycemic variability remained independently associated with increased mortality [6]. Other limitations of this study are its lack of data regarding nutritional support and corticosteroid usage before ICU admission.

Conclusions

Bolus infusion of hydrocortisone is independently associated with increased glycemic variability and increased insulin infusion rate variability in ICU patients under glycemic control aiming at blood glucose levels between 90 and 144 mg/dL. Additional studies are needed to investigate if the found associations have an affect on mortality and if continuous infusion of hydrocortisone prevents increased blood glucose variability and insulin infusion rate variability.

Abbreviations

APACHE II score: Acute physiology age and chronic health II score; BMI: Body mass index; ICU: Intensive care unit; IQR: Interquartile range; IU: International units; LOS: Length of stay; NICE: National intensive care evaluation; SAPS–II: Simplified acute physiology score II; SD: Standard deviation.

Authors' contributions

Study concept and design: RTMH, JMB, MJS. Acquisition of data: RTMH and JMB. Analysis and interpretation of data: RTMH, JMB, LDJB and MJS. Drafting of the manuscript: RTMH, MJS. Critical revision of the manuscript for important intellectual content: RTMH, JMB, LDJB, JH, NPJ, AAH, and MJS. All authors read and approved the manuscript.

Author details

[1] Department of Intensive Care Medicine, Academic Medical Center, University of Amsterdam, Meibergdreef 9, 1105 AZ Amsterdam, The Netherlands. [2] Laboratory of Experimental Intensive Care and Anesthesiology (L·E·I·C·A), Academic Medical Center, University of Amsterdam, Amsterdam, The Netherlands. [3] Department of Medical Informatics, Academic Medical Center, University of Amsterdam, Amsterdam, The Netherlands.

Acknowledgements

We express our gratitude to Mark de Jong, who exported all data from the patient data monitoring system and to Hendrik J. F. Helmerhorst for his helpful comments on the ordinal model.

Competing interests

Roosmarijn T. M. van Hooijdonk reported consulting work for Medtronic Inc., GlySure Ltd and research support from Medtronic Inc and Optiscan Biomedical—all fees and financial supports were paid to the institution. Marcus J. Schultz reported receiving consultant fees from Medtronic Inc., GlySure Ltd., Edwards Life Sciences and Roche Diagnostics and financial support from Medtronic Inc. and OptiScan Biomedical—all fees and financial supports were paid to the institution. Jan M. Binnekade, Lieuwe D. J. Bos, Janneke Horn, Nicole P. Juffermans, Ameen Abu–Hanna reported no relevant disclosures.

References

1. Dellinger RP, Levy MM, Rhodes A, Annane D, Gerlach H, Opal SM, Sevransky JE, Sprung CL, Douglas IS, Jaeschke R, Osborn TM, Nunnally ME, Townsend SR, Reinhart K, Kleinpell RM, Angus DC, Deutschman CS, Machado FR, Rubenfeld GD, Webb S, Beale RJ, Vincent J-L, Moreno R. Surviving sepsis campaign: international guidelines for management of severe sepsis and septic shock, 2012. Intensive Care Med. 2013;39:165–228.
2. Weber-Carstens S, Deja M, Bercker S, Dimroth A, Ahlers O, Kaisers U, Keh D. Impact of bolus application of low-dose hydrocortisone on glycemic control in septic shock patients. Intensive Care Med. 2007;33:730–3.
3. Loisa P, Parviainen I, Tenhunen J, Hovilehto S, Ruokonen E. Effect of mode of hydrocortisone administration on glycemic control in patients with septic shock: a prospective randomized trial. Crit Care. 2007;11:R21.
4. Schultz MJ, Harmsen RE, Spronk PE. Clinical review: strict or loose glycemic control in critically ill patients–implementing best available evidence from randomized controlled trials. Crit Care. 2010;14:223.
5. Rady MY, Johnson DJ, Patel B, Larson J, Helmers R. Corticosteroids influence the mortality and morbidity of acute critical illness. Crit Care. 2006;10:R101.
6. Mackenzie IMJ, Whitehouse T, Nightingale PG. The metrics of glycaemic control in critical care. Intensive Care Med. 2011;37:435–43.
7. Eslami S, de Keizer NF, Dongelmans DA, de Jonge E, Schultz MJ, Abu-Hanna A. Effects of two different levels of computerized decision support on blood glucose regulation in critically ill patients. Int J Med Inform. 2012;81:53–60.
8. van Hooijdonk RT, Winters T, Fischer JC, van Dongen-Lases EC, Krinsley JS, Preiser J-C, Schultz MJ. Accuracy and limitations of continuous glucose monitoring using spectroscopy in critically ill patients. Ann Intensive Care. 2014;4:8.
9. van Hooijdonk RT, Leopold JH, Winters T, Binnekade JM, Juffermans NP, Horn J, Fischer JC, van Dongen–Lases EC, Schultz MJ. Point accuracy and reliability of an interstitial continuous glucose monitoring device in critically ill patients: a prospective study. Crit Care. 2015;19.
10. Dellinger RP, Carlet JM, Masur H, Gerlach H, Calandra T, Cohen J, Gea-Banacloche J, Keh D, Marshall JC, Parker MM, Ramsay G, Zimmerman JL, Vincent J-L, Levy MM. Surviving Sepsis Campaign guidelines for management of severe sepsis and septic shock. Intensive Care Med. 2004;30:536–55.
11. Arts D, de Keizer N, Scheffer G-J, de Jonge E. Quality of data collected for severity of illness scores in the Dutch National Intensive Care Evaluation (NICE) registry. Intensive Care Med. 2002;28:656–9.
12. Knaus WA, Draper EA, Wagner DP, Zimmerman JE. APACHE II: a severity of disease classification system. Crit Care Med. 1985;13:818–29.
13. Eslami S, Taherzadeh Z, Schultz MJ, Abu-Hanna A. Glucose variability measures and their effect on mortality: a systematic review. Intensive Care Med. 2011;37:583–93.
14. Finfer S, Wernerman J, Preiser J-C, Cass T, Desaive T, Hovorka R, Joseph JI, Kosiborod M, Krinsley J, Mackenzie I, Mesotten D, Schultz MJ, Scott MG, Slingerland R, Van den Berghe G, Van Herpe T. Clinical review: consensus recommendations on measurement of blood glucose and reporting glycemic control in critically ill adults. Crit Care. 2013;17:229.
15. Krinsley JS. Association between hyperglycemia and increased hospital mortality in a heterogeneous population of critically ill patients. Mayo Clin Proc. 2003;78:1471–8.
16. Krinsley JS, Schultz MJ, Spronk PE, Harmsen RE, van Braam Houckgeest F, van der Sluijs JP, Mélot C, Preiser JC. Mild hypoglycemia is independently associated with increased mortality in the critically ill. Crit Care. 2011;15:R173.
17. McNamee R. Confounding and confounders. Occup Environ Med. 2003;60:227–34.
18. Ali NA, O'Brien JM, Dungan K, Phillips G, Marsh CB, Lemeshow S, Connors AF, Preiser J-C. Glucose variability and mortality in patients with sepsis. Crit Care Med. 2008;36:2316–21.
19. Ottens TH, Nijsten MW, Hofland J, Dieleman JM, Hoekstra M, van Dijk D, van der Maaten JM. Effect of high-dose dexamethasone on perioperative lactate levels and glucose control: a randomized controlled trial. Crit Care. 2015;19.
20. Alía I, de la Cal MA, Esteban A, Abella A, Ferrer R, Molina FJ, Torres A, Gordo F, Elizalde JJ, de Pablo R, Huete A, Anzueto A. Efficacy of corticosteroid therapy in patients with an acute exacerbation of chronic obstructive pulmonary disease receiving ventilatory support. Arch Intern Med. 2011;171:1939–46.
21. Krinsley JS, Egi M, Kiss A, Devendra AN, Schuetz P, Maurer PM, Schultz MJ, van Hooijdonk RTM, Kiyoshi M, Mackenzie IMJ, Annane D, Stow P, Nasraway SA, Holewinski S, Holzinger U, Preiser J-C, Vincent J-L, Bellomo R. Diabetic status and the relation of the three domains of glycemic control to mortality in critically ill patients: an international multicenter cohort study. Crit Care. 2013;17:R37.
22. Annane D, Cariou A, Maxime V, Azoulay E, D'honneur G, Timsit JF, Cohen Y, Wolf M, Fartoukh M, Adrie C, Santré C, Bollaert PE, Mathonet A, Amathieu R, Tabah A, Clec'h C, Mayaux J, Lejeune J, Chevret S. Corticosteroid treatment and intensive insulin therapy for septic shock in adults: a randomized controlled trial. JAMA. 2010;303:341–8.
23. Brunner R, Adelsmayr G, Herkner H, Madl C, Holzinger U. Glycemic variability and glucose complexity in critically ill patients : a retrospective analysis of continuous glucose monitoring data. Crit Care. 2012;16:R175.
24. Donati A, Damiani E, Domizi R, Botticelli L, Castagnani R, Gabbanelli V, Nataloni S, Carsetti A, Scorcella C, Adrario E, Pelaia P, Preiser J-C. Glycaemic variability, infections and mortality in a medical-surgical intensive care unit. Crit Care Resusc. 2014;16:13–23.
25. Van den Berghe G. How does blood glucose control with insulin save lives in intensive care? J Clin Invest. 2004;114:1187–95.

Automatic versus manual changeovers of norepinephrine infusion pumps in critically ill adults

Emilie Greau[1], Jean-Baptiste Lascarrou[1], Aurélie Le Thuaut[2,3], Nathalie Maquigneau[1], Yolaine Alcourt[1], Anne Coutolleau[1], Cécile Rousseau[1], Vanessa Erragne[1] and Jean Reignier[1,4,5*]

Abstract

Background: Norepinephrine is a key drug for treating shock but has a short half-life that requires continuous intravenous administration to maintain the constant plasma concentration needed to obtain a stable blood pressure. The small volume of the syringes used in power infusion pumps requires frequent changeovers, which can lead to norepinephrine flow interruptions responsible for hemodynamic instability. Changeovers from the nearly empty to the full syringe can be performed manually using the quick change technique (QC) or automatically using smart infusion pumps (SIP) that link two syringes. The purpose of our study was to evaluate the hypothesis that, compared to QC, SIP for norepinephrine changeovers was associated with less hemodynamic instability.

Methods: After information of the patient or next of kin, patients receiving norepinephrine for shock were allocated to QC or SIP changeovers. QC changeovers were performed by a nurse, who started a new loaded pump when the previous syringe was nearly empty. SIP changeovers were managed automatically by SIP workstations. The primary outcome was the proportion of changeovers followed by a ≥20 % drop in mean arterial pressure (MAP).

Results: 411 changeovers were performed, 193 in the 18 patients allocated to QC and 218 in the 32 patients allocated to SIP. Baseline patient characteristics were similar in both groups. The proportion of changeovers followed by an MAP drop ≥20 % was 12.4 % (24/193) with QC and 5.5 % (12/218) with SIP ($P = 0.01$). By multivariate analysis, two factors were independently associated with a significantly decreased risk of ≥20 % MAP drops during changeovers, namely, SIP (odds ratio, 0.47; 95 % confidence interval, 0.22–0.98) and norepinephrine dosage >0.5 μg/kg/min (odds ratio, 0.39; 95 % confidence interval, 0.19–0.81).

Conclusions: The risk of MAP drops ≥20 % during changeovers can be significantly diminished using SIPs instead of the QC method.

Keywords: Critically ill, Shock, Changeover, Catecholamines, Norepinephrine, Smart infusion pumps

Background

The management of hemodynamic failure, a key issue in intensive care, requires close and continuous monitoring and treatment. Vasoactive drugs are used to reverse vasoplegia and/or to treat heart failure in patients with persistent hemodynamic instability after volume repletion to correct hypovolemia [1–3]. Norepinephrine is currently the most widely used drug to treat vasoplegia, because of its potent and selective effects on vascular alpha receptors [4]. Similar to all other vasoconstrictors, norepinephrine has a short half-life. These features require intravenous administration at a constant flow rate, which can be achieved using a high-precision power infusion pump [5, 6].

The syringes used with power infusion pumps are small and must therefore be changed frequently. The

*Correspondence: jean.reignier@chu-nantes.fr
[5] Medical Intensive Care Unit, Nantes University Hospital, Nantes, France
Full list of author information is available at the end of the article

changeover between vasoactive drug infusion pumps (CVIP) can induce a brief change in the drug flow rate manifesting as hemodynamic instability [7]. Various methods for performing manual or automatic changeovers have been developed to prevent episodes of hemodynamic instability [6, 8]. In the quick change method (QC), a full syringe is loaded into a new pump then connected to the three-way stopcock, which is turned to open the new and close the old infusion. This new primed line is set at the same flow rate as the running pump. QC has been proven simple and effective for manual CVIP [7, 9, 10] but does not completely eliminate the risk of instability. In addition, QC generates considerable work and stress for the nurse.

Smart infusion pumps (SIP) linking two syringes have been developed to allow automatic CVIP without changing the flow rate [11]. The SIP software has a number of capabilities, including a relay feature that can link a full syringe and a nearly empty syringe, thereby limiting flow rate interruptions during CVIP while decreasing the need for nurse interventions. Compared to manual CVIP, automated CVIP using an SIP may therefore minimize episodes of hemodynamic instability. A before–after study showed reduced rates of hemodynamic incidents and decreased nurse workload with SIP compared to QC [12]. However, the available data are scant, and no randomized trials or guidelines are available.

The purpose of this prospective controlled trial was to investigate whether using a SIP for norepinephrine changeovers decreased hemodynamic instability compared to QC.

Methods

Study design and setting

This prospective controlled trial was conducted from June 2009 to February 2011 in the 18-bed adult medical-surgical intensive care unit (ICU) of the District Hospital Centre in La Roche-sur-Yon, France. The study protocol was approved by the appropriate ethics committee (Comité de Protection des Personnes de Poitiers) on April 15, 2009. According to French law, because the strategies used in both study groups are considered standard care, there was no requirement for signed informed consent. However, information of the patient or next of kin was required before inclusion in the study. The patient or next of kin could decline participation in the study at any time after being informed or included.

Patients

Adults (age > 18 years) admitted to the ICU and given norepinephrine to treat shock were eligible for inclusion. Exclusion criteria were moribund status, pregnancy or breastfeeding, infusion of another medication via the central venous port used for norepinephrine administration, absence of healthcare insurance, refusal of the patient or next of kin to participate in the study, pheochromocytoma, and carcinoid tumor.

Allocation

Eligible patients were informed about the study then enrolled by study nurses, who randomly allocated them in a 1:1 ratio to the QC or SIP method for CVIP, as described below. The random allocation sequence was generated by the clinical research unit of the La Roche Sur Yon District Hospital, using Random© (Inserm, Paris, France). No stratification was performed. Implementation of the sequence was by opaque sealed envelopes to ensure concealment.

Norepinephrine administration

Infusion lines and norepinephrine syringes were prepared according to the written protocol of the unit. The infusion lines were similar in both groups (Fig. 1). All devices used for the study were those used habitually in the unit. All ICU nurses were trained in using power infusion pumps, setting up infusion lines, and preparing norepinephrine syringes. They attended a training program specifically designed to ensure optimal quality and standardization of QC and SIP changeovers. These training programs were delivered by three highly experienced ICU nurses, who were in charge of bedside nurse training in our unit. Written standardized protocols for QC and SIP changeovers were developed, and the ability of each ICU nurse to follow them successfully was checked by the training nurses.

All study patients received continuous norepinephrine via a dedicated infusion line (BD Medical, Le Pont de Clais, France) connected to the proximal lumen of a multilumen central venous catheter (Arrow, Kingston, UK). Each Luer-Lock 60-mL syringe was loaded with an amount of norepinephrine, in mg, equal to the patient's body weight multiplied by 0.3; water for intravenous injection (Renaudin, Itxassou, France) was then added to obtain a total volume of 50 mL. The NE ampoules used in our unit to prepare the syringes contained 8 mg of NE. When the calculated NE requirement was between 23 and 25 mg, the nurses rounded to 24 mg (three ampoules) to increase the efficiency and speed of preparation at the bedside. The infusion rate in µg/kg/min was equal to 1/10 of the injection speed of the power infusion pump. Changeovers were performed when the syringe contained 5 mL or less; finally, as a safeguard, the electric infusion pump triggered a buzzer when less than 2 mL of the norepinephrine solution was left in the syringe. In both groups, a 5 % dextrose carrier of the norepinephrine infusion was used [13]. It was infused by gravity with a flow rate regulator (Fig. 1). The flow was set at 5 mL/h for all patients and checked regularly by the nurse at the bedside [14].

Changeovers in the QC group

Orchestra® power pumps were used (Fresenius Kabi, Bad Homburg, Germany). The patient's nurse prepared a new syringe with the same concentration of norepinephrine, connected it to a line and to a new power pump set at the same flow rate as the running pump, primed the line using the bolus function of the pump until a drop of norepinephrine solution was visible at the tip of the line (thereby minimizing the start-up time of the new infusion), then connected the line to the three-way stopcock. When the previous syringe contained 5 mL or less of norepinephrine solution, the nurse turned the stopcock to stop the old infusion and start the new infusion. Throughout this procedure, the patient was monitored closely by the nurse, who remained at the bedside.

Changeovers in the SIP group

The Orchestra® Base Intensive SIP workstation (Fresenius Kabi) was used. This device can manage up to six power infusion pumps and can perform automated changeovers by driving one syringe after the other at the same flow rate. The nurse presses the changeover button on the workstation, causing the display to divide into two windows, one for each syringe. The nurse then loads the new syringe containing norepinephrine solution in the same concentration as the running syringe. The new syringe is primed using the bolus function of the pump until a drop of norepinephrine solution appears at the end of the new line. Then, the new infusion line is connected to the three-way stopcock, which is then opened to both lines. After validation by the nurse, the workstation display shows the word "relay", indicating that the device is ready to perform the changeover. When the relay occurs, a buzzer sounds to let the nurse know that blood pressure should be monitored.

Data collection and follow-up

We collected the following baseline patients characteristics: age, gender, weight, body mass index, admission diagnosis, Simplified Acute Physiology Score II (SAPS II score; range from 0, lowest level of critical illness to 163, most severe level of critical illness) [15], cause of shock, Sepsis-related Organ Failure Assessment score (SOFA score; range from 0, no organ failure to 24, highest level of multiple-organ failure) [16], mechanical ventilation, ICU length of stay, and ICU and hospital mortality. For each CVIP, we collected the SOFA score, the norepinephrine dose (μg/kg/min) and concentration (mg/50 mL), blood pressure, and heart rate (HR). Noninvasive blood pressure monitoring has been proven accurate in detecting MAP drops [17], and invasive monitoring via an arterial catheter was therefore not required by the study

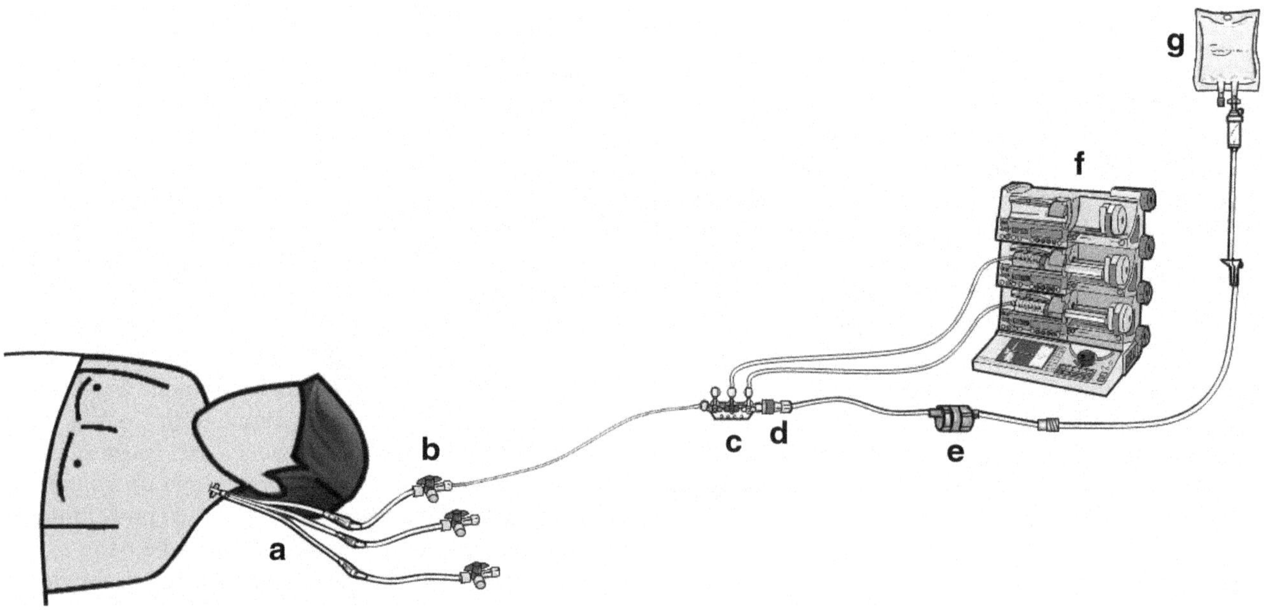

Fig. 1 Infusion line setup. **a** Multilumen central venous catheter (Arrow, Kingston, UK); **b** infusion line (BD Medical, Le Pont de Clais, France) connected to the proximal lumen of the central venous catheter; **c** perfusion ramp with a three-way stopcock (Vygon, Ecouen, France); **d** anti-reflux valve (Arrow, Kington, UK); **e** infusion rate control (CAIR LGL, Lissieu, France); **f** infusion pump; **g** Dextrose 5 % infusion set (B. Braun, Boulogne Billancourt, France)

protocol. Blood pressure was monitored continuously if the patient had an arterial catheter for another reason (Arrow, Kingston, UK) and at 1-min intervals using an automatic sphygmomanometer (Philips, DA Best, Netherlands) with an appropriately sized cuff otherwise. Maximal and minimal values of HR and MAP were recorded every 5 min over a period ranging from 15 min before to 15 min after each changeover.

Study outcome

The primary outcome was the proportion of changeovers followed by an MAP drop ≥20 % within 15 min after the changeover. The 15 min were counted starting at the stopcock turn in the QC group and the buzzer in the SIP group. Secondary outcomes were the proportions of changeovers followed by a ≥15 % MAP drop, a ≥10 % MAP drop, severe hypotension defined as MAP <50 mmHg, and a ≥20 % HR change in either direction, within 15 min after the changeover.

Sample size

We expected an MAP drop ≥20 % to occur within 15 min after 20 % of QC procedures [7]. To detect a 10 % decrease in the primary outcome in the SIP group, with α set at 0.05 and 80 % power, 200 changeovers were required in each group. All changeovers in each patient were included in the study. Patients on norepinephrine therapy usually require about 10 changeovers in all [7]. Therefore, about 40 patients in all (20 per group) were required. Because some patients require fewer than 10 changeovers and missing data may occur for some changeovers (e.g., those performed on an emergency basis), we planned to include 50 patients in all. The number of relays was checked during the enrollment phase of the study. After inclusion of 36 patients (18 in each group), 193 relays were available for analysis in the Quick Change Method compared to only 141 in the Smart Infusion Pump group. At this point, we decided to include all subsequent patients in the Smart Infusion Pump group until the required number of changeovers was reached.

Statistical analysis

Quantitative data were described as means (±standard deviation) or medians (25th–75th quartiles) and compared between changeover groups using the Student or Wilcoxon–Mann–Whitney tests, as appropriate. Qualitative data were described as *n* (%) and compared using the Pearson Chi-square test or Fisher exact test as appropriate.

A mixed-effect logistic regression model was fitted to assess factors associated with the primary outcome (≥20 % MAP drop within 15 min after the changeover). This model took the hierarchical structure of the data into account. We used a random-intercept logistic model with changeovers (level 1) nested in patients (level 2). Potential confounders related to changeover characteristics were tested. Potential confounders were identified according to the results of the univariate analysis and a previous study [12]. Covariates associated with *P* values <0.10 by univariate analysis were entered into the multivariate model. Norepinephrine concentration and dose, SOFA score, and age were forced into the final multivariate model. Odds ratios (ORs) and their 95 % confidence intervals (95 % CIs) were estimated. The same method was used to analyze ≥20 % HR variations and other secondary outcomes.

All comparisons were two-sided, and *P* values <0.05 were considered significant. The data were analyzed using Stata statistical software version 13.0 (StataCorp LP, College Station, TX, USA).

Results

The 50 included patients had 411 changeovers, 193 in the 18 patients allocated to QC and 218 in the 32 patients allocated to SIP (Fig. 2). The median number of changeovers per patient was 6 [3–12] in the QC group and 3 [1–11] in the SIP group (*P* = 0.07). All patients had at least 1 changeover. The only patient characteristic that differed significantly between the two groups was ICU stay length, which was longer in the QC group (Table 1). Table 2 compares the baseline characteristics in the two changeover groups; the norepinephrine dose and HR were significantly higher in the SIP group than in the QC group.

Primary outcome

MAP dropped by ≥20 % in 24/193 (12.4 %) QC changeovers and 12/218 (5.5 %) SIP changeovers (*P* = 0.01). Multivariate analysis identified two factors independently associated with a significant decrease in the risk of ≥20 % MAP drops, namely, SIP (OR, 0.47; 95 % CI, 0.22–0.98) and norepinephrine dose >0.5 μg/kg/min (OR, 0.39; 95 % CI, 0.19–0.81) (Table 3).

Secondary outcomes

Overall, changeovers were associated with a significant MAP increase within the first 5 min, in both groups (QC group, from 78 ± 14 to 80 ± 14 mmHg, *P* = 0.03; SIP group, from 77 ± 13 to 78 ± 14 mmHg, *P* = 0.004) (Fig. 3). These increases were not significantly different between the two groups (*P* = 0.22). MAP increased by more than 20 % in a single QC patient and none of the SIP patients.

MAP drops ≥15 % occurred within 15 min after 40 (20.7 %) QC changeovers and 21 (9.6 %) SIP changeovers (*P* = 0.002). Similarly, MAP drops ≥10 % were

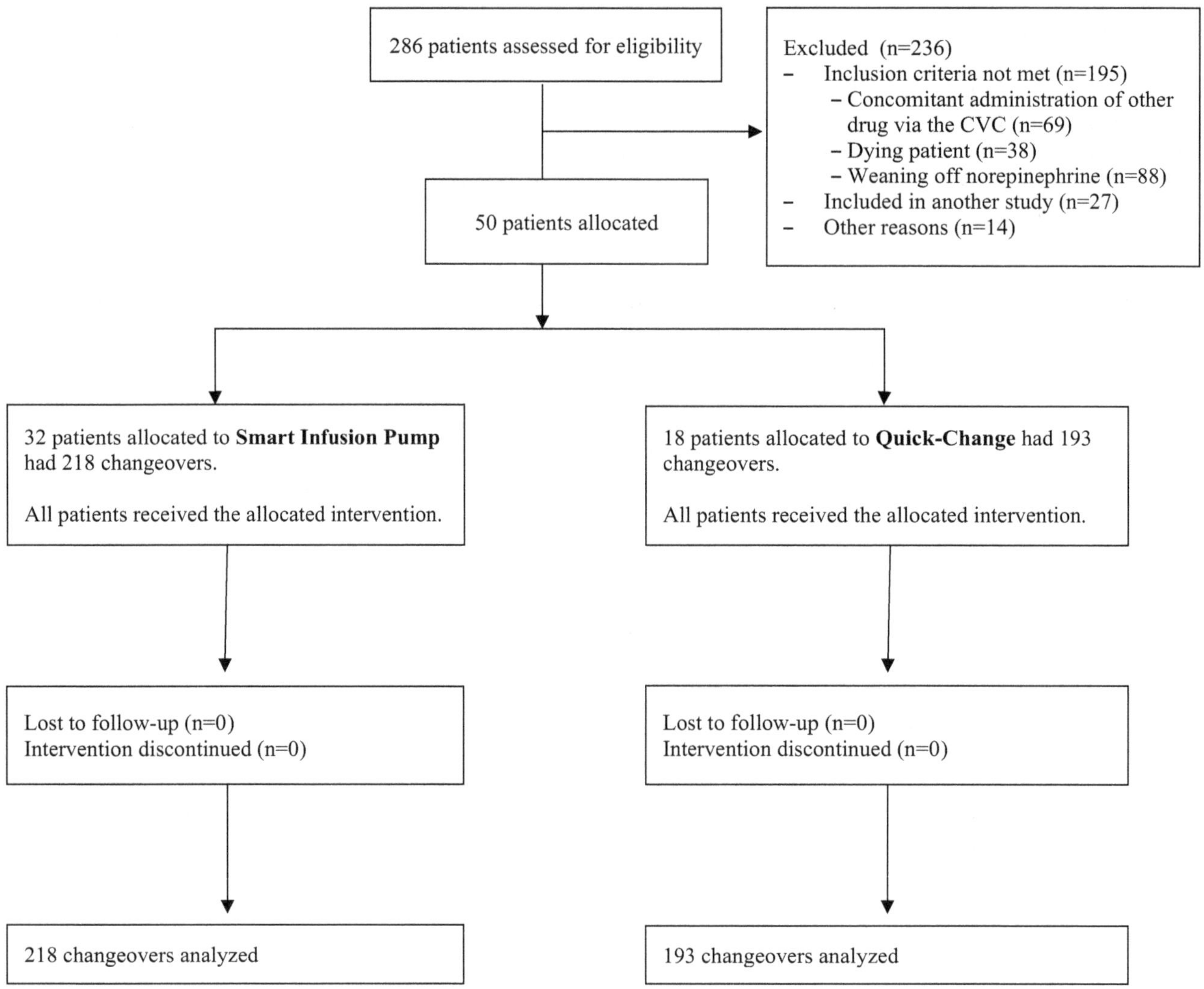

Fig. 2 Flowchart

significantly more common with QC than with SIP (34.2 vs. 24.3 %, $P = 0.03$). However, severe hypotension (MAP < 50 mmHg) occurred in similar proportions of patients in the two groups (4.7 % with QC and 4.1 % with SIP, $P = 0.79$).

HR changes ≥20 % occurred within 15 min after 15 (7.8 %) changeovers in the QC group (10 increases and 5 decreases) and 6 (2.8 %) changeovers in the SIP group (5 increases and 1 decrease) ($P = 0.03$). By multivariate analysis, the changeover method was not independently associated with HR variations (Table 4).

Discussion

We report the first prospective controlled trial designed to compare automated norepinephrine syringe changeovers using an SIP to manual changeovers using QC, in critically ill adults with shock. Our main finding is that SIP changeovers were associated with lower rates of hypotension than changeovers managed manually by the nurse using the QC technique.

Norepinephrine syringe changeovers are among the most important and stressful procedures required by the management of shock. There is a risk of decreased drug delivery during the changeovers [6, 8], with hypotension and clinical deterioration. Several methods have been developed to shorten the changeover period, thereby limiting the risks to the patient. However, few studies of these methods have been published. Manual changeover methods include the QC and the double infusion pump (DIP) technique. With both methods, the nearly empty syringe and the new full syringe, set at the same flow rate, are connected to the catecholamine line of the central

Table 1 Patient characteristics

	Quick change method (*n* = 18)	Smart infusion pump (*n* = 32)	*P* value
Age (years), mean ± SD	63.3 ± 13.4	68.1 ± 12.8	0.22
Gender (male), *n* (%)	14 (77.8 %)	25 (78.1 %)	0.98
Weight (kg), mean ± SD	77.7 ± 14.1	86.5 ± 19.9	0.10
Body mass index (kg/m^2), mean ± SD	27.7 ± 5.5	29.9 ± 5.0	0.36
Admission diagnosis, *n* (%)			0.26
Cardiac arrest	2 (11.1 %)	3 (9.4 %)	
Circulatory failure	9 (50 %)	9 (28.1 %)	
Acute respiratory failure	3 (16.7 %)	14 (43.8 %)	
Trauma	0	1 (3.1 %)	
Other	4 (22.2 %)	5 (15.6 %)	
Surgical patient, *n* (%)	8 (44.4 %)	8 (25.0 %)	0.16
SAPS II, mean ± SD	64.1 ± 19.3	65.9 ± 18.6	0.75
Method of arterial pressure monitoring			0.72
Automatic sphygmomanometer	3 (16.7)	8 (25.0)	
Invasive arterial line	15 (83.3)	24 (75.0)	
Cause of shock, *n* (%)			0.78
Sepsis	14 (77.8 %)	24 (75.0 %)	
Hemorrhage	2 (11.1 %)	2 (6.4 %)	
Other	2 (11.1 %)	5 (16.1 %)	
SOFA score at inclusion, mean ± SD	12.5 ± 4.0	11.3 ± 2.7	0.21
Mechanical ventilation, *n* (%)	17 (94.4 %)	29 (90.6 %)	0.63
ICU length of stay (days), median (IQR)	15 [9–34]	9 [3–25.5]	0.03
ICU mortality, *n* (%)	5 (27.8 %)	13 (40.6 %)	0.36
Hospital mortality, *n* (%)	5 (27.8 %)	14 (43.7 %)	0.26

SAPS II Simplified Acute Physiology Score, version II, *SOFA* Sequential Organ Failure Assessment, *ICU* intensive care unit, *IQR* inter-quartile range

Table 2 Baseline characteristics in the two changeover groups

	Quick change method (*n* = 193)	Smart infusion pump (*n* = 218)	*P* value
Age in years, mean ± SD	64.9 ± 12.2	65.7 ± 15.0	0.71
Male, *n* (%)	177 (91.7 %)	204 (93.6 %)	0.47
Weight, mean ± SD	78.8 ± 15.5	81.6 ± 18.5	0.84
Body mass index (kg/m^2), mean ± SD	26.7 ± 5.7	28.6 ± 4.2	0.13
Cause of shock, *n* (%)			0.34
Sepsis	176 (91.2 %)	194 (90.6 %)	
Hemorrhage	10 (5.2 %)	7 (3.3 %)	
Other	7 (3.6 %)	13 (6.1 %)	
SOFA score, mean ± SD	13.3 ± 3.1	12.9 ± 3.1	0.2
Mechanical ventilation, *n* (%)	186 (96.4 %)	215 (98.6)	0.14
Dose of NE, µg/kg/min, median [IQR]	0.6 [0.3–1.2]	0.8 [0.4–2.0]	<0.001
Concentration of NE, mg/50 mL, mean ± SD	25.1 ± 6.9	24.8 ± 6.3	0.34
Heart rate at baseline	99.3 ± 22.1	107.2 ± 18.9	<0.001
Mean arterial blood pressure at baseline	78.2 ± 13.8	76.8 ± 13.4	0.31

SOFA Sequential Organ Failure Assessment, *NE* norepinephrine, *IQR* inter-quartile range

venous catheter via a three-way stopcock, which is used to close the running infusion and open the new infusion at the same time. With QC, a brief interruption in the drug infusion may occur if the new line is not perfectly primed and/or the old syringe empties before the stopcock is turned to the new syringe and/or a delay occurs

Table 3 Multivariate analysis to identify factors independently associated with mean arterial pressure (MAP) drops ≥20 % versus baseline

	OR [95 % CI]	*P* value
SIP changeover	0.47 [0.22–0.98]	0.04
Concentration of NE	0.95 [0.89–1.02]	0.19
Dose of NE >0.5 μg/kg/min	0.39 [0.19–0.81]	0.01
SOFA score at baseline	1.12 [0.99–1.26]	0.08
Age	1.00 [0.97–1.91]	0.85

OR odds ratio, *95 % CI* 95 % confidence interval, *SIP* smart infusion pump, *NE* norepinephrine, *SOFA* Sequential Organ Failure Assessment

while turning the stopcock. Theoretically, none of these problems can occur with the DIP method, in which there is an overlap between the two syringes with a gradual decrease in the flow rate of the old syringe and a commensurate gradual increase in the flow rate of the new syringe. However, neither method is well standardized, a shortcoming that can result in flow rate variations, stress, human error, and hemodynamic instability. Previous studies found no significant differences in the risk of hemodynamic instability between QC and DIP [7, 9, 10]. Compared to DIP, QC is less time-consuming and therefore associated with a lower workload. We consequently chose QC as the comparator to SIP in our trial. SIPs were designed to drive syringe pumps and changeovers automatically according to specific algorithms to standardize drug delivery and decrease the nurse workload, thereby reducing the risk of error and improving the quality of care. However, their use remains controversial [11]. In some studies, the use of SIPs failed to improve drug safety [18, 19], due to the complexity of the SIP algorithm and settings. This complexity requires specific training of the nurses, which has been shown to decrease unwanted hemodynamic events after changeovers [7]. As indicated previously, all the nurses in our unit received in depth training and familiarization with both changeover methods. In a recent study, the use of an SIP for CVIP decreased the frequency of adverse hemodynamic events compared to QC [12]. However, the nonrandomized before–after design of this study limits the interpretation of the results, as effects of time and other confounding factors cannot be excluded. Moreover, the patients received a variety of vasoactive drugs including norepinephrine, epinephrine, and dobutamine, whose different effects on α- and β-adrenergic receptors produce different changes in vascular tone, HR, and myocardial contractility [4] and, therefore, in blood flow and blood pressure. Thus, the variations in hemodynamic variables observed in this study [12] may be related to the changeover, drug effects, or both. In our trial, only norepinephrine was used. Norepinephrine chiefly induces vasoconstriction and is considered the vasopressor of choice for most critically ill patients with shock [1, 2, 20]. Last, in addition to the device or changeover technique, a major issue is standardization of the circuit to eliminate variations in dead volume, compliance, resistance, and flow rate [21]. In our study, the perfusion lines were set up in a standardized manner and in the same way in all study patients. In the light of these considerations, we are confident that the between-group differences in our study were ascribable only to the changeover technique.

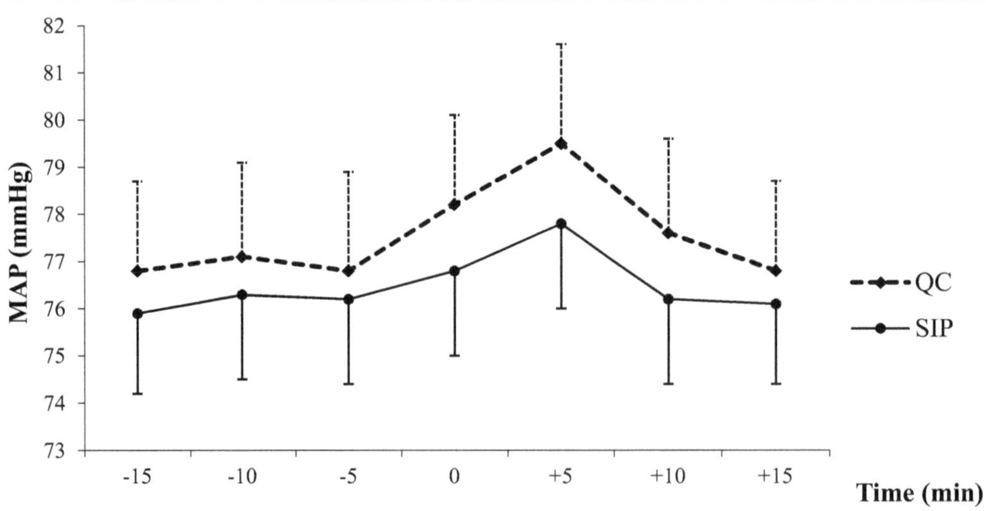

Fig. 3 MAP variations before, during, and after norepinephrine changeovers. *MAP* mean arterial pressure, *QC* quick change, *SIP* smart infusion pump. Variations in mean values of MAP from 15 min before to 15 min after changeovers in both groups. T0 was just before changeover initiation

Table 4 Multivariate analysis to identify factors independently associated with heart rate (HR) changes ≥20 % in either direction versus baseline

	OR [95 % CI]	*P* value
SIP changeover	0.42 [0.12–1.40]	0.16
Concentration of NE	1.01 [0.92–1.11]	0.80
Dose of NE >0.5 μg/kg/min	0.37 [0.13–1.06]	0.06
SOFA score at baseline	1.03 [0.98–1.08]	0.26
Age	1.18 [0.97–1.42]	0.09

OR odds ratio, *95 % CI* 95 % confidence interval, *SIP* smart infusion pump, *NE* norepinephrine, *SOFA* Sequential Organ Failure Assessment

The main finding from our trial is that using an SIP for norepinephrine syringe changeovers significantly decreased the frequency of MAP drops. This result is consistent with the above-mentioned before–after study, in which adverse hemodynamic events were also less common with SIP than with QC [12]. However, in contrast to previous studies, our trial did not include all adverse hemodynamic events (MAP drop, MAP elevation, and HR variation) in the primary endpoint [7, 12]. Instead, our primary endpoint was an MAP drop ≥20 %. A key goal of shock management is correction of the hypotension followed by prevention of further hypotensive episodes potentially responsible for decreased tissue perfusion. Current guidelines on shock recommend maintaining MAP at 65 mmHg or higher but do not indicate a maximum MAP value that should not be exceeded [2, 3]. Interestingly, as shown in Fig. 3, baseline MAP values in both groups were above the 65-mmHg minimal value indicated in our local shock management protocol. Moreover, MAP increased very slightly but significantly in both changeover groups. These findings are consistent with previous studies and reflect safety behaviors [7, 22] manifesting as a reluctance to decrease the norepinephrine flow rate even when the MAP target is reached in severely ill and unstable ICU patients. During changeovers, the mean MAP increase was also related to the brief increase in the norepinephrine flow rate due to the brief overlap between the nearly empty and full syringes. There is no evidence that moderate MAP increases have deleterious effects. A recent large randomized controlled trial in patients with septic shock found no significant differences in outcomes between the group with a high MAP target of 85–90 mmHg and the group with a standard MAP target of 65–70 mmHg [22]. Another finding from our study is that a norepinephrine dose >0.5 μg/kg/min was associated with a lower frequency of MAP drops. Thus, compared to lower flow rates, a high flow rate of norepinephrine protected against the small variations that may occur during changeovers. It is thus conceivable that maintaining a higher flow rate and using a more diluted norepinephrine solution may prevent MAP variations during changeovers in patients receiving low norepinephrine doses. However, higher flow rates may require a greater number of changeovers, and thereby increasing the risk of hemodynamic incidents. Last, norepinephrine has little effect on HR, which was therefore not included in our primary outcome. Our results consistently showed that the changeover method was not independently associated with HR variations.

Limitations of the trial include its single-center design, which may restrict the general applicability of the results. However, the devices and changeover methods used were very similar to those reported previously. Moreover, the patient characteristics reflected the overall population of patients with shock admitted to nonspecialized ICUs. Last, the prospective design strongly limits the risk of bias and allows the conclusion that using an SIP is causally related to a lower frequency of changeover-related hypotension. We are thus confident in the reliability and general applicability of our data. A second limitation of the trial is that, as indicated in the methods section, we stopped the randomization process when we found an imbalance between the two groups and we subsequently included all patients in the SIP group, to obtain similar numbers of changeovers in the two groups. We do not believe this fact significantly weakens our data, for the following reasons: (1) most patients were randomized, (2) consecutive patients were included, (3) all patients met predefined inclusion criteria, and (4) the multivariate analysis clearly demonstrated that the changeover method was independently associated with the occurrence of MAP variations. A third limitation is that we did not assess nurse workload, as our aim was to focus on potential benefits to patients. Although nurse workload is subjective, a previous non-randomized study showed a decrease in nurse's workload with SIP use [12]. A fourth limitation of our study may lie in the method used to calculate the amount of norepinephrine in the syringe for each individual patient. Indeed, doses calculations may lead to errors. However, this method has been used for many years in our ICU. Thus, all the nurses have considerable experience with it, and we are confident that the risk of error was very low. Moreover, although smart pumps could calculate doses in μg/kg/min, they were not used in the QC group. We therefore used the calculation method in both groups to avoid concerns about possible differences in norepinephrine concentrations. Last, our trial was not designed to assess the potential impact of the changeover method on patient outcomes. A far larger number of patients would have been required to assess possible effects on mortality. However, maintenance of hemodynamic stability was associated with improved patient outcomes in previous work and is a key goal of critical care [23]. Thus, our trial can be viewed as an important first step in demonstrating that SIPs improve the quality of care. Our results support the conduct of a large trial designed to assess the impact of SIP norepinephrine changeovers on patient outcomes.

Conclusion

This prospective controlled trial supports the use of SIPs for norepinephrine changeovers in critically ill adults with shock. Compared to QC, SIP changeovers are associated with improved hemodynamic stability.

Abbreviations

ICU: intensive care unit; MAP: mean arterial pressure; NE: norepinephrine; QC: quick change; SIP: smart infusion pump.

Authors' contributions

EG and JR were responsible for the study concept and design; EG, JBL, YA, NM, AC and JR for data acquisition; EG, JBL and JR for data analysis and interpretation; ALT for the statistical analysis; EG, JBL, ALT, and JR for drafting the manuscript; and JBL and JR for interpreting the data and critically revising the manuscript for important intellectual content. All authors read and approved the final manuscript.

Author details

[1] Medical-Surgical Intensive Care Unit, District Hospital Center, La Roche-sur-Yon, France. [2] Clinical Research Unit, District Hospital Center, La Roche-sur-Yon, France. [3] Délégation à la Recherche Clinique et à l'Innovation, CHU Hôtel Dieu, 44093 Nantes Cedex, France. [4] UPRES EA-3826, Clinical and Experimental Therapies for Infections, University of Nantes, Nantes, France. [5] Medical Intensive Care Unit, Nantes University Hospital, Nantes, France.

Acknowledgements

We thank A. Wolfe, MD, for assistance in preparing and reviewing the manuscript. We thank also Johanna Chupin for designing Fig. 1. This study was funded solely by institutional and departmental sources.

Competing interests

The authors declare that they have no competing interests.

References

1. Bougle A, Harrois A, Duranteau J. Resuscitative strategies in traumatic hemorrhagic shock. Ann Intensive Care. 2013;3(1):1. doi:10.1186/2110-5820-3-1.
2. Dellinger RP, Levy MM, Rhodes A, Annane D, Gerlach H, Opal SM, et al. Surviving Sepsis Campaign: international guidelines for management of severe sepsis and septic shock, 2012. Intensive Care Med. 2013;39(2):165–228. doi:10.1007/s00134-012-2769-8.
3. Levy B, Bastien O, Benjelid K, Cariou A, Chouihed T, Combes A, et al. Experts' recommendations for the management of adult patients with cardiogenic shock. Ann Intensive Care. 2015;5(1):52. doi:10.1186/s13613-015-0052-1.
4. Hollenberg SM. Vasoactive drugs in circulatory shock. Am J Respir Crit Care Med. 2011;183(7):847–55. doi:10.1164/rccm.201006-0972CI.
5. Monnet X, Lefrant JY, Teboul JL. Field 6. Safety practices for haemodynamic procedures (administration of vasoactive drugs, vascular and cardiac catheterization). French-speaking Society of Intensive Care. French Society of Anesthesia and Resuscitation. Ann Fr Anesth Reanim. 2008;27(10):e91–9. doi:10.1016/j.annfar.2008.09.012.
6. Trim JC, Roe J. Practical considerations in the administration of intravenous vasoactive drugs in the critical care setting: the double pumping or piggyback technique-part one. Intensive Crit Care Nurs. 2004;20(3):153–60. doi:10.1016/j.iccn.2004.02.006.
7. Argaud L, Cour M, Martin O, Saint-Denis M, Ferry T, Goyatton A, et al. Changeovers of vasoactive drug infusion pumps: impact of a quality improvement program. Crit Care. 2007;11(6):R133. doi:10.1186/cc6209.
8. Morrice A, Jackson E, Farnell S. Practical considerations in the administration of intravenous vasoactive drugs in the critical care setting. Part II—how safe is our practice? Intensive Crit Care Nurs. 2004;20(4):183–9. doi:10.1016/j.iccn.2004.04.008.
9. Arino M, Barrington JP, Morrison AL, Gillies D. Management of the changeover of inotrope infusions in children. Intensive Crit Care Nurs. 2004;20(5):275–80. doi:10.1016/j.iccn.2004.06.003.
10. de Barbieri I, Frigo AC, Zampieron A. Quick change versus double pump while changing the infusion of inotropes: an experimental study. Nurs Crit Care. 2009;14(4):200–6. doi:10.1111/j.1478-5153.2009.00333.x.
11. Murdoch LJ, Cameron VL. Smart infusion technology: a minimum safety standard for intensive care? Br J Nurs. 2008;17(10):630–6. doi:10.12968/bjon.2008.17.10.29476.
12. Cour M, Hernu R, Benet T, Robert JM, Regad D, Chabert B, et al. Benefits of smart pumps for automated changeovers of vasoactive drug infusion pumps: a quasi-experimental study. Br J Anaesth. 2013;111(5):818–24. doi:10.1093/bja/aet199.
13. Genay S, Decaudin B, Scoccia S, Barthelemy C, Debaene B, Lebuffe G, et al. An in vitro evaluation of infusion methods using a syringe pump to improve noradrenaline administration. Acta Anaesthesiol Scand. 2015;59(2):197–204. doi:10.1111/aas.12439.
14. Ténière A, Omrani S, Odouard E, Szostek AS, Piriou V, Cabelguenne D. Comparaison in vitro des dispositifs de perfusion : précision et fiabilité du débit, régulateur versus pince à roulette du perfuseur (In vitro comparison of infusion devices: accuracy and reliability of flow, infusion control device versus IV set). Anesth Reanim. 2015;1:108–17.
15. Le Gall JR, Lemeshow S, Saulnier F. A new Simplified Acute Physiology Score (SAPS II) based on a European/North American multicenter study. JAMA. 1993;270(24):2957–63.
16. Vincent JL, Moreno R, Takala J, Willatts S, De Mendonca A, Bruining H, et al. The SOFA (Sepsis-related Organ Failure Assessment) score to describe organ dysfunction/failure. On behalf of the Working Group on Sepsis-Related Problems of the European Society of Intensive Care Medicine. Intensive Care Med. 1996;22(7):707–10.
17. Lakhal K, Ehrmann S, Runge I, Legras A, Dequin PF, Mercier E, et al. Tracking hypotension and dynamic changes in arterial blood pressure with brachial cuff measurements. Anesth Analg. 2009;109(2):494–501. doi:10.1213/ane.0b013e3181a8d83a.
18. Nuckols TK, Bower AG, Paddock SM, Hilborne LH, Wallace P, Rothschild JM, et al. Programmable infusion pumps in ICUs: an analysis of corresponding adverse drug events. J Gen Intern Med. 2008;23(Suppl 1):41–5. doi:10.1007/s11606-007-0414-y.
19. Rothschild JM, Keohane CA, Cook EF, Orav EJ, Burdick E, Thompson S, et al. A controlled trial of smart infusion pumps to improve medication safety in critically ill patients. Crit Care Med. 2005;33(3):533–40.
20. De Backer D, Biston P, Devriendt J, Madl C, Chochrad D, Aldecoa C, et al. Comparison of dopamine and norepinephrine in the treatment of shock. N Engl J Med. 2010;362(9):779–89. doi:10.1056/NEJMoa0907118.
21. Peterfreund RA, Philip JH. Critical parameters in drug delivery by intravenous infusion. Expert Opin Drug Deliv. 2013;10(8):1095–108. doi:10.1517/17425247.2013.785519.
22. Asfar P, Meziani F, Hamel JF, Grelon F, Megarbane B, Anguel N, et al. High versus low blood-pressure target in patients with septic shock. N Engl J Med. 2014;370(17):1583–93. doi:10.1056/NEJMoa1312173.
23. Beck V, Chateau D, Bryson GL, Pisipati A, Zanotti S, Parrillo JE, et al. Timing of vasopressor initiation and mortality in septic shock: a cohort study. Crit Care. 2014;18(3):R97. doi:10.1186/cc13868.

3

The passive leg raising test to guide fluid removal in critically ill patients

Xavier Monnet[1,2,4*], Flora Cipriani[1,2], Laurent Camous[1,2], Pierre Sentenac[1,2], Martin Dres[1,2], Evguenia Krastinova[2,3], Nadia Anguel[1,2], Christian Richard[1,2] and Jean-Louis Teboul[1,2]

Abstract

Background: To investigate whether haemodynamic intolerance to fluid removal during intermittent renal replacement therapy (RRT) in critically ill patients can be predicted by a passive leg raising (PLR) test performed before RRT.

Methods: We included 39 patients where intermittent RRT with weight loss was decided. Intradialytic hypotension was defined as hypotension requiring a therapeutic intervention, as decided by the physicians in charge. Before RRT, the maximal increase in cardiac index (CI, pulse contour analysis) induced by a PLR test was recorded. RRT was then started.

Results: Ultrafiltration rate was similar in patients with and without intradialytic hypotension. Thirteen patients presented intradialytic hypotension, while 26 did not. In patients with intradialytic hypotension, it occurred 120 min [interquartile range 60–180 min] after onset of RRT. In the 26 patients without intradialytic hypotension, the PLR test induced no significant change in CI. Conversely, in patients with intradialytic hypotension, PLR significantly increased CI by 15 % [interquartile range 11–36 %]. The PLR-induced increase in CI predicted intradialytic hypotension with an area under the ROC curve of 0.89 (95 % interval confidence 0.75–0.97) ($p < 0.05$ from 0.50). The best diagnostic threshold was 9 %. The sensitivity was 77 % (95 % confidence interval 46–95 %), the specificity was 96 % (80–100 %), the positive predictive value was 91 % (57–100 %), and the negative predictive value was 89 % (72–98 %). Compared to patients without intolerance to RRT, CI decreased significantly faster in patients with intradialytic hypotension, with a slope difference of −0.17 L/min/m^2/h.

Conclusion: The presence of preload dependence, as assessed by a positive PLR test before starting RRT with fluid removal, predicts that RRT will induce haemodynamic intolerance.

Keywords: Passive leg raising, Renal replacement therapy, Ultrafiltration, Volume responsiveness, Acute kidney injury, Hypotension

Background

Removing fluid is a common therapeutic option in patients with acute circulatory failure and/or acute respiratory distress syndrome (ARDS), especially at the late phase of disease [1, 2]. This is based on the evidence that the cumulative fluid balance is an independent factor that increases mortality in patients with septic shock [3] and ARDS [4], especially in the case of acute kidney injury [5]. Fluid overload may impair the function of many organs, including the kidneys [6]. Along with the prediction of preload unresponsiveness, which prevents administration of ineffective fluid boluses, fluid removal contributes to reducing the fluid balance. Compared to a liberal strategy of fluid administration, a conservative strategy including fluid removal prompted extubation in ARDS patients [7]. The net fluid removal by renal replacement therapy (RRT) was shown to decrease the intra-abdominal pressure, the cardiac preload and the extravascular lung water [8].

However, the risk of fluid removal is to remove too much fluid and to impair the haemodynamic condition. Intradialytic hypotension is obviously deleterious [9] and

*Correspondence: xavier.monnet@aphp.fr
[4] Service de réanimation médicale, Centre Hospitalier Universitaire de Bicêtre, 78, rue du Général Leclerc, 94270 Le Kremlin-Bicêtre, France
Full list of author information is available at the end of the article

alters renal recovery in patients with acute renal failure [10, 11]. Also, in cases when it leads to premature termination of RRT, intradialytic hypotension reduces the dose of dialysis and the volume of fluid removal [9, 12].

Decrease in cardiac output as an adverse effect of excessive fluid removal should occur in the case of preload dependence, i.e. when changes in cardiac preload physiologically result in changes in cardiac output. The aim of this study was to test whether the presence of preload dependence can predict intolerance to fluid removal performed with ultrafiltration in patients under RRT. Passive leg raising (PLR) was used to test preload dependence.

Patients and methods

Patients

The study was conducted in the 15-bed medical intensive care of a university hospital. It was approved by the institutional review board of our institution (Comitě pour la Protection des Personnes Ile-de-France VII). Informed consent was obtained from all patients or next of kin.

Patients were enrolled under the following conditions:

1. Episode of acute circulatory failure, in its acute or resolution phase, defined by (1) systolic blood pressure <90 mmHg (or a decrease >50 mmHg in previously hypertensive patients) or the need for norepinephrine, (2) urine output <0.5 mL/kg/h for at least 2 h, (3) tachycardia >100 beats/min, (4) skin mottling or (5) blood lactate >2 mmol/L. The resolution phase of circulatory failure was defined by a decrease of the dose of norepinephrine for more than 24 h.
2. Monitoring by a PiCCO2 device (Pulsion Medical Systems, Munich, Germany) already in place.
3. Decision by the physician in charge to perform intermittent RRT with weight loss.
4. Haemodynamic stability, as defined by no volume expansion, no increase in the dose of catecholamines and no change in mean arterial pressure >10 mmHg during the last 3 h.

Patients were excluded if they presented intracranial hypertension (which is a contraindication to the PLR test), if RRT was interrupted for non-haemodynamic reasons and if ventilation and sedation modalities were changed during the study period.

Transpulmonary thermodilution and pulse contour analysis

All patients had an internal jugular vein catheter and a thermistor-tipped arterial catheter (PV2024 Pulsion Medical Systems, Munich, Germany) in the femoral artery connected to the PiCCO2 device. The dialysis catheter was in the femoral position, contralateral to the arterial catheter. Three cold boluses were used when performing transpulmonary thermodilution [13]. This allowed us to measure cardiac index (CI) (through transpulmonary thermodilution and pulse contour analysis), global end-diastolic volume and extravascular lung water (both through transpulmonary thermodilution) [14].

Global end-diastolic volume corresponds to the volume of the four cardiac chambers at end diastole and is a marker of cardiac preload [15]. Extravascular lung water is the volume of water that is contained in the interstitium, the intracellular compartment, the lymphatic fluid, the surfactant and the alveoli [16, 17]. Echocardiography was performed at the time of inclusion.

It has been already reported that extracorporeal circulation of blood during RRT does not alter the reliability of transpulmonary thermodilution measurements [18, 19], even for blood pump flows as high as 350 mL/min [19], even though this has been reported during continuous and not intermittent RRT. All values were indexed by the ideal and not the actual body weight, so that indexation in itself could not change the variables due to the simple weight loss induced by fluid removal.

RRT modalities

Intermittent RRT was performed according to the current practice of our unit. It was performed with the AK200-TS device (Gambro, Lund, Sweden) by using AN69-ST membranes (Hospal, Meyzieu, France). In our unit, besides intermittent RRT, we also use continuous RRT, which is preferred in cases of haemodynamic instability. Patients receiving continuous RRT were not included in the study.

Patients had a 14F dual-lumen catheter inserted in the femoral or jugular veins (with 25- and 14-cm catheter lengths, CS-26142-F and CS-12142-F, Arrow Intl, Reading, PA, respectively). Both lines of the circuit filled with heparinised 0.9 % saline were simultaneously connected to the catheter. Circuit anticoagulation was performed with enoxaparin (4000 IU in the circuit at the beginning of dialysis), except if unfractionated heparin was already intravenously administered for another reason. In the case of high haemorrhagic risk, anticoagulation was not performed, but the circuit was flushed with 100 mL of saline every 30 min. No fluid was systematically infused at the induction of haemodialysis.

Purified (reverse osmosis) water and bicarbonate-based dialysate were used. According to our practice, dialysate sodium concentration was set at 145 mmol/L, except in the case of severe dysnatremia. Potassium concentration was set at 3 mmol/L, except in the case of severe hyperkalaemia. Dialysate temperature was 36 °C. Dialysate flow rate was 500 mL/min in all sessions, and blood flow rate was 200–300 mL/min. The duration of intermittent RRT and the volume of fluid removed were planned by the physicians in charge of the patient.

Study design

Patients were included when RRT with ultrafiltration was planned and the RRT modalities were fixed. The study protocol stipulated that these modalities must not be changed by the participation of the patient to the study and by the results of the PLR test.

At baseline, before connecting the patient to the RRT circuit, a first set of haemodynamic variables was recorded, including heart rate, blood pressure, CI (measured by transpulmonary thermodilution), global end-diastolic volume and extravascular lung water. A PLR test was then performed as it has been previously described [20]. Briefly, the patient was moved from the semi-recumbent position to a PLR position, with legs elevated at 45° and the trunk horizontal. This was achieved by moving the bed without touching the patient. The peak CI value (measured by pulse contour analysis) during the PLR test was recorded. It is usually attained within one minute [21]. Transpulmonary thermodilution was not performed during PLR because, due to the time required by the repeated bolus injections, it could miss the maximal change in CI, which may decrease after having reached its peak value in some patients [20].

The patient was moved back to the semi-recumbent position. After stabilisation of CI, intermittent RRT was started. Immediately after the beginning of RRT (H0) and at each of the *n* hours until the end of RRT (H1 to Hn), haemodynamic variables were recorded again, including heart rate, blood pressure, CI (measured by transpulmonary thermodilution), global end-diastolic volume and extravascular lung water. Clinicians in charge were not blind for the result of the PLR test.

Intolerance to intermittent RRT

Haemodynamic intradialytic hypotension was defined as the occurrence of one episode of hypotension requiring one or more of the following interventions from the clinicians in charge: interruption of fluid removal, introduction of norepinephrine or increase in its dose, administration of volume expansion or interruption of RRT. Hypotension was defined as a mean arterial pressure lower than 65 mmHg [22], except in patients with a previous medical history of chronic hypertension. In this case, hypotension was defined by a mean arterial pressure lower than 80 mmHg. In all patients, a set of haemodynamic measurements was recorded at the time of hypotension before any further intervention. In patients where RRT was interrupted, a set of haemodynamic measurements was also recorded immediately after blood restitution. For better clarity of data presentation in patients with intradialytic hypotension, analysis was stopped at the time of hypotension, even if this did not lead to the interruption of RRT (i.e. if hypotension led to the introduction/increase in the dose of norepinephrine or the stop of fluid removal).

Statistical analysis

The normality of data distribution was tested with the Anderson–Darling test. Data are expressed as median [interquartile range] or *n* (frequency in %), as appropriate. The primary analysis consisted in predicting the occurrence of intradialytic hypotension by the means of the PLR test performed before RRT. Receiver operating characteristic (ROC) curves were constructed to test the ability of PLR-induced changes in CI and of CI at baseline to predict intradialytic hypotension. The areas under the ROC curves (AUC) were compared using the DeLong's test. AUC, sensitivities, specificities, positive and negative predictive values are expressed as the values [95 % confidence interval]. The best value of PLR-induced changes in CI and arterial pulse pressure (PP) for predicting intradialytic hypotension was determined as the one providing the best Youden index.

A secondary analysis consisted in describing the time course of different variables in patients with and without intolerance to RRT. The dynamics of the variables was modelled using linear mixed-effect models with a random intercept and slope and compared [23]. Mixed-effect models that we used are currently the best way to explore longitudinal data with repeated measurements over time. Mixed models take into account the correlation between measurements in a given subject and more importantly use the whole information (i.e. all the measurements), providing a greater power than when the outcome is dichotomised as, for example, in logistic regression analysis. The models included both fixed and random effects for the intercept and slope. In multivariate analysis, the model was adjusted on age, fluid removal and initial systolic arterial pressure.

The sample size was estimated by considering a predicted mean value of CI at a baseline of 3 L/min/m^2, a standard deviation of CI at a baseline of 1 L/min/m^2, a PLR-induced change in CI of 20 % in patients with intradialytic hypotension [24] and an incidence of intradialytic hypotension of 33 %, with an α-risk of 5 % and a β-risk of 20 %. Eventually, the sample size was estimated to be 26 cases of well-tolerated RRT and 13 cases poorly tolerated RRT. Statistical analysis was performed with MedCalc 8.1.0.0 software (Mariakerke, Belgium). Mixed model analyses were performed with STATA software (release 13; StataCorp., College Station, Texas, USA).

Results

Patient characteristics

Four patients were excluded because RRT was interrupted due to filter clotting and three others because the dose of sedative drugs was increased during the study period.

Among the 39 remaining patients, six were under chronic intermittent haemodialysis before ICU admission. Eight patients had a renal transplant. No patient received antihypertensive treatment at the time of the study. The characteristics of the 26 patients without intradialytic hypotension and of the 13 patients with intradialytic hypotension are described in Table 1. RRT settings in both groups are shown in Table 2. No patient presented clinical signs of intra-abdominal hypertension. No patient received dobutamine. Mortality in the intensive care unit was 54 % in both groups of patients.

Outcome of RRT

At mixed-effects model analysis, the global end-diastolic volume decreased in patients with and without intradialytic hypotension with similar slopes (−11 and −22 mL/m^2/h, respectively, p = 0.40). Apart from global end-diastolic volume, in the 26 patients without intradialytic hypotension, no significant change in haemodynamic variables was observed during RRT (Table 3). In the 13 patients where intradialytic hypotension occurred, the time between the start of RRT and hypotension was 120 [60–180] min (Table 4). In these patients at H2, the decrease in CI (21 ± 15 %) was significantly lower than the decrease in arterial pulse pressure (11 ± 11 %) (p < 0.001). This was also the case for the decrease in stroke volume index (18 ± 16 %).

The slopes of mean and diastolic arterial pressure and of CI differed significantly between patients with and without intradialytic hypotension. The slope differences in mean arterial pressure, diastolic arterial pressure, stroke volume index and CI were −4 mmHg/h, p = 0.02, −3 mmHg/h, p = 0.04, −2.2 L/min/m^2, p < 0.01 and −0.17 L/min/m^2/h, p = 0.02, respectively (Additional file 1: Table SDC2). No slope difference was found when comparing between-group changes in heart rate and systolic arterial pressure over time.

In 10 of the 13 patients with intradialytic hypotension, the decision was taken to stop RRT (Table 4). In these cases, blood restitution induced a significant increase in global end-diastolic volume, CI and mean arterial pressure (Additional file 1: Table SDC1). Norepinephrine was increased in three other patients with intradialytic hypotension. In all 13 cases, this treatment resolved hypotension.

Differences at baseline between patients with and without intradialytic hypotension

The CI at baseline was significantly lower in patients with than in patients without intradialytic hypotension (3.0 [2.3–3.2] vs. 3.5 [2.7–4.2] L/min/m^2, respectively, p = 0.03, Table 3; Fig. 1).

Patients with and without intradialytic hypotension did not differ at baseline in any variables except CI, including heart rate, systolic and mean arterial pressures, global end-diastolic volume, proportion of patients receiving norepinephrine and dose of norepinephrine in patients receiving this drug (Tables 1, 3). The settings of intermittent RRT at baseline were similar in both groups of patients (Table 2).

Prediction of intradialytic hypotension

As shown in Table 3 and Fig. 2, in the 26 patients without intradialytic hypotension, the PLR test did not induce any significant change in CI. Conversely, in patients with intradialytic hypotension, PLR significantly increased CI by 20 ± 16 % (p = 0.001, Table 3; Fig. 2).

PLR-induced changes in CI predicted the occurrence of intradialytic hypotension with an AUC under the ROC curve of 0.89 (95 % confidence interval 0.75–0.97) (p < 0.05 from 0.50) (Fig. 3; Additional file 1: Table SDC3). The best diagnostic threshold was 9 %. It provided a sensitivity of 77 % (95 % confidence interval 46–95 %), a specificity of 96 % (95 % confidence interval 80–100 %), a positive predictive value of 91 % (95 % confidence interval 57–100 %) and a negative predictive value of 89 % (95 % confidence interval 72–98 %). Three false negatives were observed. In these patients, the volume of fluid that had been removed was 2420, 2750 and 3500 mL.

As shown in Fig. 3 and Additional file 1: Table SDC3, the area under the ROC curves constructed for the value of CI, stroke volume and global end diastolic at baseline was significantly lower than that of PLR-induced changes in CI. This was also the case for the PLR-induced changes in arterial pulse pressure (Fig. 3; Additional file 1: Table SDC3).

Discussion

In this study, we observed that preload dependence, as assessed by the PLR test, was higher in patients who presented haemodynamic intolerance to fluid removal during intermittent RRT than in patients who well tolerated fluid removal. A PLR-induced increase in CI at baseline by more than 9 % predicted intradialytic hypotension with a good specificity and a good positive predictive value.

Table 1 Patient characteristics

	Patients without intradialytic hypotension ($n = 26$)	Patients with intradialytic hypotension ($n = 13$)	p value
Age (years)	63 [49–69]	63 [54–80]	0.17
Male gender (no, %)	17 (65 %)	8 (59 %)	0.99
Simplified Acute Physiology Score II	41 [46–55]	49 [45–53]	0.49
Previous chronic renal failure (no, %)	10 (40 %)	5 (38 %)	0.82
Previous chronic arterial hypertension (no, %)	8 (30 %)	5 (40 %)	0.79
Aetiology of acute circulatory failure (no, %)			
Septic	20 (77 %)	10 (77 %)	0.69
Cardiogenic	6 (23 %)	3 (23 %)	0.69
Incidence of shock diagnosis criteria at the initial phase			
Systolic arterial pressure <90 mmHg	26 (100 %)	13 (100 %)	–
Decrease >50 mmHg in previously hypertensive patients	0 (0 %)	1 (8 %)	0.68
Need for norepinephrine administration	26 (100 %)	13 (100 %)	–
Urine output <0.5 mL/kg/h for at least 2 h	26 (100 %)	12 (92 %)	0.68
Heart rate >100 beats/min	20 (77 %)	13 (100 %)	0.16
Skin mottling	8 (31 %)	6 (46 %)	0.57
Blood lactate >2 mmol/L	26 (100 %)	11 (85 %)	0.21
Left ventricular ejection fraction (%)	50 [30–60]	45 [35–52]	0.57
Modalities of ventilation			
Invasive mechanical ventilation (no, %)	11 (42 %)	6 (46 %)	0.91
Tidal volume (mL/kg)	6 [6–7]	7 [6–7]	0.34
PEEP (cmH_2O)	7 [6–10]	7 [7–11]	0.22
Plateau pressure (cmH_2O)	17 [16–19]	18 [16–24]	0.31
Respiratory rate (min^{-1})	20 [15–20]	20 [20–21]	0.71
Non-invasive mechanical ventilation (no, %)	6 (23 %)	0 (0 %)	0.16
No mechanical ventilation (no, %)	9 (35 %)	7 (54 %)	0.43
Acute respiratory distress syndrome (no, %)	10 (38 %)	6 (46 %)	0.89
Blood urea nitrogen (mmol/L)	32 [28–34]	30 [29–31]	0.25
Patients receiving norepinephrine (no, %)	9 (35 %)	7 (54 %)	0.43
Dose of norepinephrine (μg/kg/min)	0.15 [0.04–0.25]	0.24 [0.21–0.32]	0.69
Lactate (mmol/L)	1.1 [0.9–1.1]	0.9 [0.9–1.1]	0.38
Days in the ICU before inclusion (days)	13 [6–28]	11 [5–18]	0.67

Values are expressed as median [interquartile range] or number and frequency in %

There was no significant difference between patients with and patients without intradialytic hypotension

PEEP positive end-expiratory pressure; *RRT* renal replacement therapy

Table 2 Settings of intermittent renal replacement therapy at baseline

	Patients without intradialytic hypotension ($n = 26$)	Patients with intradialytic hypotension ($n = 13$)	p value
Planned duration (h)	4.0 [4.0–5.3]	6.0 [4.0–6.0]	0.08
Rate of fluid removal (mL/h)	1000 [660–1000]	660 [500–1000]	0.53
Dialysate sodium concentration (mmol/L)	145 [144–145]	145 [144–145]	0.40
K^+ in dialysate (mmol/L)	3.0 [2.0–3.0]	3.0 [3.0–3.0]	0.53
Temperature (°C)	36 [36–36]	36 [36–36]	–

Values are expressed as median [interquartile range] or number and frequency in %

There was no significant difference between patients with and patients without intradialytic hypotension

RRT renal replacement therapy

Table 3 Changes in haemodynamic variables

	Baseline	PLR	(% change from baseline)	H1	H2	H3	H4	H5	H6
Number of patients at this time of the study									
Patients without intra-dialytic hypotension	26	26		26	26	25	23	8	7
Patients with intradialytic hypotension	13	13		13	9	5	2	0	0
Heart rate (beats/min)									
Patients without intra-dialytic hypotension	93 [81–106]	91 [79–101]	0 [-2–1]	90 [78–104]	93 [78–103]	91 [81–109]	89 [78–107]	97 [84–110]	97 [94–119.00]
Patients with intradialytic hypotension	95 [90–98]	95 [91–97]	0 [1–1]	91 [90–99]	93 [73–102]	89 [68–96]	103 [96–111]	–	–
Systolic arterial pressure (mmHg)*									
Patients without intra-dialytic hypotension	130 [120–151]	134 [120–151]	0 [0–3]	125 [115–153]	131 [118–148]	128 [113–150]	130 [110–149]	117 [109–140]	97 [94–119.00]
Patients with intradialytic hypotension	117 [102–131]	120 [111–130]	0 [0–3]	112 [108–120]	105 [102–108]	108 [98–109]	105 [92–119]	–	–
Mean arterial pressure (mmHg)									
Patients without intra-dialytic hypotension	87 [82–98]	90 [82–102]	0 [-1–3]	84 [78–95]	90 [80–96]	90 [76–96]	86 [79–94]	82 [74–92]	67 [66–61.00]
Patients with intradialytic hypotension	87 [79–89]	88 [82–92]	2 [-1–5]	81 [69–84]	75 [69–83]	68 [68–85]	78 [72–84]	–	–
Diastolic arterial pressure (mmHg)*									
Patients without intra-dialytic hypotension	64 [57–73]	64 [58–75]	0 [0–4]	62 [56–69]	65 [57–71]	65 [52–72]	61 [58–67]	63 [56–68]	57 [53–60.00]
Patients with intradialytic hypotension	65 [63–71]	68 [60–71]	1 [0–4]	63 [46–70]	59 [54–63]	51 [48–61]	62 [21–63]	–	–
Cardiac index (L/min/m^2)*									
Patients without intra-dialytic hypotension	3.5 [2.7–4.2]	3.6 [2.9–4.1]	2 [0–5]	3.4 [2.6–3.8]	3.1 [2.6–3.8]	3.4 [2.2–3.8]	3.1 [2.6–3.7]	2.8 [2.5–3.4]	2.6 [2.4–2.9]
Patients with intradialytic hypotension	3.0 [2.3–3.2]	3.5 [3.1–4.0]	15 [11–36]	2.4 [1.7–2.8]	2.3 [1.6–2.3]	1.5 [1.4–2.1]	1.9 [1.5–2.2]	–	–
Global end-diastolic volume (mL/m^2)									
Patients without intra-dialytic hypotension	765 [654–834]			716 [609–786]	685 [597–786]	707 [588–846]	712 [626–772]	812 [652–921]	865 [632–935]
Patients with intradialytic hypotension	700 [626–749]			693 [570–709]	641 [584–710]	500 [500–663]	539 [503–574]	–	–
Extravascular lung water (mL/kg)									
Patients without intra-dialytic hypotension	11 [8–16]			11 [8–15]	9 [8–15]	8 [8–14]	8 [7–12]	7 [6–9]	9 [6–11]
Patients with intradialytic hypotension	8 [7–14]			8 [7–15]	8 [7–13]	6 [5–7]	5 [5–6]	–	–

Table 3 continued

	Baseline	PLR (% change from baseline)	H1	H2	H3	H4	H5	H6
Cardiac function index (min^{-1})								
Patients without intradialytic hypotension	4.5 [3.5–5.4]		4.4 [4.1–5.2]	4.7 [3.9–5.6]	4.1 [3.8–5.1]	4.8 [4.0–5.0]	4.0 [3.8–4.1]	3.5 [3.0–4.4]
Patients with intradialytic hypotension	4 [3.5–5.0]		4.1 [2.9–5.0]	3.4 [2.5–4.1]	4.3 [3.4–5.2]	4.3 [4.0–4.5]	–	–
Volume of fluid removed (mL)								
Patients without intradialytic hypotension	–	–	1000 [660–1000]	2000 [1320–2000]	3000 [1860–3000]	4000 [2480–4000]	3300 [2900–5000]	4980 [3240–6000]
Patients with intradialytic hypotension	–	–	660 [500–1000]	2000 [1320–2000]	1980 [1500–3000]	3000 [2500–3500]	–	–
Body temperature								
Patients without intradialytic hypotension	37.6 [37.0–38.3]	–	37.6 [37.0–38.3]	37.6 [36.9–38.3]	37.3 [36.6–38.0]	37.2 [36.4–38.0]	37.2 [36.8–37.8]	37.2 [36.8–37.8]
Patients with intradialytic hypotension	37.5 [36.9–37.9]	–	37.5 [36.9–37.9]	37.4 [36.7–37.9]	37.6 [36.6–38.2]	37.0 [36.8–37.3]	–	–

Values were recorded before (baseline) and during PLR. Afterwards, they were recorded 1, 2, 3, 4, 5 and 6 h after starting renal replacement therapy (H1–H6)

Values are expressed as median [interquartile range] or number and frequency in %

PLR passive leg raising

* $p < 0.05$ for these variables, the slope from H1 to the end of renal replacement therapy or intolerance was significantly different from 1 and was higher in patients with no versus patients with intradialytic hypotension

Table 4 Haemodynamic variables at the time of intolerance to renal replacement therapy ($n = 13$)

	Before renal replacement therapy	At the previous record before intradialytic hypotension	At the time of intradialytic hypotension
Time elapsed since the onset of RRT (min)	–	120 [60–180]	130 [100–220]
Volume removed (mL)	–	1980 [1320–2000]	2000 [1000–3000]
Heart rate (beats/min)	95 [89–98]	91 [88–98]	97 [90–104]
Systolic arterial pressure (mmHg)	117 [102–131]	108 [100–111]	90 [76–95]
Mean arterial pressure (mmHg)	87 [79–89]	68 [66–76]	62 [52–65]*
Diastolic arterial pressure (mmHg)	65 [63–71]	57 [48–53]	47 [43–53]*
Cardiac index (L/min/m^2)	3.0 [2.3–3.2]	2.1 [1.5–2.5]	1.7 [1.2–2.1]*
Global end-diastolic volume (mL/m^2)	700 [626–749]	651 [500–728]	600 [554–619]
Extravascular lung water (mL/kg)	8 [7–14]	7 [6–8]	8 [7–12]
Cardiac function index (min^{-1})	4 [3.5–5.0]	3.7 [3.4–5.0]	3.4 [2.6–4.9]
Dose of norepinephrine (μg/kg/min) (in 5 patients)	0.24 [0.21–0.32]	0.24 [0.21–0.32]	0.24 [0.21–0.32]
Decision			
Interruption of RRT (no, %)	–	–	10 (77 %)
Increase of norepinephrine (no, %)	–	–	3 (23 %)

Values are expressed as median [interquartile range] or number and frequency in %

RRT renal replacement therapy

* $p < 0.05$ versus at the previous record before hypotension

Excessive fluid removal is the main cause of intradialytic hypotension [9, 25]. Based on physiology, one could make the hypothesis that this impairment may occur in the specific condition of preload responsiveness, i.e. if the heart is working on the steep and initial part of the cardiac function curve [26]. In such conditions, a decrease in preload induces a decrease in cardiac output and then in blood pressure.

Consistent with this hypothesis, we observed that the risk of intradialytic hypotension during fluid removal was associated with the presence of preload dependence at baseline, while the rate of fluid removal was similar in patients with and without intradialytic hypotension. Moreover, a positive PLR test before RRT identified patients who were likely to present intradialytic hypotension. A 9 % increase in CI during the PLR test was the threshold providing the best Youden index. Clinicians may choose the threshold depending on whether they want to favour sensitivity or specificity (Fig. 3).

Nowadays, in order to decide to undertake ultrafiltration or not, clinicians likely take into account some criteria like baseline levels of arterial pressure, cardiac output, heart rate, cardiac preload (assessed by the global end-diastolic volume in our study). They also likely take into account the fact that the patient receives norepinephrine and the dose of norepinephrine. What our study shows is that intradialytic hypotension was not predicted by any of these criteria that are commonly used. Except the PLR-induced changes in CI, CI was the only variable that differed at baseline between patients with and without intradialytic hypotension. Nonetheless, we found that the prediction of intolerance to fluid removal that it provided was significantly poorer than that provided by the PLR test. It was the same for stroke volume index. The global end-diastolic volume did neither predict intradialytic hypotension. This is consistent with the fact that, although it is a reliable marker of preload [15, 27–29], it does not detect preload responsiveness [24, 28, 30]. These facts suggest that our study actually brings a valuable answer to a common question remained pending until now.

Our results suggest that the PLR test can be used to guide fluid removal in critically ill patients. The positive predictive value and the specificity were good, meaning that a positive PLR test incites to not remove fluid. For a 9 % increase in CI, the PLR test predicted intradialytic hypotension with a good specificity but a lower sensitivity, especially with false-negative cases. An explanation could be that the ability of the PLR test to detect preload responsiveness is not perfect. Another explanation could be that preload responsiveness may be absent at baseline in some patients but could appear later, along with fluid removal. Accordingly, the volume of fluid removed was particularly high in the three false positives we observed. A third explanation for the false negatives could be that, besides excessive fluid removal, vasodilation may contribute to some cases of intradialytic hypotension [9, 25].

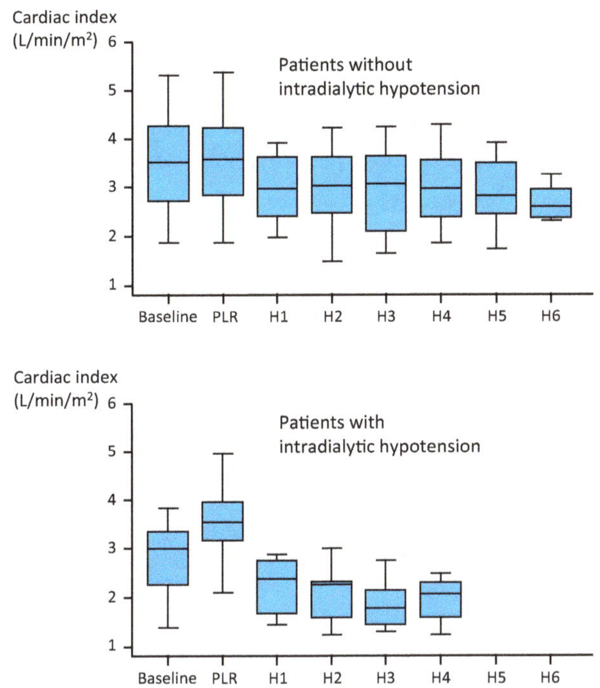

Fig. 1 Changes in cardiac index at different study times in patients with and without intolerance to renal replacement therapy (RRT). *PLR* passive leg raising. The *central box* represents the values from lower to upper quartiles. The *middle line* represents the median. The *vertical line* extends from the minimum to the maximum values

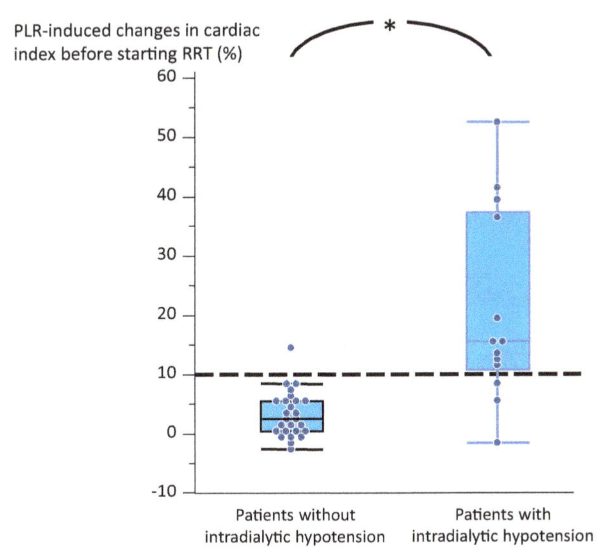

Fig. 2 Changes in cardiac index induced by passive leg raising (PLR) test performed before starting renal replacement therapy (RRT) in patients with and without intradialytic hypotension. *$p < 0.05$ versus patients with intradialytic hypotension

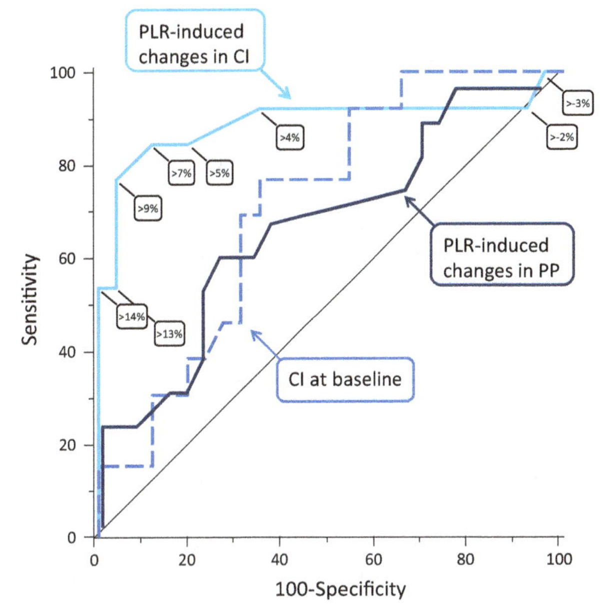

Fig. 3 Receiver operating characteristic curves describing the ability of the changes in cardiac index (CI) induced by passive leg raising (PLR, with corresponding thresholds), the changes in arterial pulse pressure (PP) induced by PLR and the value of cardiac index at baseline to predict the occurrence of intradialytic hypotension

Our study should be regarded as a proof of the concept that the risk of intradialytic hypotension in patients with acute circulatory failure is associated with the presence of preload dependence. In a next step, prospective studies should compare strategies where the decision to remove fluid during RRT would be based on the assessment of preload dependence or not, with the occurrence of intradialytic hypotension as an end point. More generally, this would offer the opportunity to decide fluid removal on standardised protocols. In this regard, an interesting study showed that protocolised fluid removal with continuous RRT was associated with large negative fluid balances in patients, while standard fluid balance prescription did not result in a substantial negative fluid balance [31].

We chose to investigate fluid removal performed only by intermittent RRT and not by other means. Indeed, with diuretics, the volume of removed fluid is variable and this would make the investigation complex. Also, we did not test continuous RRT since it is not in our practice to use this technique in haemodynamically stable patients. The majority of our patients were in the resolving phase of circulatory failure. Even though our findings should be the same at earlier phases of shock, the decision to reduce cardiac preload is less often taken at the initial phase of haemodynamic resuscitation.

We defined intolerance to fluid removal on changes in mean arterial pressure. Nevertheless, since the sympathetic system tends to maintain mean arterial pressure stable when CI changes [32], changes in CI occurred earlier than changes in mean arterial pressure in our patients. For instance, at H2 in patients with intradialytic hypotension, the decrease in mean arterial pressure was 14 ± 11 %, while the decrease in CI was 21 ± 15 % ($p < 0.05$). Assessing whether haemodynamic intolerance to fluid removal should be defined on CI rather than on mean arterial pressure was out of the purpose of this study.

We decided to leave the ultrafiltration rate at the discretion of the attending clinician. In theory, one could suspect that patient characteristics at baseline would have influenced this choice. Nevertheless, the study protocol stipulated that the choice of ultrafiltration rate should be taken before the PLR test and should not be changed afterwards. Also, it is unlikely that other factors like heart rate, the presence of norepinephrine infusion and the rate of this infusion for instance would have significantly influenced the choice of ultrafiltration rate. Indeed, in such a case, such characteristics would have been significantly different between patients with and without intradialytic hypotension. Except for CI at baseline, this was not the case.

One limitation of the present research is that, for feasibility reasons, we did not perform the PLR test at each time point of the study. It is likely that a continuous assessment of preload dependence would avoid the occurrence of intradialytic hypotension, but this has yet to be investigated. Another limitation is that we did not monitor the changes in blood urea nitrogen or plasma sodium concentration during dialysis, while their variations may influence the haemodynamic tolerance of dialysis [9]. Nevertheless, the facts that their levels at baseline were similar in both groups and that the rate of dialysate flow was also similar suggest that the changes of these variables were similar in patients with and without intradialytic hypotension. A limitation of our study could also reside in the fact that we did not measure the intra-abdominal pressure, although it may have an impact on the phenomena we observed [33, 34]. Another limitation is that the PLR test was not performed in a blind manner. Finally, in this study, we did not compare two strategies of fluid removal, one in which it would be guided by the PLR test and another one in which it would not. This should be performed by further investigations.

In conclusion, the presence of preload dependence, as assessed by a positive PLR test before starting RRT, predicts whether fluid removal by ultrafiltration will induce haemodynamic intolerance or not.

Key messages

- Haemodynamic intolerance to fluid removal during RRT is associated with the presence of preload dependence.
- A positive PLR test before fluid removal predicts the occurrence of subsequent hypotension during RRT.

Abbreviations

CI: cardiac index; PLR: passive leg raising test; RRT: renal replacement therapy.

Authors' contributions

XM conceived the study, performed analysis and interpretation of the data and drafted the manuscript. FC and LC performed the collection of data, contributed to analysis and interpretation of the data. PS, MD and NA contributed to the collection of data. EK supervised the statistical analysis. CR helped draft the manuscript. J-LT participated in the study design, performed analysis and interpretation of the data and helped draft the manuscript. All authors read and approved the final manuscript.

Author details

[1] Service de réanimation médicale, Hôpital de Bicêtre, Hôpitaux universitaires Paris-Sud, 78, rue du Général Leclerc, 94270 Le Kremlin-Bicêtre, France. [2] Faculté de médecine Paris-Sud, Inserm UMR S_999, Univ Paris-Sud, 63, rue Gabriel Péri, 94270 Le Kremlin-Bicêtre, France. [3] Service de santé publique, Hôpital de Bicêtre, Hôpitaux universitaires Paris-Sud, 78, rue du Général Leclerc, 94270 Le Kremlin-Bicêtre, France. [4] Service de réanimation médicale, Centre Hospitalier Universitaire de Bicêtre, 78, rue du Général Leclerc, 94270 Le Kremlin-Bicêtre, France.

Acknowledgements

The authors warmly thank Dr. Antoine RACHAS for his help in statistical reviewing.

Competing interests

Profs. Jean-Louis Teboul and Xavier Monnet are members of the Medical Advisory Board of Pulsion Medical Systems. Dr. Dres gave some lectures for Pulsion Medical Systems. The authors declare that they have no competing interests.

References

1. Lira A, Pinsky MR. Choices in fluid type and volume during resuscitation: impact on patient outcomes. Ann Intensive Care. 2014;4:38.
2. Marik PE. Iatrogenic salt water drowning and the hazards of a high central venous pressure. Ann Intensive Care. 2014;4:21.
3. Vincent JL, Sakr Y, Sprung CL, Ranieri VM, Reinhart K, Gerlach H, et al. Sepsis in European intensive care units: results of the SOAP study. Crit Care Med. 2006;34:344–53.
4. Jozwiak M, Silva S, Persichini R, Anguel N, Osman D, Richard C, et al. Extravascular lung water is an independent prognostic factor in patients with acute respiratory distress syndrome. Crit Care Med. 2013;41:472–80.
5. Payen D, de Pont AC, Sakr Y, Spies C, Reinhart K, Vincent JL. A positive fluid balance is associated with a worse outcome in patients with acute renal failure. Crit Care. 2008;12:R74.
6. Prowle JR, Kirwan CJ, Bellomo R. Fluid management for the prevention and attenuation of acute kidney injury. Nat Rev Nephrol. 2014;10:37–47.

7. Wiedemann HP, Wheeler AP, Bernard GR, Thompson BT, Hayden D, deBoisblanc B, et al. Comparison of two fluid-management strategies in acute lung injury. N Engl J Med. 2006;354:2564–75.
8. De Laet I, Deeren D, Schoonheydt K, Van Regenmortel N, Dits H, Malbrain ML. Renal replacement therapy with net fluid removal lowers intra-abdominal pressure and volumetric indices in critically ill patients. Ann Intensive Care. 2012;2(Suppl 1):S20.
9. Schortgen F. Hypotension during intermittent hemodialysis: new insights into an old problem. Intensive Care Med. 2003;29:1645–9.
10. Manns M, Sigler MH, Teehan BP. Intradialytic renal haemodynamics—potential consequences for the management of the patient with acute renal failure. Nephrol Dial Transplant. 1997;12:870–2.
11. Augustine JJ, Sandy D, Seifert TH, Paganini EP. A randomized controlled trial comparing intermittent with continuous dialysis in patients with ARF. Am J Kidney Dis. 2004;44:1000–7.
12. Palmer BF, Henrich WL. Recent advances in the prevention and management of intradialytic hypotension. J Am Soc Nephrol. 2008;19:8–11.
13. Monnet X, Persichini R, Ktari M, Jozwiak M, Richard C, Teboul JL. Precision of the transpulmonary thermodilution measurements. Crit Care. 2011;15:R204.
14. Sakka SG, Reuter DA, Perel A. The transpulmonary thermodilution technique. J Clin Monit Comput. 2012;26:347–53.
15. Michard F, Alaya S, Zarka V, Bahloul M, Richard C, Teboul JL. Global end-diastolic volume as an indicator of cardiac preload in patients with septic shock. Chest. 2003;124:1900–8.
16. Sakka SG. Extravascular lung water in ARDS patients. Minerva Anestesiol. 2013;79:274–84.
17. Jozwiak M, Teboul JL, Monnet X. Extravascular lung water: recent advances and clinical applications. Ann Intensive Care. 2015;5(1):38.
18. Sakka SG, Hanusch T, Thuemer O, Wegscheider K. The influence of veno-venous renal replacement therapy on measurements by the transpulmonary thermodilution technique. Anesth Analg. 2007;105:1079–82.
19. Dufour N, Delville M, Teboul JL, Camous L, Favier du Noyer A, Richard C, et al. Transpulmonary thermodilution measurements are not affected by continuous veno-venous hemofiltration at high blood pump flow. Intensive Care Med. 2012;38:1162–8.
20. Monnet X, Teboul JL. Passive leg raising: five rules, not a drop of fluid! Crit Care. 2015;19:18.
21. Monnet X, Rienzo M, Osman D, Anguel N, Richard C, Pinsky MR, et al. Passive leg raising predicts fluid responsiveness in the critically ill. Crit Care Med. 2006;34:1402–7.
22. Asfar P, Meziani F, Hamel JF, Grelon F, Megarbane B, Anguel N, et al. High versus low blood-pressure target in patients with septic shock. N Engl J Med. 2014;370:1583–93.
23. Fitzmaurice G, Laird N, Ware J. Applied longitudinal analysis. 2nd ed. Hoboken: Wiley; 2011.
24. Monnet X, Osman D, Ridel C, Lamia B, Richard C, Teboul JL. Predicting volume responsiveness by using the end-expiratory occlusion in mechanically ventilated intensive care unit patients. Crit Care Med. 2009;37:951–6.
25. Daugirdas JT. Pathophysiology of dialysis hypotension: an update. Am J Kidney Dis. 2001;38:S11–7.
26. Marik PE, Monnet X, Teboul JL. Hemodynamic parameters to guide fluid therapy. Ann Intensive Care. 2011;1:1.
27. Malbrain ML, De Potter TJ, Dits H, Reuter DA. Global and right ventricular end-diastolic volumes correlate better with preload after correction for ejection fraction. Acta Anaesthesiol Scand. 2010;54:622–31.
28. Reuter DA, Felbinger TW, Moerstedt K, Weis F, Schmidt C, Kilger E, et al. Intrathoracic blood volume index measured by thermodilution for preload monitoring after cardiac surgery. J Cardiothorac Vasc Anesth. 2002;16:191–5.
29. Reuter DA, Goetz AE. Differentiating "volumetric preload monitoring" and assessing "fluid responsiveness". Anesth Analg. 2006;102:651–2.
30. Trepte CJ, Haas SA, Nitzschke R, Salzwedel C, Goetz AE, Reuter DA. Prediction of volume-responsiveness during one-lung ventilation: a comparison of static, volumetric, and dynamic parameters of cardiac preload. J Cardiothorac Vasc Anesth. 2013;27:1094–100.
31. Ganter CC, Hochuli R, Bossard M, Etter R, Takala J, Uehlinger DE, et al. Forced fluid removal in critically ill patients with acute kidney injury. Acta Anaesthesiol Scand. 2012;56:1183–90.
32. Monnet X, Letierce A, Hamzaoui O, Chemla D, Anguel N, Osman D, et al. Arterial pressure allows monitoring the changes in cardiac output induced by volume expansion but not by norepinephrine*. Crit Care Med. 2011;39:1394–9.
33. Kirkpatrick AW, Roberts DJ, De Waele J, Jaeschke R, Malbrain ML, De Keulenaer B, et al. Intra-abdominal hypertension and the abdominal compartment syndrome: updated consensus definitions and clinical practice guidelines from the World Society of the Abdominal Compartment Syndrome. Intensive Care Med. 2013;39:1190–206.
34. Malbrain ML, Peeters Y, Wise R. The neglected role of abdominal compliance in organ–organ interactions. Crit Care. 2016;20:67.

4

Accuracy and limitations of continuous glucose monitoring using spectroscopy in critically ill patients

Roosmarijn TM van Hooijdonk[1*], Tineke Winters[1], Johan C Fischer[2], Edmée C van Dongen-Lases[2], James S Krinsley[3], Jean-Charles Preiser[4] and Marcus J Schultz[1,5]

Abstract

Background: OptiScanner devices, continuous glucose monitoring devices that perform automated blood draws via a central venous catheter and create plasma through centrifugation, measure plasma glucose levels through mid-infrared spectroscopy at the bedside. The objective of this study was to determine accuracy and practicality of the devices in critically ill patients attempting glycemic control.

Methods: The plasma glucose level was measured by the devices and in comparative plasma samples using Yellow Springs Instrument (YSI) plasma analyzers. After adding several previously unrecognized interferences in the interference library, we reanalyzed the mid-infrared signals and compared the resulting plasma glucose level with the reference value. Results are presented in Clarke error grids, glucose prediction errors and Bland-Altman plots and expressed as correlation coefficients.

Results: We analyzed 463 comparative samples from 71 patients (median 6 (4 to 9) samples per patient). After calibrating the system, a Clarke error grid showed 100% of the values in zones A or B. The glucose predictor error demonstrated that 86% of the glucose values < 75 mg/dL were within ± 15 mg/dL of the YSI results and 95% ≥ 75 mg/dL were within 20% of the comparative YSI results. Bland-Altman plot showed a bias of −0.6 with limit of agreement of −24.6 to 23.3. The Pearson correlation coefficient was 0.93 and R^2 was 0.87. In one third of the patients the devices had to be disconnected prematurely (that is before planned disconnection) because of repeated occlusion alarms suggesting blood draw errors.

Conclusion: The devices needed calibration for several previously unrecognized interferences. Thereafter, accuracy of the device to measure plasma glucose levels in 'our cohort' of critically ill patients improved, but external validation is highly recommended. The automated blood draw system of the devices needs further improvement to make this device of value for clinical use (trial registration (Netherlands Trial Register): NTR2864).

Keywords: Glucose; Spectroscopy; Point-of-care; Monitoring; ICU

Background

Critically ill patients often receive insulin infusion [1,2], although concerns with the risk of hypoglycemia and failure to show a positive impact on patient outcome has altered the frequency of use. Intense monitoring of the blood glucose level is a prerequisite for efficient and safe insulin infusion [1,2]. At present, ICU nurses monitor the blood glucose level through intermittent manually obtained blood samples for glucose measurements in central laboratories or at the bedside using different types of point-of-care analyzers [3].

Today's blood glucose monitoring suffers from a variety of error sources that can put ICU patients at risk for insulin titration inaccuracies [4]. Moreover, intermittent glucose monitoring lacks sufficient trending, while immediate feedback and predictability of the effects of insulin could have the potential to improve titration of

* Correspondence: r.t.vanhooijdonk@amc.uva.nl
[1]Department of Intensive Care, Academic Medical Center, University of Amsterdam, Room, Meibergdreef 9, 1105 AZ, Amsterdam, the Netherlands
Full list of author information is available at the end of the article

insulin in ICU patients [5]. Also, ICU nurses usually take > 2 mL of blood with every blood draw and the time consumed is estimated to be as high as five minutes with each draw and subsequent measurement [6], which makes intense monitoring impractical if not impossible. Automated continuous glucose monitoring (CGM) could overcome several of these problems.

OptiScanner devices (OptiScan Biomedical Corporation, Hayward, CA, USA), devices that perform automated blood draws via central venous catheters and create plasma through automatic centrifugation, measure the plasma glucose level every 15 minutes through mid-infrared spectroscopy at the bedside [7]. In a pre-clinical animal study, this device accurately measured the glucose level along hypoglycemic, euglycemic and hyperglycemic ranges [7]. Similar results came from a study with diabetic volunteers [8], and a study of frozen and stored plasma samples from critically ill patients [9]. We hypothesized that the devices provide accurate glucose level measurements in ICU patients. In this study we tested the accuracy of the devices in a cohort of critically ill patients treated according to a glucose control guideline targeting blood glucose levels between 90 and 144 mg/dL (ICU-A in [10]).

Methods

Study design and informed consent

This was an investigator-initiated observational study testing the accuracy of the devices in critically ill patients. OptiScan Biomedical Corporation sponsored part of the study, identified interferences and updated the interference library. The company had no influence on study design, the final analysis and the writing of this manuscript. The Institutional Review Board of the Academic Medical Center (AMC), Amsterdam, the Netherlands, approved the study protocol. Patients or next of kin had to provide written informed consent before the start of any procedure of the study. Analysis of paired data followed the analysis plan as published at [http://www.trialregister.nl/] (NTR2864).

Study location

The study was performed in a 32-bed mixed medical-surgical ICU in a university hospital (AMC), a closed format department with patients under the direct care of an ICU team. The nurse to patient ratio is 1:2. All beds are equipped with a patient data management system (MetaVision®, iMDsoft, Tel Aviv, Israel) in which all clinical and laboratory data are stored.

Study population

Patients were eligible for inclusion if they were aged ≥ 18 years, had an expected ICU length of stay of > three days at time of enrollment and an Acute Physiology and Chronic Health Evaluation (APACHE) II [11] score ≥ 10, had an existing arterial line, and had an existing central venous catheter (CVC) with a free lumen available. Both patients who received insulin infusion and patients who did not receive insulin infusion could be included in the study. Patients were excluded if they had received any investigational product or if they had received treatment with an investigational device within the previous 30 days or were pregnant. For practical reasons, patients in isolation for colonization with multi-resistant bacteria were excluded from participation.

ICU nurses performed glucose control with insulin, following a local guideline targeting at blood glucose levels between 90 and 144 mg/dL (ICU-A in [10]). The local guideline for glucose control advised starting continuous infusion of insulin when the blood glucose level > 144 mg/dL. Insulin was exclusively given by continuous intravenous infusion with only a bolus of insulin given when the blood glucose level exceeded > 360 mg/dL. Subcutaneous insulin is never used. Insulin infusion adjustments were made using sliding scales [10]. Insulin infusion was stopped and boluses of dextrose were given when the blood glucose level declined < 61 mg/dL. According to the local guideline for glucose control, glucose levels were to be measured at least every four hours, but for the study the study protocol dictated that comparative glucose levels were to be measured every two hours. Glucose levels used for insulin adjustment were measured in arterial blood samples using RapidLab 1265 blood gas analyzers (Siemens Healthcare Diagnostics, The Hague, the Netherlands), located in the ICU.

OptiScanner

The device withdraws approximately 2.6 mL of blood every 15 minutes. From this, a sample of approximately 0.1 mL is extracted, heparinized, converted to plasma and analyzed by a mid-infrared spectrometer. For this, after each draw, the device centrifuges the sample, and a measurement is conducted on the plasma component using spectral analysis. This spectroscopy technique is based on the characteristic absorption of vibrational nodes of different molecules, including glucose. Mid-infrared spectroscopy can be used because the glucose spectral peaks are in the mid-infrared region [7]. After measurement, the device automatically flushes the sample to sealed waste containers, cleaning the micro-cuvette in the process. The remaining approximate 2.5 mL of blood is returned back to the patient with a small amount of saline (less than 2.0 mL). There is no heparin in the blood that is returned to the patient. The devices have an onboard interference library which includes drugs and endogenous substances that is used to subtract out interferences.

Study procedures

One device was connected to the proximal port of an existing CVC for up to 24 hours in the first 65 patients, and for up to 72 hours in the last 10 patients. Every 15 minutes, the device withdrew blood and measured the plasma glucose level. These results were not visible for ICU nurses and staff, but were downloaded to a computer after disconnection of the device. Comparative arterial blood draws were taken every two hours, at the same time as the device was drawing venous blood, starting from approximately 8 am until 10 pm. Comparative glucose levels in plasma were measured immediately with the YSI 2300 STAT Plus (Yellow Springs Instrument, Yellow Springs, OH, USA) and with the RapidLab 1265 blood gas analyzers (Siemens Healthcare Diagnostics, The Hague, the Netherlands). The results of the blood gas analyzers were available for the nurses for insulin titration.

Dealing with new interfering substances

An interfering substance was suspected if we found significant discrepancies between paired fixed-wavelength mid-infrared glucose measurements and YSI readings. OptiScan Biomedical Corporation then analyzed the source documentation to identify what substances could have affected the spectra. Pure spectra of the identified interferences were then isolated and subsequently proven to interfere in separate laboratory experimentation by OptiScan Biomedical Corporation. If subsequently verified, the interference was added to the interference library. First, the updated interference library was tested in the already collected spectroscopies. Thereafter, the interference library was updated to the onboard database and used in subsequent patients.

The onboard interference library was updated twice during the study, that is after inclusion and analysis of patient 28 and patient 63, and once after inclusion of the last patient. We thus had accrued three different interference libraries during the study, and one new interference library at the end of the study. After adding all validated interferences in the interference library, the mid-infrared spectroscopies were reanalyzed by OptiScan Biomedical Corporation, calculating a new glucose value for every collected spectroscopy.

Statistical analysis

In two patients, we detected frequent non-physiological glucose changes, defined as increases and/or decreases of the glucose level more than 80 mg/dL in consecutive device-readings while insulin infusion rates were not altered. These non-physiological glucose changes were caused by simultaneous intravenous infusion of 5% dextrose in one patient, and parenteral nutrition in another patient via another lumen of the CVC. Therefore these two patients were excluded for analysis. Figure 1 shows an example of a patient without interferences and a patient with non-physiological glucose changes in a patient who received parenteral nutrition via another lumen of the CVC used for sampling by the device.

We report data as means (± SD) or medians (IQR) where appropriate. In order to be considered for the statistical analysis, each patient needed to have at least two consecutive and successfully analyzed blood draws.

Clarke error grid (CEG) analyses were used to show the percentage of paired values falling within predefined zones. The CEG is divided in ten zones: in the two zones A the device results are < 20% of the YSI results, which is seen as clinical acceptable, or the results are < 70 mg/dL; in the two zones B the device results deviate > 20% from the YSI result, but deviations are seen as clinically acceptable because they are considered only to cause benign insulin titration errors; in the zones C to E the deviations become increasingly unacceptable; in zones D potentially dangerous hypoglycemia or hyperglycemia are left undetected, and in zones E device results lead to opposite treatment decisions, that is the device suggests

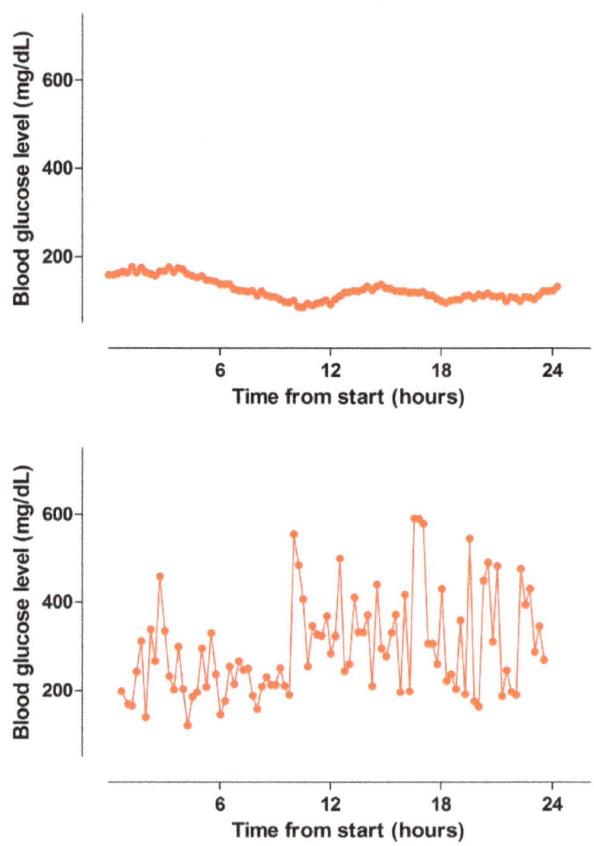

Figure 1 An example of a patient without interferences (upper panel) and of a patient with non-physiological glucose changes caused by simultaneous infusion of parenteral nutrition (lower panel).

hypoglycemia while the YSI shows hyperglycemia, or *vice versa* [12].

For each pair of device and YSI results, the glucose prediction error was defined as (device result – YSI result). The percentage of paired data points with glucose prediction errors are presented according to the current International Standards Organization standard (ISO15197), with the percentage of data points specified that fall within ± 15 mg/dL of the YSI results for YSI glucose level of < 75 mg/dL, and within ± 20% of the YSI results for YSI glucose level ≥ 75 mg/dL. The higher the percentages, the better accuracy for YSI results < 75 mg/dL, or ≥ 75 mg/dL.

Bland-Altman plot with bias (mean difference between the device and YSI measurements) and limits of agreement (bias ± 1.96 x standard deviation of the bias) were used to show agreement between the device and YSI measurements [13]. The limit of agreement shows the band in which 95% of the device results deviate from the mean difference between the YSI and device results. The smaller the bias and limit of agreement, the better agreement between the YSI and device results [13].

The results of the device were regressed on the results of the YSI using unweighted least squares. The linearity between the device and the YSI over the study measurement range were assessed by the Pearson correlation coefficient and coefficient of determination, R^2.

To assess if the occurrence of occlusion alarms was related to the insertion site of the CVC, patients were divided into groups based on the location of their CVC (jugular, femoral or subclavian). The Chi-square test was used to compare the different locations with and without alarms. A *P*-value < 0.05 was considered statistically significant.

Analyses were performed using IBM SPSS Statistics 20 (IBM, Armonk, New York, United States). R (version: 2.15.1; R Foundation for Statistical Computing, Vienna, Austria) was used for CEG, glucose prediction error, Bland-Altman plot and linearity tests.

Results

Patients

We included 75 patients (Figure 2). Two patients from whom non-physiological blood glucose changes were noted and two patients, from whom we could not collect the minimum number of two consecutive blood draws, were excluded from the analysis.

Patient characteristics and metrics of glucose control are shown in Tables 1 and 2. The median connection time was 22.9 (11.4 to 24) hours for patients planned to be connected up to 24 hours and 28.4 (3.2 to 63.3) for the final ten patients planned to be connect up to 72 hours. In total, we used 101 cartridges (median 1 (1 to 2) per patient planned to be connected up to 24 hours; median 1 (1 to 2.25) per patient connected up to 72 hours).

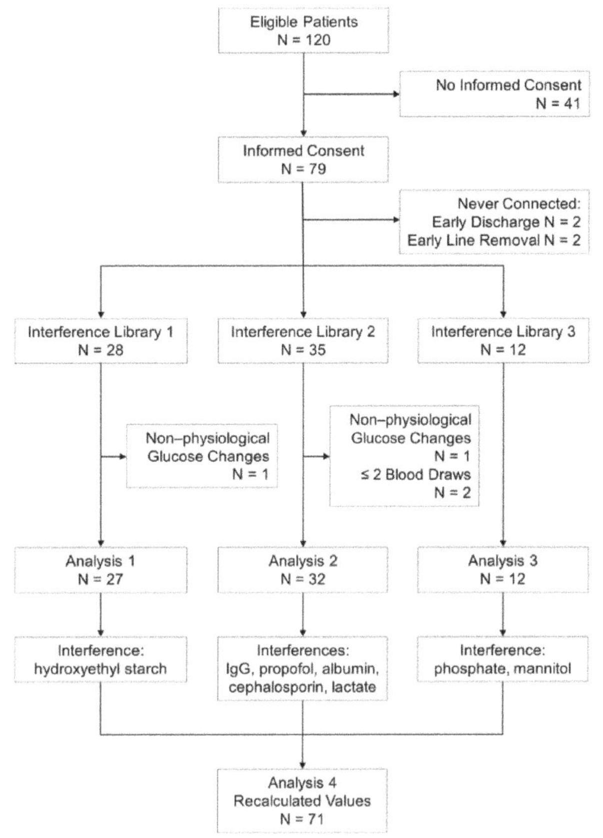

Figure 2 CONSORT diagram of the study.

Accuracy of devices in critically ill patients

We collected 168 paired samples in 27 patients using interference library 1, 168 paired samples in 32 patients using interference library 2, and 98 paired samples in 12 patients using interference library 3. CEGs (Figure 3), glucose predictor error (Figure 3) and Bland-Altman plot (Figure 3) demonstrated that the accuracy of the device improved with the two updates of the interference libraries. Indeed, the percentage of paired samples in zones B and C of the CEG decreased with successive updates. In accordance, the glucose prediction errors and Bland-Altman plots showed an improved accuracy and a smaller bias and limits of agreement. The Pearson correlation coefficient and R^2 increased from 0.80 and 0.63 (with interference library 1), to 0.82 and 0.67 (with interference library 2) and 0.93 and 0.88 (with interference library 3).

With the recalculated values we analyzed all paired samples (Figure 3). The correlation coefficient was 0.93 and R^2 was 0.87. The accuracy of the results of the final 12 patients was consistent with the reanalysis by OptiScan Biomedical Corporation of the overall study population.

Table 1 Patient characteristics

Age (years), median (IQR)	65 (55 to 73)
Male gender, number (%)	44 (62)
Admission diagnosis, number (%)	
Medical	42 (59.2)
Surgical	18 (40.8)
Unplanned admission	56 (78.9)
APACHE II scores, median (IQR)_	21 (16 to 26)
SAPS II, median (IQR)	43 (36 to 54)
ICU LOS (days), median (IQR)	10 (5 to 20)
Hospital LOS (days), median (IQR)	20 (12 to 34)
ICU mortality, number (%)	16 (22.5)
Hospital mortality, number (%)	20 (28.2)
Central venous catheter insertion site, number (%)	
Femoral	30 (42.3)
Jugular	30 (42.3)
Subclavian	11 (15.5)
Type of central venous catheter, number (%)	
Trilumen	23 (32.4)
Quad lumen	48 (67.6)

Abbreviations: *APACHE* Acute Physiology and Chronic Health Evaluation, *BMI* body-mass index, *ICU* intensive care unit, *IQR* interquartile range, *LOS* length of stay, *SAPS* Simplified Acute Physiology Score.

Table 2 Measures of blood glucose control

Number of measurements	484
Blood glucose level - mg/dL (median (IQR))	130.3 (113.0 to 147.3)
Blood glucose level - mg/dL (mean ± SD)	134.3 ± 35.0
Number of measurements per patient (median, IQR)	6 (4 to 9)
Severe hypoglycemia < 40 mg/dL - measurements, number (%)	0
Severe hypoglycemia < 40 mg/dL - patients, number (%)	0
Mild hypoglycemia < 75 mg/dL - measurements, number (%)	8 (1.7%)
Mild hypoglycemia < 75 mg/dL - patients, number (%)	5 (7.0%)
Mild hyperglycemia > 150 mg/dL - measurements, number (%)	110 (22.7%)
Mild hyperglycemia > 150 mg/dL - patients, number (%)	36 (50.7%)
Severe hyperglycemia > 180 mg/dL - measurements, number (%)	42 (8.7%)
Severe hyperglycemia > 180 mg/dL - patients, number (%)	13 (18.3%)

Data consider the period of the study to be from when the OptiScanner® was connected.

New interferences

We found the following interferences; 6% hydroxyethyl starch (Venofundin®, B Braun, Melsungen, Germany); 20% human albumin (Albuman®, Sanquin, Amsterdam, the Netherlands, immunoglobulin G (Nanogam®, Sanquin, Amsterdam, the Netherlands), propofol (Propofol-®Lipuro, B Braun, Melsungen, Germany), cephalosporin (including cefotaxim and ceftazidim), lactate (infusion fluid containing lactate used for continuous veno-venous hemofiltration), mannitol and infusion of phosphate (Figure 1).

Practicality of the devices in critically ill patients

The device was prematurely disconnected (that is, before 24 hours in the first 65 patients, or before 72 hours in the remaining 10 patients) in 8 patients because of early patient discharge, death, or the necessity to use the lumen of the CVC for infusion of medication, and in 26 patients because of device errors (two patients) or problems with withdrawal of blood from the central venous line. In 32 patients occlusion alarms occurred, suggesting that the devices could not draw blood from the CVC (Table 3). In eight patients this alarm was solved through flushing the connection system. In 24 patients, this alarm could not be solved and the device was disconnected. The occurrence of occlusion alarms was independent of the insertion site of the CVC (femoral versus jugular versus subclavian) or type of CVC (trilumen versus quad lumen).

In 18 out of 101 (18%) cartridges an error occurred, mandating replacement of the cartridge. Twelve cartridge failures occurred prior to connecting the device to the patient, that is during the systems initial self-diagnostic check of the system. After connection, in four cases there was a problem with the fluidics system within the cartridge; in one case blood could not be drawn and in one case there was a problem with loading heparin into the cartridge. A system error, mandating a reset of the system, occurred three times. In all cases this happened before connection of the device to the patient. We could not further determine what actually happened, because the logging capabilities failed to analyze this error.

Discussion

The present study shows that the device, after calibration for previously unrecognized interferences, had a better accuracy for measuring plasma glucose levels in critically ill patients. However, in a significant number of patients the devices had to be disconnected prematurely because of occlusion alarms, which could not easily be overcome by flushing the system.

The results of the present investigation confirm findings from previous studies with the same devices. One study of otherwise healthy diabetic patients showed 99%

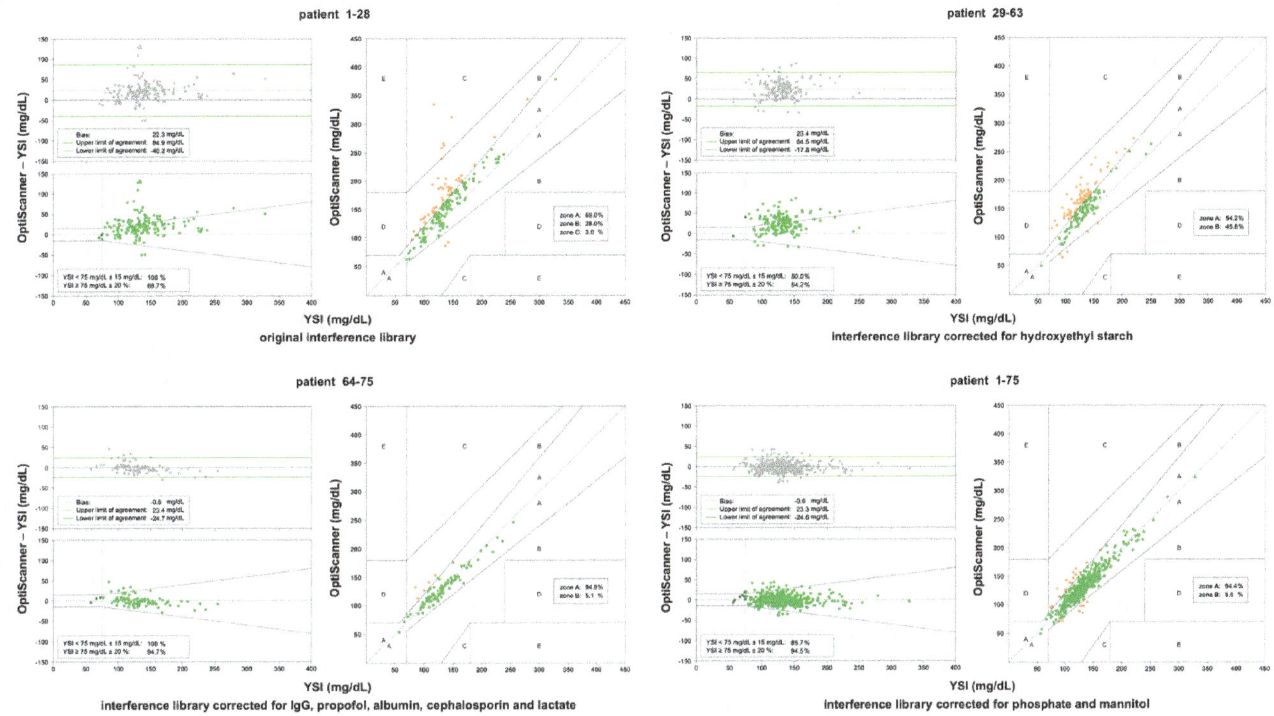

Figure 3 Bland-Altman plot (upper left panels), glucose prediction error (left lower panels) and Clarke error grid (right panels) for patients 1 to 28 using interference library 1 (left upper box), for patients 29 to 63 using interference library 2 (right upper box) and patients 64 to 75 using interference library 3 (left lower box). The paired samples of all patients together (that is, patients 1 – 28 + 29 – 63 + 64 –75) were recalculated using interference library 4 (right lower box).

Table 3 Occlusion alarms

	Number (%) of patients	Number (%) of cartridges
Total alarms	32 (45%)	36 (36%)
Per insertion site		
Femoral	14 (47%)	17 (42%)
Jugular	12 (40%)	13 (30%)
Subclavian	6 (55%)	6 (35%)
Per type of central venous catheter		
Trilumen	14 (61%)	15 (52%)
Quad lumen	18 (38%)	21 (29%)
Alarms leading to disconnection	24 (34%)	24 (24%)
Per insertion site		
Femoral	12 (40%)	12 (29%)
Jugular	8 (27%)	8 (19%)
Subclavian	4 (37%)	4 (24%)
Per type of central venous catheter		
Trilumen	11 (48%)	11 (38%)
Quad lumen	13 (27%)	13 (18%)

of data in zones A or B of the CEG analysis [8]. Another study testing *ex vivo* point accuracy of the same devices using frozen plasma samples from a series of ICU patients found a correlation coefficient of 0.94 [9]. While the device was designed for critically ill patients it had not yet been tested *in vivo*, and specifically, in critically ill patients at the ICU bedside. The present study expands the experience with the devices and shows that the devices could perform accurate glucose level measurements.

The accuracy of the device improved after adding interferences to the interference library. Indeed, after adding the interferences as identified in this study cohort, all paired samples were in zones A and B.

The total percentage of paired data values outside the glucose prediction error of the device is around 6%, less accurate than most of the blood gas analyzers [14]. Several different continuous glucose monitoring devices are being developed, using dissimilar sampling techniques and sensors [1]. The reports on accuracy of other continuous glucose monitoring devices show comparable accuracies, with 95 to 100% of the paired measurements in zone A and B of the CEG [12,13,15-18].

Even though numerous interferences were already identified in previous studies [7-9], several new ones were identified. We were not surprised to find interferences, although we did not expect to find such commonly used substances as interferences. This is probably explained by the fact that the devices were previously only *ex vivo* tested in an ICU patient cohort. Furthermore, this cohort was in another continent, where other medications and infusion fluids are used [10]. The finding of commonly used medications as interferences shows the importance of external validation in different continents and countries, and maybe even hospitals. Therefore, caution is needed with the implementation of devices.

Additionally, we encountered cartridge errors, and system errors which occurred before connection of the device to the patient. We had to disconnect the device frequently because of occlusion alarms, suggesting that the device could not draw a blood sample. Sometimes occlusion alarms could be easily overcome by flushing the connection system. If not, manipulation of the CVC was needed to facilitate blood draws. We are uncertain whether these problems may persist in daily clinical practice.

Notably, results from two patients with simultaneous glucose infusion via another port of the CVC were excluded in the analysis. While simultaneous glucose infusion via the same infusion system that is used for measuring glucose levels should be avoided, the finding clearly shows the risk of erroneous readings.

Any device that uses a CVC has the potential to increase the risk of catheter-associated blood stream infections, especially when blood is retracted repeatedly through the CVC. In addition, the latter could also cause clotting in the lumen. We explicitly looked for these clinically important complications but did not find them in this cohort of patients. It should be noted, though, that this study is too small to draw firm conclusions regarding the risk of blood stream infections or clotting. Also, we did not find a difference in occurrence of occlusion alarms between insertion site or type of catheters. In some cases of occlusion, alarms were solved by manipulation of the CVC. It should be noted, though, that the need for manipulation of the CVC could be a shortcoming of the device. Second, it should be noted that nurses were allowed to disconnect the device at any moment an occlusion alarm occurred in the absence of the investigators. However, it is unknown what happens if repeated occlusion alarms occur and are resolved, that is whether this promotes clotting of the lumen. This needs to be investigated in future studies.

One limitation of the study is that we only collected paired glucose measurements during working hours, which could have prevented us from finding additional interferences (for example, medications that are only infused during the night). Furthermore, this was a single-center study. Also, it is possible that additional interferences could be found when the devices are used in other patient populations.

In addition, the number of paired glucose measurements per patient was small. An additional limitation of the study is that most data points were in a narrow glucose range - we only had 8 of the 484 paired measurements < 75 mg/dL and 42 of the 484 paired measurements > 180 mg/dL. We did not have the opportunity to assess the ability of the device to detect severe hypoglycemia (that is, < 40 mg/dL) as it did not occur during conduct of the study. Here, the low incidence of hypoglycemia suggests that the nurses were experts in insulin titration. Indeed, the nurses had experience with the insulin infusion guideline for many years. In addition, the blood glucose target in the local guideline is higher compared to that in the original Leuven studies, which could also have affected the incidence of severe hypoglycemia. Furthermore, because nurses were aware that the devices monitored the blood glucose level in their patients frequently, it could be that they titrated insulin more precisely. Finally, the nurses had access to all blood glucose levels, thus also the extra ones taken for the study. As such, nurses could also better prevent severe hypoglycemia.

Conclusion

The blood glucose measuring devices we used needed calibration for several previously unrecognized interferences. Thereafter, accuracy of the device for measuring plasma glucose levels in 'our cohort' of critically ill patients improved, but external validation is highly recommended. Also, the automated blood draw system of these devices needs further improvement to make them of value for clinical use.

Abbreviations

AMC: Academic Medical Center; APACHE: Acute Physiology and Chronic Health Evaluation; BMI: body-mass index; CEG: Clarke error grid; CGM: continuous glucose monitoring; CVC: central venous catheter; IQR: interquartile range; LOS: length of stay; SAPS: Simplified Acute Physiology Score; SD: standard deviation; YSI: Yellow Springs Instrument.

Competing interest

Roosmarijn TM van Hooijdonk reported consulting work for Medtronic Inc., GlySure Ltd and research support from Medtronic Inc. and OptiScan Biomedical. Tineke Winters reported consulting work for Medtronic Inc., GlySure Ltd and OptiScan Biomedical. James S Krinsley reports receiving consultant fees from Medtronic Inc., Edwards Life Sciences, Roche Diagnostics, OptiScan Biomedical and Alere and research support from OptiScan Biomedical. Jean-Charles Preiser reported receiving consultant fees from Medtronic Inc., Edwards Life Sciences and OptiScan Biomedical. Johan C Fischer and Edmée C van Dongen-Lases reported no relevant disclosures. Marcus J Schultz reported receiving consultant fees from Medtronic Inc., GlySure Ltd., Edwards Life Sciences and Roche Diagnostics and financial support from Medtronic Inc. and OptiScan Biomedical - all fees and financial supports were paid to the institution. The AMC Medical Research BV received €60.000 for covering personnel and laboratory costs associated with performing this trial. OptiScan Biomedical provided the OptiScanner devices and cartridges free of charge. The investigators were free to make a publication and had no restrictions made by OptiScan Biomedical. OptiScan Biomedical was only allowed to check the publication for company proprietary information. The authors declare that they have no competing interests.

Authors' contributions

Study concept and design: RTMvH, TW, JCF, ECD-L and MJS. Acquisition of data: RTMvH, TW and MJS. Analysis and interpretation of data: RTMvH and MJS. Drafting of the manuscript: RTMvH and MJS. Critical revision of the manuscript for important intellectual content: RTMvH, TW, JCF, ECvD-L, JSK, J-CP and MJS. All authors read and approved the final manuscript.

Author details

[1]Department of Intensive Care, Academic Medical Center, University of Amsterdam, Room, Meibergdreef 9, 1105 AZ, Amsterdam, the Netherlands. [2]Department of Clinical Chemistry, Academic Medical Center, University of Amsterdam, Amsterdam, the Netherlands. [3]Division of Critical Care, Stamford Hospital, Columbia University College of Physicians and Surgeons, Stamford, CT, USA. [4]Department of Intensive Care, Erasme University Hospital, Brussels, Belgium. [5]Laboratory of Experimental Intensive Care and Anesthesiology (LEICA), Academic Medical Center, University of Amsterdam, Amsterdam, the Netherlands.

References

1. Jacobi J, Bircher N, Krinsley J, Agus M, Braithwaite SS, Deutschman C, Freire AX, Geehan D, Kohl B, Nasraway SA, Rigby M, Sands K, Schallom L, Taylor B, Umpierrez G, Mazuski J, Schunemann H: **Guidelines for the use of an insulin infusion for the management of hyperglycemia in critically ill patients.** *Crit Care Med* 2012, **40:**3251–3276.
2. Schultz MJ, Harmsen RE, Spronk PE: **Clinical review: strict or loose glycemic control in critically ill patients - implementing best available evidence from randomized controlled trials.** *Crit Care* 2010, **14:**223.
3. Finfer S, Wernerman J, Preiser JC, Cass T, Desaive T, Hovorka R, Joseph JI, Kosiborod M, Krinsley J, Mackenzie I, Mesotten D, Schultz MJ, Scott MG, Slingerland R, Van den Berghe G, Van Herpe T: **Clinical review: consensus recommendations on measurement of blood glucose and reporting glycemic control in critically ill adults.** *Crit Care* 2013, **17:**229.
4. Dungan K, Chapman J, Braithwaite SS, Buse J: **Glucose measurement: confounding issues in setting targets for inpatient management.** *Diabetes Care* 2007, **30:**403–409.
5. Miller M, Skladany MJ, Ludwig CR, Guthermann JS: **Convergence of continuous glucose monitoring and in-hospital tight glycemic control: closing the gap between caregivers and industry.** *J Diabetes Sci Technol* 2007, **1:**903–906.
6. Aragon D: **Evaluation of nursing work effort and perceptions about blood glucose testing in tight glycemic control.** *Am J Crit Care* 2006, **15:**370–377.
7. Magarian P, Sterling B: **Plasma-generating glucose monitor accuracy demonstrated in an animal model.** *J Diabetes Sci Technol* 2009, **3:**1411–1418.
8. Jax T, Heise T, Nosek L, Gable J, Lim G, Calentine C: **Automated near-continuous glucose monitoring measured in plasma using mid-infrared spectroscopy.** *J Diabetes Sci Technol* 2011, **5:**345–352.
9. Krinsley J, Bochicchio K, Calentine C, Bochicchio G: **Glucose measurement of intensive care unit patient plasma samples using a fixed-wavelength mid-infrared spectroscopy system.** *J Diabetes Sci Technol* 2012, **6:**294–301.
10. Eslami S, de Keizer NF, Dongelmans DA, de Jonge E, Schultz MJ, Abu-Hanna A: **Effects of two different levels of computerized decision support on blood glucose regulation in critically ill patients.** *Int J Med Inform* 2012, **81:**53–60.
11. Knaus WA, Draper EA, Wagner DP, Zimmerman JE: **APACHE II: a severity of disease classification system.** *Crit Care Med* 1985, **13:**818–829.
12. Mulavisala K, Gopal P, Crane B, Mackenzie A: **Preliminary ICU experience of a novel intravascular blood glucose sensor.** *Crit Care* 2012, **16:**P175. Abstract.
13. Schierenbeck F, Owall A, Franco-Cereceda A, Liska J: **Evaluation of a continuous blood glucose monitoring system using a central venous catheter with an integrated microdialysis function.** *Diabetes Technol Ther* 2013, **15:**26–31.
14. Inoue S, Egi M, Kotani J, Morita K: **Accuracy of blood-glucose measurements using glucose meters and arterial blood gas analyzers in critically ill adult patients: systematic review.** *Crit Care* 2013, **17:**R48.
15. Bird S, Macken L, Flower O, Bass F, Hammond N, Webb S, Kennedy N, Baker A, Yarad E, Chau C, Librande M, Strasma P, Finfer S: **Continuous arterial and venous glucose monitoring by quenched chemical fluorescence in ICU patients after cardiac surgery.** *Crit Care* 2013, **17:**P461. Abstrac.
16. Nasraway SA, Ehsan A, Melanson AM, Menzie W, Trieu MQ, Berlin J, Hurley J, Krystyniak K, Segal S: **Accuracy of a novel non-invasive transdermal continuous glucose monitor in critically ill patients.** *Crit Care Med* 2012, **40:**S305. Abstract.
17. De Block C, Manuel YKB, Van Gaal L, Rogiers P: **Intensive insulin therapy in the intensive care unit: assessment by continuous glucose monitoring.** *Diab Care* 2006, **29:**1750–1756.
18. Goldberg PA, Siegel MD, Russell RR, Sherwin RS, Halickman JI, Cooper DA, Dziura JD, Inzucchi SE: **Experience with the continuous glucose monitoring system in a medical intensive care unit.** *Diab Technol Ther* 2004, **6:**339–347.

5

Caring for the critically ill patients over 80

Bertrand Guidet[1,2,3*], Helene Vallet[3,4], Jacques Boddaert[2,4], Dylan W. de Lange[5], Alessandro Morandi[6,7], Guillaume Leblanc[8,9], Antonio Artigas[10] and Hans Flaatten[11,12]

Abstract

Background: There is currently no international recommendation for the admission or treatment of the critically ill older patients over 80 years of age in the intensive care unit (ICU), and there is no valid prognostic severity score that includes specific geriatric assessments.

Main body: In this review, we report recent literature focusing on older critically ill patients in order to help physicians in the multiple-step decision-making process. It is unclear under what conditions older patients may benefit from ICU admission. Consequently, there is a wide variation in triage practices, treatment intensity levels, end-of-life practices, discharge practices and frequency of geriatrician's involvement among institutions and clinicians. In this review, we discuss important steps in caring for critically ill older patients, from the triage to long-term outcome, with a focus on specific conditions in the very old patients.

Conclusion: According to previous considerations, we provide an algorithm presented as a guide to aid in the decision-making process for the caring of the critically ill older patients.

Introduction

In the past 20 years, there has been an increase in the elderly population admitted to the intensive care unit (ICU) [1, 2]. Currently, the median age of critically ill patients approaches 65 years in many countries, and the proportion of the very old (80 years or over) critically ill patients will increase faster than any other cohort in the ICUs [3]. Intensive care unit resources use in the very old patients carries a high burden on healthcare costs [4, 5]. In a Canadian study, the average cost of an ICU admission of patients 80 years or over was $31,679 [4]. Undeniably, caring for older patients frequently poses ethical and practical challenges both prior to and during ICU admission [6]. Such decision making requires an in-depth understanding of aging and its consequences on normal organ function, together with close communication with family and other caregivers [7].

*Correspondence: bertrand.guidet@aphp.fr
[1] Assistance Publique - Hôpitaux de Paris (AP-HP), Service de Réanimation Médicale, Hôpital Saint-Antoine, 184 rue du Faubourg Saint-Antoine, 75012 Paris, France
Full list of author information is available at the end of the article

In this review, we will discuss important steps in caring for the critically ill patients 80 years or over, from the triage to discharge, long-term rehabilitation or palliative care. We will highlight recent researches and advances in this field and propose an algorithm that can be used as a guide in the decision-making process for the caring of the critically ill older patients (Fig. 1).

Characterization of an old patient: lessons to be learnt from geriatricians

Aging

There is no consensual definition of aging [8]. The World Health Organization considers anyone over 65 years old as "elderly." However, in the ICU, we commonly characterize patients 80 years or over as "very old." Aging is a complex transition that includes a physiological and cognitive vulnerability, making the individual more prone to diseases and acute medical events, leading to further decrease in reserve capacities, loss of functional independency and ultimately to death (Fig. 2).

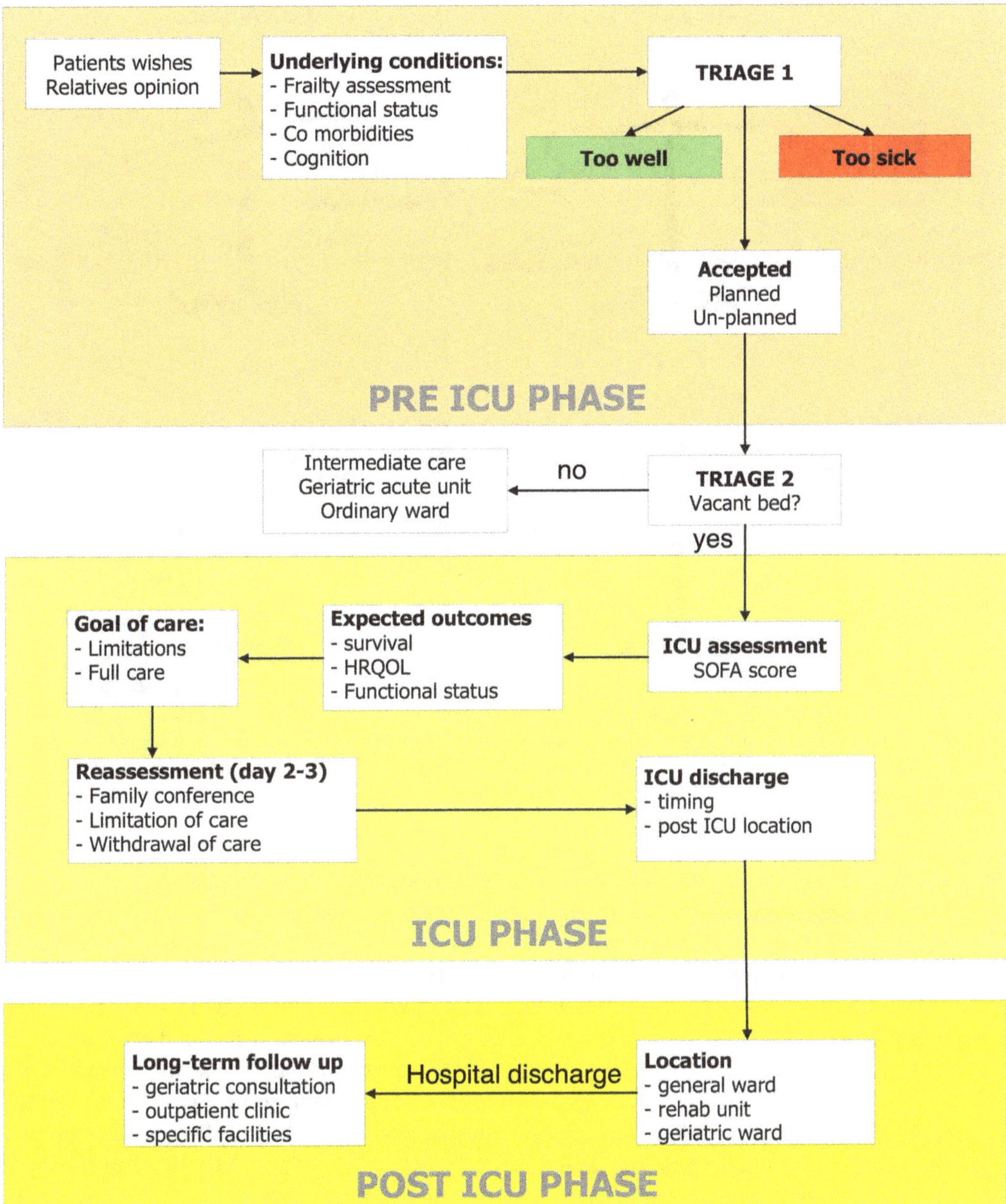

Fig. 1 Algorithm for critically ill patients over 80y

Comorbidities

The proportion of patients with comorbidities and the number of comorbidities per patients increase with age. The mean number of comorbidities per patients is 2.6 ± 2.2 in patients 65–84 years old and 3.6 ± 2.3 in patients 85 years or over [9]. The most common comorbidities are hypertension, diabetes, chronic obstructive pulmonary disease, cardiac failure, cancer and cognitive impairment [9, 10]. Comorbidities are associated with an increased mortality [11], loss in physical independency and an increase in hospitalization rates [12]. In ICUs, comorbidities are associated with higher in-hospital [13, 14] and long-term mortality rates [15]. The Charlson comorbidity index (Table 1) has been validated in critically ill patients and is predictive of mortality [15, 16].

Physiological changes leading to the decrease in reserve capacities have been extensively described [17–20]. Advanced age leads to an alteration in respiratory physiology (loss of elastic lung tissue, increased anteroposterior diameter of the chest, decreased muscle

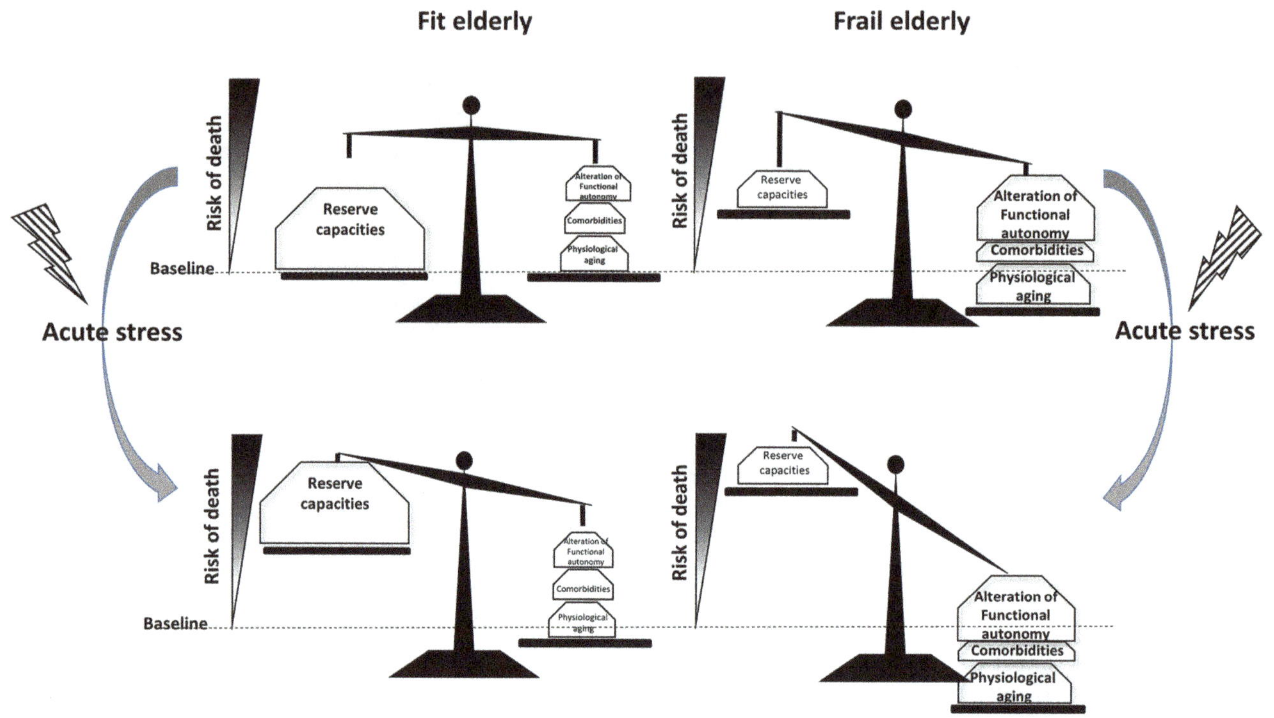

Fig. 2 Impact of acute stress on fit or frail elderly. Physiological aging, comorbidities and functional dependency are the main components of frailty syndrome, leading to decrease in reserve capacities. At baseline, impact of frailty on survival is slight but its weight dramatically grows in case of acute stress (all medical events leading to ICU admission) and increase the risk of death comparatively to the fit elderly

strength and sensitivity of respiratory centers to hypoxemia and hypercapnia) leading to increased risk of acute respiratory failure and mortality. The combination of immunosuppression and "inflamm-aging," called "immunosenescence," results in higher rates of viral reactivation and infection susceptibility and severity.

Malnutrition

Malnutrition affects 12–45% of hospitalized older patients and is associated with longer hospital length of stay, poor physical independency, poor quality of life and higher mortality [21, 22]. Furthermore, malnutrition importantly contributes to "frailty" [23]. In critically ill patients, malnutrition and negative protein–energy balance are associated with higher ICU length of stay, mortality, rate of acquired infection and length of mechanical ventilation [24].

Cognitive impairment

Prevalence of preexisting cognitive impairment at ICU admission ranges from 6 to 43% [25, 26]. In the ICU, cognitive impairment is a strong risk factor for delirium [27, 28], which is associated with increased mortality and with subsequent further cognitive and executive function decline [25, 29].

Functional decline and frailty

General assessment of baseline functional status is crucial. Several scales estimate physical dependency, like the Activities of Daily Living scale and Instrumental Activities of Daily Living scale (Table 1) [30, 31]. In clinical practice, a simplified version of Instrumental Activities of Daily Living scale is used [32].

The "frailty syndrome" is defined as an individual's inherent vulnerability leading to difficulties to overcome acute stress [33, 34]. The frailty model includes areas such as physiological functioning, comorbidities, functional impairment and social difficulties [34, 35]. An easy-to-use Clinical Frailty Scale (CFS) was proposed in 2008, ranking patients in nine group from "very fit" to "terminally ill" (Table 1) (Additional file 1) [36, 37]. An increased CFS is associated with a higher risk of mortality [36]. Furthermore, frailty is associated with a higher risk of falls, worsening mobility and institutional care [38]. A recent meta-analysis concludes that there is a higher risk of not returning to home and a higher risk of in-hospital and long-term mortality in frail patients admitted to the ICU [33]. In the VIP1 study, which included 5132 critically ill patients ≥ 80 years from 311 European ICUs, frailty (CFS > 4) was present in 43.1% and was independently related to ICU (22.2%) and 30-day mortality (35.8%) [39].

Table 1 Summary of main scales used in geriatric evaluation

Comorbidities	
Charlson comorbidity index [16]	Age (years old)
	50–59 (1 point)
	60–69 (2 points)
	70–79 (3 points)
	≥ 80 (4 points)
	Diabetes
	Uncomplicated (1 point)
	End-organ damage (2 points)
	Liver disease
	Mild (1 point)
	Moderate to severe (3 points)
	Malignancy
	Any leukemia, lymphoma or localized solid tumor (2 points)
	Metastatic solid tumor (6 points)
	AIDS (6 points)
	Moderate-to-severe renal disease (2 points)
	Congestive heart failure (1 point)
	Myocardial infarction (1 point)
	Chronic pulmonary disease (1 point)
	Peripheral vascular disease (1 point)
	Cerebrovascular disease (1 point)
	Dementia (1 point)
	Hemiplegia (2 points)
	Connective tissue disease (1 point)
	Peptic ulcer disease (1 point)
Functional autonomy	
ADL scale [30]	Bathing (independent: 1 point; partially dependent: 0,5 point; totally dependent: 0 point)
	Dressing (independent: 1 point; partially dependent: 0,5 point; totally dependent: 0 point)
	Toileting (independent: 1 point; partially dependent: 0,5 point; totally dependent: 0 point)
	Transfer (independent: 1 point; partially dependent: 0,5 point; totally dependent: 0 point)
	Continence (independent: 1 point; partially dependent: 0,5 point; totally dependent: 0 point)
	Feeding (independent: 1 point; partially dependent: 0,5 point; totally dependent: 0 point)
Scale from 0 (totally dependent) to 6 (independent)	
IADL scale [31]	Ability to use telephone
	Operates telephone on own initiative; looks up and dials numbers (1 point)
	Dials a few well-known numbers (1 point)
	Answers telephone, but does not dial (1 point)
	Does not use telephone at all (0 point)

Table 1 (continued)

	Shopping
	Takes care of all shopping needs independently (1 point)
	Shops independently for small purchases (0 point)
	Needs to be accompanied on any shopping trip (0 point)
	Completely unable to shop (0 point)
	Food preparation
	Plans, prepares and serves adequate meals independently (1 point)
	Prepares adequate meals if supplied with ingredients (0 point)
	Heats and serves prepared meals or prepares meals but does not maintain adequate diet (0 point)
	Needs to have meals prepared and served (0 point)
	Housekeeping
	Maintains house alone with occasion assistance (heavy work) (1 point)
	Performs light daily tasks such as dishwashing, bed making (1 point)
	Performs light daily tasks, but cannot maintain acceptable level of cleanliness (1 point)
	Needs help with all home maintenance tasks (1 point)
	Does not participate in any housekeeping tasks (0 point)
	Laundry
	Does personal laundry completely (1 point)
	Launders small items, rinses socks, stockings, etc. (1 point)
	All laundry must be done by others (0 point)
	Mode of transportation
	Travels independently on public transportation or drives own car (1 point)
	Arranges own travel via taxi, but does not otherwise use public transportation (1 point)
	Travels on public transportation when assisted or accompanied by another (1 point)
	Travel limited to taxi or automobile with assistance of another (0 point)
	Does not travel at all (0 point)
	Responsibility for own medications
	Is responsible for taking medication in correct dosages at correct time (1 point)
	Takes responsibility if medication is prepared in advance in separate dosages (0 point)
	Is not capable of dispensing own medication (0 point)

Table 1 (continued)

	Ability to handle finances
	Manages financial matters independently (budgets, writes checks, pays rent and bills, goes to bank); collects and keeps track of income (1 point)
	Manages day-to-day purchases, but needs help with banking, major purchases, etc. (1 point)
	Incapable of handling money (0 point)
Scale from 0 (low function/dependent) to 8 (high function/independent)	
Frailty	
Rockwood Clinical Frailty Scale [36]	1. Very fit—People who are robust, active, energetic and motivated. These people commonly exercise regularly. They are among the fittest for their age
	2. Well—People who have no active disease symptoms but are less fit than category 1. Often, they exercise or are very active occasionally, e.g., seasonally
	3. Managing well—People whose medical problems are well controlled, but are not regularly active beyond routine walking
	4. Vulnerable—While not dependent on others for daily help, often symptoms limit activities. A common complaint is being "slowed up," and/or being tired during the day
	5. Mildly frail—These people often have more evident slowing and need help in high-order IADLs (finances, transportation, heavy housework, medications). Typically, mild frailty progressively impairs shopping and walking outside alone, meal preparation and housework
	6. Moderately frail—People need help with all outside activities and with keeping house. Inside, they often have problems with stairs and need help with bathing and might need minimal assistance (cuing, standby) with dressing
	7. Severely frail—Completely dependent for personal care, from whatever cause (physical or cognitive). Even so, they seem stable and not at high risk of dying (within ~ 6 months)
	8. Very severely frail—Completely dependent, approaching the end of life. Typically, they could not recover even from a minor illness
	9. Terminally ill—Approaching the end of life. This category applies to people with a life expectancy

AIDS Acquired Immunodeficiency Syndrome, *ADL* activity of daily living, *IADL* Instrumental Activities of Daily Living

Medications: a special concern in old patients

The problem of medication and its biodisponibility in old patients have been well described since 1980 [40, 41]. Polypharmacy and inappropriate medications prescription among older patients are receiving increasing attention [42, 43] as it frequently leads to adverse outcomes [44, 45]. In particular, acute hospitalizations pose an increased risk of inappropriate prescription because of newly prescribed medications, the presence of multiple prescribers, inadequate medication reconciliation and a lack of care coordination [46].

Medications typically intended for short-term use during acute illness are sometimes continued after discharge without a documented indication [47]. While it is possible that these drugs were appropriately started during an acute illness in the ICU, most should have been discontinued at ICU or hospital discharge [48]. A common complication of critical illness is an increase in psychological symptoms, sleep cycle alterations, delirium and cognitive impairment, which is associated with increased prescription of specific medications, such as antipsychotics or benzodiazepines [45, 49, 50]. Despite the lack of reliable evidence supporting their use in the ICU, antipsychotics are routinely used in critically ill patients [51]. One potential drawback of antipsychotic use in the ICU is their continuation after the transition to other clinical settings, including discharge from the hospital [52]. Between 12 and 32% of older ICU survivors are discharged with an antipsychotic despite the fact that the majority of these patients were no longer delirious [48, 52–54]. Antipsychotics may even increase the risk of long-term mortality, especially in patients with dementia [55]. The use of these drugs has strongly been discouraged by the American Geriatrics Society and National Institute for Clinical Excellence because of their potential harmful effects [56].

Benzodiazepines and sedative hypnotics are commonly used to treat insomnia and agitation in older adults despite significant risks. Benzodiazepine administration was found to be an independent risk factor for delirium [50, 57]. Clinicians should use alternatives known to reduce the daily number of benzodiazepines such as use of dexmedetomidine or propofol [58, 59].

Early detection of inappropriate medication prescriptions may prevent adverse drug events and improve geriatric care [60, 61]. Different criteria are available to support a multidisciplinary team in medications evaluation such as the Beers Criteria for Potentially Inappropriate Medications Use in Older Adults [62]; the STOPP (Screening Tool of Older Persons' potentially inappropriate Prescriptions) and START (Screening Tool to Alert doctors to the Right Treatment) criteria [63].

Triage: a multidisciplinary approach including the patient's wishes

Intensive care unit triage is triggered by a formal or informal contact from a referring physician to a consultant physician. Both physicians, together with the patient and relatives, should consider the potential benefit from an ICU admission. If there is potential benefit considered, the patient should be proposed for admission to the ICU. If the benefit of an ICU admission is considered to be low, other options may be considered, from admission to a high-dependency unit or intermediate care to treatment on a regular or palliative care ward. It should be emphasized that there is often a mismatch between the clinicians' assessment and the patient's wishes [64]. Multidisciplinary collaboration in the decision-making process is strongly advocated [65]. More specifically for the very old, all healthcare providers who can help to improve the decision-making process for the benefit of the patient should be involved. Several important aspects should be considered by clinicians in the decision-making process: self-reflective and empowering leadership by physicians; practice and culture of open interdisciplinary reflection; culture of not avoiding end-of-life decisions; culture of mutual respect within the interdisciplinary team; active involvement of nurses in end-of-life care and decision making; active decision making by physicians; and practice and culture of ethical awareness.

Many patients are triaged by the emergency physician or the treating physician on the ward before the ICU consultation. This "hidden triage" is often not captured by studies focusing only on patients proposed for ICU admission [66]. However, even when proposed for ICU admission many old patients are declined. In a single-center study, 73.3% (132/180) of older patients referred for ICU admission were declined [67]. Similar data were recently found in a Norwegian multicenter study [68]. In the ICE-CUB 1 study [66], the ICU admission rate in critically ill older patients was only 14.4% after being triaged by the emergency physician and the intensivist. It is remarkable to notice that in these three studies, the long-term mortality was inferior to 100% in patients considered too sick for an ICU admission. On the other hand, the mortality was far from 0% in patients considered too well for an ICU admission (Table 2). These results suggest over- and under-utilization of ICUs. However, in the large multicenter observational Eldicus study ($n=6796$ patients), 82% of all patients were admitted, while nearly half of the patients (49%) were ≥ 65 years. Although a higher proportion of older patients were refused ICU admission, the survival benefit of admitted versus non-admitted patient seemed to increase with age [69].

Advanced directives should be available for older patients

When an ICU admission is considered, clinicians must ensure that invasive procedures consistent with intensive care are in accordance with the patient's wishes. Patient physical dependency and previous documented decisions about end of life must be respected. However, very often realistic advanced healthcare directives have not been discussed before ICU admission. Whenever this is the situation, there are three possibilities:

- The patient has a normal cognition and is able to consent to care. Usually such conversation should be undertaken in the presence of the family or caregivers.
- Frequently, the old patients are unable to consent to care. In that case, physicians must discuss the intensity of care with the surrogate decision makers (family or caregivers). The main question is not what the surrogate decision maker think about and ICU admission, but what they know about the patient's wishes and how the patient would have responded to being admitted to intensive care.
- In emergency situations, there is no time for information retrieval from the surrogate decision makers and treatments are usually started without informed consent. In most countries, it is then possible to withdraw life-sustaining therapies (LSTs) when more information is available [70] (see small case story in Additional file 2).

Level of treatment during the intensive care unit stay

When an older patient has been admitted to the ICU, the most appropriate treatment should be given. However, this does not necessarily mean maximal treatment. If, during the shared decision-making process, certain treatments such as invasive mechanical ventilation are thought to be disproportional to the chances of survival

Table 2 Results from three studies of pre ICU triage in very old patients

Patients triaged	Hospital mortality (%)	Long-term mortality (%)
Garrouste-Ortegas [67]		At 1 year
Admission ($n=48$)	62.5	70.8
Too sick ($n=79$)	70.8	87.3
Too well ($n=51$)	17.6	47
Boumendil [109]		At 6 months
Admission ($n=316$)	32.7	47.5
Too sick ($n=821$)	58	81.1
Too well (1339)	10.1	33.1
Andersen [68]		At 1 year
Admission ($n=250$)	44	60
Too sick ($n=52$)	67.3	88.5
Too well ($n=46$)	34.8	50

or certain treatments are refused by the patient, these treatments should not be imposed upon the patient [64]. However, to give a patient a fair chance all other treatments should be applied. The ethical climate has also been found to have an impact on treatment-limitation decisions and time until death [71].

Severity of the disease

The severity scores have a poor discrimination in old patients [3] because they do not consider any geriatric assessment. A Canadian study developed a prediction tool for futility of ICU care although this study experienced extremely high observed mortality in the higher percentiles of risk [72].

Withholding and withdrawing treatment

Older patients often receive a lower level of treatment intensity than their younger counterparts. For example, the prevalence of limitations of life-sustaining therapies increased with age in surgical population [73–75]. In addition, decisions to withhold LST were made earlier during the ICU stay in comparison with younger patients [13, 76]. In patients without improvement of their clinical situation, the therapeutic intensity level may no longer be in accordance with the patients' chances of long-term survival with acceptable quality of life, and a clinical decision might need to be made. Obviously, the timing of such a decision is arbitrary, but most agree that the older patient should be offered an "ICU trial" that lasts long enough to observe possible improvements [77]. Life-sustaining therapies limitation is not equivalent to end-of-life decision. In the VIP1 study including more than 5000 patients $\geq$ 80 years, the ICU and 30-day mortality rates were, respectively, 29% and 53% in the withholding group, and 82% and 93% in the withdrawing group [70]. In another study, ICU and hospital mortality rates were 56% and 69% despite a decision to withhold or withdraw LST [78].

For patients with withholding or withdrawing of LST, an important goal is to achieve the most comfortable death [78]. Family members reported that the "patient be comfortable and suffer as little as possible" was their most important value and "the belief that life should be preserved at all costs" was their least important value considered in making treatment decisions [79]. Mobile palliative care team could be very useful to help in the decision process and even to propose admission in a palliative unit.

In a recent study focusing on patients older than 80, LST limitation was common (27.2%) but with important regional differences [70]. In the Northern region, 45.2% had LST withdrawn compared with 12.8% in the Eastern region.

Apart from patient-related factors, other reasons to limit LSTs might play a role. Apparently, the ICU bed availability is associated with the timing of limitations of LSTs. Patients admitted in ICUs with a lower bed availability had a shorter time to do-not-resuscitate decisions and patients who had do-not-resuscitate decisions had shorter time to death [80]. In the VIP1 study, there was no relation between number of ICU beds and percentage of LST limitations. Percentage of LST limitations was higher in countries with high growth domestic product and was lower in more religious countries [70].

Situations with specificities related to age

Acute respiratory failure (ARF) was the most frequent reason for urgent ICU admission in the VIP1 study (25%). Mechanical ventilation is responsible for a large percentage of ICU costs [81]. Experimental studies suggest that aging is also associated with an increased susceptibility to ventilator-induced lung injury [82]. The high mortality could be related to delays in diagnosis and treatment [83] since the presenting signs and symptoms may not be primarily respiratory such as delirium and cognitive impairment.

The incidence of acute respiratory distress syndrome (ARDS) increases markedly with age, which is largely determined by a higher incidence of sepsis in the very old [84]. Several studies have shown that age is independently associated with mortality in patients requiring mechanical ventilation and in ARDS [85, 86]. Age was also associated with longer duration of mechanical ventilation, ICU length of stay and mortality in ARDSNet database [87]. Long-term sequelae have been described after ARDS and are more frequent and severe in older patients. The ability to sustain spontaneous respiration after extubation is lower in patients older than 70 years, mainly due to the inability to clear tracheobronchial secretions and a higher incidence of nosocomial pneumonia [87].

Sepsis The incidence of sepsis increases with age. Additional risks include: subtle clinical presentations, institutionalization, use of invasive devices, multiple medications, reduced renal function and poor nutritional status. In the elderly population, sepsis is a major cause of morbidity and mortality, with almost 60% of septic patients being over 65 years of age [88].

Typically, younger patients with sepsis demonstrated fever, tachycardia and capillary vasodilatation. Older patients often exhibit few of these clinical symptoms but may present with an altered mental status, making early recognition rather challenging. Elderly patients often present with heart failure, arrhythmias and arterial hypertension. They have a lower cardiac compliance, whereas the renal perfusion is more cardiac flow dependent; thus, the management of fluid therapy is more sensitive. A predefined volume administration (30 mL/kg) is inappropriate in most patients. Fluid bolus (250 ml at 5- to 10-min intervals) and further evaluation to test whether goals are reached is a reasonable option.

Scheduled surgery should be considered apart from other stays Postoperative patients after planned surgery have a much better long-term survival than acute or emergency admissions [39, 89]. Obviously, patients after elective surgery represent a highly selected population of older patients. These patients tend to be younger, less frail and with a lower SOFA score on the first day of admission than patients after emergency admission [39]. In the VIP1 study, postoperative elective ICU admissions ($n = 906$) accounted for 17.7% of all admission and 24.6% of ICU stays shorter than 24 h. Most of the patients were not frail, and the 1-month mortality was much lower than for acutely admitted patients [39]. In a study by Bagshaw, 72% of critically ill patients over 80 years admitted to the ICU were discharged home after elective surgery [13]. Long-term prognostic is much better for scheduled surgery compared to urgent admission [90].

No validated score is currently available to predict the need of perioperative ICU admission in the older patients. In a study of 275 patients aged 65 years or over undergoing intermediate- or high-risk elective surgery, a multidimensional frailty model (composed of the Charlson comorbidity index, dependence in activities of daily living, dementia, risk of delirium, short mid-arm circumference and malnutrition) predicted mortality rates more accurately than the ASA classification (84% sensitivity and 69% specificity). High-risk patients (defined as a multidimensional frailty score > 5) showed increased postoperative mortality risk and longer hospital LOS [91]. In contrast, the urgent surgical patients requiring ICU admission are as severely ill as medical patients need more organ support and have longer hospital LOS (see Additional file 3).

Timing and location of ICU discharge are keys elements for the outcome

Risk factors for in-hospital mortality after ICU discharge include age, comorbidities and severity of illness [92], in addition to organizational factors, such as discharge time and the availability of step-down facilities [93, 94]. Older patients discharged from the ICU are particularly vulnerable to poor handovers due to their complicated physiology and the substantial decrease in monitoring when these patients are transferred from the ICU to a general ward [95, 96]. However, studies have failed to show an impact of discharge protocol on hospital mortality [96], although none tested the discharge location as a potential variable of interest [95]. Except for acute geriatric units (AGUs), geriatric expertise is usually not available on a regular basis in other wards. To illustrate this, of the participants of the VIP1 study [39], one-third disagreed that a consultation of a geriatrician should be sought when deciding to discharge an elderly patient [97]. Yet, due to their expertise in the field of multimorbidities and acute stress in older patients, geriatricians make a more comprehensive assessment of old patients that may lead to better care and orientation decisions in these patients. Including a geriatrician in shared decision making for old critically ill older patients may improve their outcome. However, no large-scale study supports this hypothesis.

In a cohort of 1283 French patients of ≥ 75 years, 40.3% of the patients were transferred to a geriatric unit after an emergency department visit [98]. Four factors were related to admission to a geriatrics unit: cognitive disorder, "failure to thrive" syndrome, depression or loss of Activities of Daily Living. However, considerable nationwide variations were observed underlying the need to clarify and reinforce this discipline in the emergency healthcare system. A small-scale, single-center study illustrates the beneficial effect of geriatric intervention on the functional dependency of 45 older patients after discharge from a medical/surgical ICU [99]. Although physical function was usually recovered rapidly, the degree of recovery depended on the patient's previous physical dependency.

Inclusion of geriatric consultations has proven valuable in other areas of medicine. Studies have documented that for postoperative older patients, mainly after hip fracture, geriatric unit admission offers a benefit as compared to surgical unit admission [100]. Postoperative admission to a dedicated geriatric unit reduced both re-admission rate and 6-month mortality. After adjustment for comorbidities, risk ratio of death at 6 months was of 0.43 (95% CI 0.25–0.73, $P = 0.002$) [101].

Long-term outcomes are the best criteria to judge appropriateness of decision (admission, LST during the ICU stay)

Predicting long-term survival and quality of life is difficult [102]. The outcome of an older patient admitted to the ICU is dependent on: previous comorbidities, diagnosis at admission, severity of the acute illness at the time, course of the disease during the ICU stay, limitations of LSTs and age itself. There is a confounding factor in the data reporting the long-term survival and quality of life, since patients might have died of limitation of LST.

The quality of life and recovery has been shown to be poorer in elderly patients ventilated for more than 7 days, with higher proportion of debilities [103]. Similar finding were reported for neurocognitive problems such as PTSD or cognitive impairment [25].

A higher proportion of older patients will be expected to wish limitation of care when having a critical illness. Outcome in terms of survival (Fig. 3), physical function at 1 year [104] and quality of life [105] in elderly ICU survivors are often reported to be significantly lower than in their younger counterparts (Table 3).

Older patients surviving the ICU often suffer from sequels, including increased long-term mortality [89], poor quality-adjusted survival [107], cognitive impairment and functional disability [25, 106–108]. Many of these events occur beyond the scope of intensive care. However, it is of outmost importance to try to predict the functional outcome (Table 3) of this very elderly patient group [102] as their focus is less on "longevity" but more on "quality of life." The very old ICU patient is at risk of complications resulting from heavy sedation, prolonged ventilation, immobilization, insufficient nutrition, etc. Ultimately this leads to functional decline. In a prospective study, including 2646 older patients, among the survivors after 6 months only one-third was independent for all activities listed in Katz's scale, while 16.2% were unable to perform at least one activity that they had been able to perform at the time of the ED visit [109]. The pessimistic conclusion was that, at 6 months after the ED visit, 63% of patients had either died or experienced functional deterioration. This is corroborated by a recent Canadian study in older patients with ICU LOS of more than 24 h. The survivors reported significantly worse physical functioning after 3, 6 and 12 months compared with age- and gender-matched controls [104]. In the ICE-CUB 2 study, including 3036 patients (mean age 85 years), the ADL scale decreased in at least one domain in 64% of the patients at 6 months [110]. However, other studies find that only 28–37% did not restore their previous functional dependency, evaluated on activity of daily living at 3, 6 and 12 months [111, 112]. At 12 months, 50% of survival patients recovered their previous ADL, IALD and physical capacities [104, 113]. Furthermore, 72–77% of patients return at home after ICU [13, 112, 114]. It is interesting to point at the lack of data concerning comparison of functional dependency recovery between "young" and "old" patients, while almost 25% of "young" patients do not restore their functional dependency after ICU [115].

A decline in functional performance is accompanied by a decrease in health-related quality of life (HRQoL) as demonstrated in the ICE-CUB 2 study [110]. In an UK study [116], the physical and the mental component of HRQoL short-form questionnaire (SF36) did not improve from 6 to 12 months after ICU discharge. In a Scandinavian study, the HRQoL was lower for the very elderly than for younger patients, although 97% of the elderly survivors lived at home and 88% of them considered their QoL satisfactory or good after hospital discharge [117]. Indeed, other studies show that the long-term HRQoL appears to be similar to age-matched populations [67, 112, 114, 118]. Ultimately, in the worse scenario the patients are at risk of loss of function, inability to return home, requirement for a nursing home and/or remain bed bound for the rest of their lives.

Quality-adjusted life years

Kaarlola et al. [117] showed that the QALYs derived from ICU admission of patients 80 years or over would be a median of 4.1 years, in the 65- to 79-year-old group it would be 10.2 years and in patients less than 65 years it would be 22 years.

House caregivers

One of the most neglected groups is the caregivers of the very old ICU survivors. After hospital discharge, many patients still need help in many activities of daily living, often provided by family members or partners. This radically changes their role from "loved one" to "caregiver." However, many of the family members of surviving older

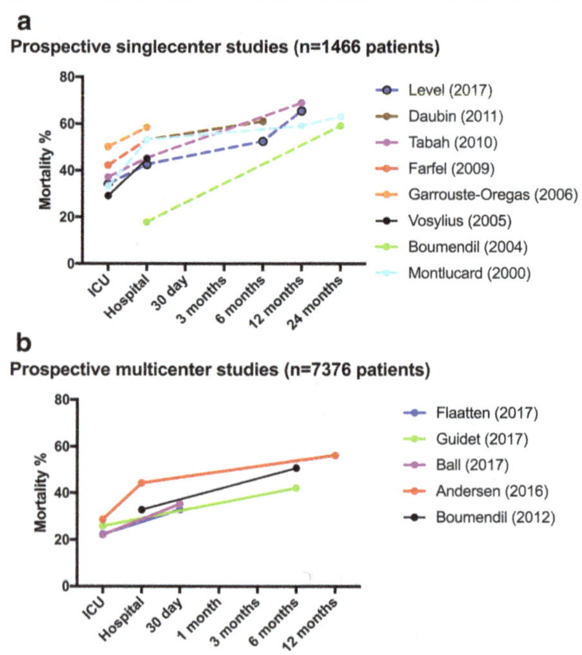

Fig. 3 Mortality. **a** Represents mortality rates in critically ill elderly patients following admission to the ICU at ICU and hospital discharge, at 30-day and 3, 6, 12 and 24 months in single-center studies from 2000 to 2017. **b** Represents mortality rates in critically ill elderly patients following admission to the ICU at ICU and hospital discharge, at 30-day and 3, 6, 12 and 24 months in multicenter studies from 2012 to 2017

Table 3 Long-term functional outcome

References	Tool	Design	Age-group	Patient followed	Main results	Comparison with baseline data (ICU admission)
Kass [123]	ADL	Prospective and retrospective	> 80 years	38/105 (36.1%)	Nonsignificant decline of ADL score at 1 year	Yes
Chelluri [124]	ADL	Prospective	> 75 years, 65–74 years)	96 18/54 (33%) 20/43 (46.5%)	No difference between two age-groups at 1, 6, 12 months	Yes Method?
Broslawski [125]	ADL, IADL, GDS	Prospective	> 70 years	27/45 (60%)	Changes at 6 months related to ICU LOS and severity but not to age	Yes Method?
Montuclard [126]	ADL	Retrospective	> 70 years with 30 days of MV	30/75 (40%)	Decrease in all domains except feeding at 6 months	Retrospective estimation by the patient
Udekwu [127]	ADL	Retrospective	> 70 years	342/672 (50.8%)	At 21 months, significant decrease in ADL with more dependent patients	Yes Method?
Garrouste-Orgeas [37]	ADL	Prospective	≥ 80 years	9/48 (18%)	No change	Retrospective estimation by the patient
Kaarlola [119]	EQ-5D SF-36	Retrospective (in survivors)	65–69 years 70–74 years 75–79 years 80–94 years	114 117 91 50	More than 50% assessed their overall health status as satisfactory. Largest % in those ≥ 80	No
Tabah [128]	ADL	Prospective	≥ 80 years	23/106 (21%)	No change 74% of patients were fully independent	Prospective estimation by the patient or relatives
Boumendil [109]	ADL	Prospective	≥ 80 years	162/329	At 6 months 16.2% were unable to perform at least one activity that they had been able to perform at the time of the ED visit	Prospective estimation by the patient or relatives
Andersen [129]	EQ-5D	Retrospective	≥ 80	58/395	HRQOL comparable with a comparison group (1 year)	
Andersen 2017 [68]	EQ-5D	Prospective	≥ 80	62/250	Lower HRQOL than a comparison group (1 year)	Compared with a age and gender reference population $n = 179$
Heyland [104]	SF-36 (physical function)	Prospective	≥ 80	505/610	50% dead and 26% achieved physical recovery at 12 months	PF compared with baseline values at admission
Level 2017 [130]	ADL, Barthel index	Prospective	≥ 75	65/188	83% of 1-year survivors lived in their own home	ADL compared with baseline at admission
Guidet [110]	ADL	Prospective	≥ 75 years	1528/3036	Selection criteria: preserved baseline ADL (median 6) At 6 months, decrease in ADL of 0.5 points	Prospective estimation by the patient or relatives

critically ill patients are old themselves. As such, they can be considered as "the second victim" and may suffer from the same cognitive and even functional decline as the ICU survivors. For example, in a general ICU population 67% of the caregivers reported depressive symptoms, which remained in 43% at a follow-up of 1 year [119]. Variables that were significantly associated with worse mental health outcomes in caregivers were greater effect of patient care on other activities, less social support, and therefore less sense of control over life. Post-traumatic stress disorder (PTSD) and strain are seen in 21% of the caregivers [120]. A randomized trial, where caregivers provided respiratory physiotherapy at home, showed improvement of the cardiorespiratory status of the patients and their HRQoL (as measured with the EuroQoL 5D methodology) [121, 122]. While the majority of the above-mentioned studies were not specifically designed for the very elderly patient group, it seems logical that the perceived strain, depressive symptoms and HRQoL will also translate to this group of caregivers.

Conclusions and algorithm

In this review, we have given an up-to-date review of the present knowledge about caring for the older ICU patients. This specific group will in the future certainly claim their rights to receive high-quality health care including intensive care. The outcome of the very old has improved over the past decades but remains poorer than for younger patients. Several factors account for this high mortality and more related to underlying disease than age by itself. Advanced care planning will become more and more important in the future because of the increasing number of admission in combination with technological innovation. We summarized in a table, the keys elements that should be considered when deciding to admit a patient older than 80 in ICU (Table 4). There are still many unresolved questions [3] (Table 4), and it is important to get answers to these unresolved issues before the huge « age-tsunami » reaches the hospitals within 10–15 years.

Table 4 Key messages and *unresolved issues*

Triage
Seek for advance directives—*How promoting diffusion?*
Every time it is possible, ask the patient about his/her wishes
If the patient is unable to communicate, seek for relatives/family wishes
Try to estimate the immediate and long-term risk of death considering
Patient baseline characteristics:
Age
Functional status (Clinical Frailty Scale, frailty phenotype, Performance status)
Comorbidities including cancer
Nutritional status and protein–energy balance
Cognitive and psychiatric disorders
Type of admission: scheduled versus urgent
Reason for admission
Acute severity—*a specific score tailored to old patient should be available*
Mobilize geriatric expertise if possible—*impact should be proved by interventional studies*
Define a goal of care anticipating second evaluation after few ICU days—*Impact on triage, mortality, LOS, LST limitation?*
If the patient is denied ICU admission consider palliative care
During the ICU stay
Organ support guidelines might not be appropriate for old patients—*Interventional studies focusing on older adults*
Fluid loading
Ventilator settings
Weaning strategy
Special attention to medication with high risk of
Overdose
Interaction
Consider LST limitation in case of poor response to initial treatment—*Harmonize practice within and between countries*
ICU discharge—*Intervention that should be tested in prospective trials*
Patients are seen by a geriatrician after ICU discharge
They are discharged to specialized geriatric unit
Discuss timing
Long-term outcomes
Test the impact of early rehabilitation on mortality, HRQOL and functional status
Consider the burden for the house caregivers

Abbreviations

ICU: Intensive care unit; ADL: Activities of Daily Living; IADL: Instrumental Activities of Daily Living; CFS: Clinical Frailty Scale; ICE-CUB: Intensive Care for Elderly-CUB Rea Network; APACHE: Acute Physiology and Chronic Health Evaluation; SAPS: Simplified Acute Physiology Score; SOFA: Sequential Organ Failure Assessment; LST: life-sustaining treatments; ARF: acute respiratory failure; ARDS: acute respiratory distress syndrome; STOPP: Screening Tool of Older Persons' Potentially Inappropriate Prescriptions; START: Screening Tool to Alert doctors to the Right Treatment; VIP: Very elderly intensive care patient; ED: emergency department; HRQoL: health-related quality of life; QALYs: quality-adjusted life years; PTSD: post-traumatic stress disorder.

Authors' contributions

All authors contributed to the writing of the manuscript and approved the final version.

Author details

[1] Assistance Publique - Hôpitaux de Paris (AP-HP), Service de Réanimation Médicale, Hôpital Saint-Antoine, 184 rue du Faubourg Saint-Antoine, 75012 Paris, France. [2] Sorbonne Universités, Université Pierre et Marie Curie - Paris 06, Paris, France. [3] INSERM, UMR_S 1136, Institute Pierre Louis d'Épidémiologie et de Santé Publique, 75013 Paris, France. [4] Assistance Publique - Hôpitaux de Paris (AP-HP), Service de gériatrie, Hôpital Pitié salpêtrière, 75013 Paris, France. [5] Department of Intensive Care, University Medical Center Utrecht, University Utrecht, Utrecht, The Netherlands. [6] Department of Rehabilitation Hospital Ancelle di Cremona, Cremona, Italy. [7] Geriatric Research Group, Brescia, Italy. [8] Division of Critical Care Medicine, Department of Anesthesiology and Critical Care Medicine, Université Laval, Québec City, QC, Canada. [9] Centre de recherche du CHU de Québec – Université Laval, Population Health and Optimal Health Practices Research Unit (Trauma – Emergency – Critical Care Medicine), Université Laval, Québec City, QC, Canada. [10] Department of Intensive Care Medecine, CIBER EnfermedadesRespiratorias, Corporacion Sanitaria Universitaria Parc Tauli, Autonomous University of Barcelona, Sabadell, Spain. [11] Department of Anaesthesia and Intensive Care, Haukeland University Hospital, Bergen, Norway. [12] Department of Clinical Medicine, University of Bergen, Bergen, Norway.

Competing interests

The authors declare that they have no competing interests.

Funding

No funding for this review.

References

1. Flaatten H. Intensive care in the very old: are we prepared? Acta Anaesthesiol Scand. 2007;51(5):519–21.
2. Laake JH, Dybwik K, Flaatten HK, Fonneland I-L, Kvåle R, Strand K. Impact of the post-World War II generation on intensive care needs in Norway. Acta Anaesthesiol Scand. 2010;54(4):479–84.
3. Flaatten H, de Lange DW, Artigas A, Bin D, Moreno R, Christensen S, et al. The status of intensive care medicine research and a future agenda for very old patients in the ICU. Intensive Care Med. 2017;43(9):1319–28.
4. Chin-Yee N, D'Egidio G, Thavorn K, Heyland D, Kyeremanteng K. Cost analysis of the very elderly admitted to intensive care units. Crit Care. 2017;21(1):109.
5. Angus DC. Admitting elderly patients to the intensive care unit—is it the right decision? JAMA. 2017;318(15):1443–4.
6. Nguyen Y-L, Angus DC, Boumendil A, Guidet B. The challenge of admitting the very elderly to intensive care. Ann Intensive Care. 2011;1(1):29.
7. Leblanc G, Boumendil A, Guidet B. Ten things to know about critically ill elderly patients. Intensive Care Med. 2017;43(2):217–9.
8. Hennessy D, Juzwishin K, Yergens D, Noseworthy T, Doig C. Outcomes of elderly survivors of intensive care: a review of the literature. Chest. 2005;127(5):1764–74.
9. Barnett K, Mercer SW, Norbury M, Watt G, Wyke S, Guthrie B. Epidemiology of multimorbidity and implications for health care, research, and medical education: a cross-sectional study. Lancet. 2012;380(9836):37–43.
10. Salive ME. Multimorbidity in older adults. Epidemiol Rev. 2013;35:75–83.
11. Menotti A, Mulder I, Nissinen A, Giampaoli S, Feskens EJ, Kromhout D. Prevalence of morbidity and multimorbidity in elderly male populations and their impact on 10-year all-cause mortality: the FINE study (Finland, Italy, Netherlands, Elderly). J Clin Epidemiol. 2001;54(7):680–6.
12. Wolff JL, Starfield B, Anderson G. Prevalence, expenditures, and complications of multiple chronic conditions in the elderly. Arch Intern Med. 2002;162(20):2269–76.
13. Bagshaw SM, Webb SAR, Delaney A, George C, Pilcher D, Hart GK, et al. Very old patients admitted to intensive care in Australia and New Zealand: a multi-centre cohort analysis. Crit Care. 2009;13(2):R45.
14. Zampieri FG, Colombari F. The impact of performance status and comorbidities on the short-term prognosis of very elderly patients admitted to the ICU. BMC Anesthesiol. 2014;14:59.
15. Stavem K, Hoel H, Skjaker SA, Haagensen R. Charlson comorbidity index derived from chart review or administrative data: agreement and prediction of mortality in intensive care patients. Clin Epidemiol. 2017;9:311–20.
16. Charlson ME, Pompei P, Ales KL, MacKenzie CR. A new method of classifying prognostic comorbidity in longitudinal studies: development and validation. J Chronic Dis. 1987;40(5):373–83.
17. Marik PE. Management of the critically ill geriatric patient. Crit Care Med. 2006;34(9 Suppl):S176–82.
18. Zeleznik J. Normative aging of the respiratory system. Clin Geriatr Med. 2003;19(1):1–18.
19. Hughes VA, Frontera WR, Roubenoff R, Evans WJ, Singh MAF. Longitudinal changes in body composition in older men and women: role of body weight change and physical activity. Am J Clin Nutr. 2002;76(2):473–81.
20. Marzetti E, Leeuwenburgh C. Skeletal muscle apoptosis, sarcopenia and frailty at old age. Exp Gerontol. 2006;41(12):1234–8.
21. Abd Aziz NAS, Teng NIMF, Abdul Hamid MR, Ismail NH. Assessing the nutritional status of hospitalized elderly. Clin Interv Aging. 2017;12:1615–25.
22. Neumann SA, Miller MD, Daniels L, Crotty M. Nutritional status and clinical outcomes of older patients in rehabilitation. J Hum Nutr Diet. 2005;18:129–36.
23. Walston J, Hadley EC, Ferrucci L, Guralnik JM, Newman AB, Studenski SA, et al. Research agenda for frailty in older adults: toward a better understanding of physiology and etiology: summary from the American Geriatrics Society/National Institute on Aging Research Conference on Frailty in Older Adults. J Am Geriatr Soc. 2006;54(6):991–1001.
24. Thibault R, Pichard C. Nutrition and clinical outcome in intensive care patients. Curr Opin Clin Nutr Metab Care. 2010;13(2):177–83.
25. Pandharipande PP, Girard TD, Jackson JC, Morandi A, Thompson JL, Pun BT, et al. Long-term cognitive impairment after critical illness. N Engl J Med. 2013;369(14):1306–16.
26. Pisani MA, Inouye SK, McNicoll L, Redlich CA. Screening for preexisting cognitive impairment in older intensive care unit patients: use of proxy assessment. J Am Geriatr Soc. 2003;51(5):689–93.
27. Elie M, Cole MG, Primeau FJ, Bellavance F. Delirium risk factors in elderly hospitalized patients. J Gen Intern Med. 1998;13(3):204–12.
28. Schor JD, Levkoff SE, Lipsitz LA, Reilly CH, Cleary PD, Rowe JW, et al. Risk factors for delirium in hospitalized elderly. JAMA. 1992;267(6):827–31.
29. Ouimet S, Kavanagh BP, Gottfried SB, Skrobik Y. Incidence, risk factors and consequences of ICU delirium. Intensive Care Med. 2007;33(1):66–73.
30. Katz S, Akpom CA. 12. Index of ADL. Med Care. 1976;14(5 Suppl):116–8.
31. Lawton MP, Brody EM. Assessment of older people: self-maintaining and instrumental activities of daily living. The Gerontologist. 1969;9(3):179–86.
32. Barberger-Gateau P, Commenges D, Gagnon M, Letenneur L, Sauvel C, Dartigues JF. Instrumental activities of daily living as a screening tool for cognitive impairment and dementia in elderly community dwellers. J Am Geriatr Soc. 1992;40(11):1129–34.
33. Muscedere J, Waters B, Varambally A, Bagshaw SM, Boyd JG, Maslove D, et al. The impact of frailty on intensive care unit outcomes: a systematic review and meta-analysis. Intensive Care Med. 2017;43(8):1105–22.
34. Clegg A, Young J, Iliffe S, Rikkert MO, Rockwood K. Frailty in elderly people. Lancet. 2013;381(9868):752–62.
35. Cruz-Jentoft AJ, Kiesswetter E, Drey M, Sieber CC. Nutrition, frailty, and sarcopenia. Aging Clin Exp Res. 2017;29(1):43–8.
36. Rockwood K, Song X, MacKnight C, Bergman H, Hogan DB, McDowell I, et al. A global clinical measure of fitness and frailty in elderly people. CMAJ. 2005;173(5):489–95.
37. http://geriatricresearch.medicine.dal.ca/clinical_frailty_scale.htm.
38. Fried LP, Ferrucci L, Darer J, Williamson JD, Anderson G. Untangling the concepts of disability, frailty, and comorbidity: implications for improved targeting and care. J Gerontol A Biol Sci Med Sci. 2004;59(3):255–63.
39. Flaatten H, De Lange DW, Morandi A, Andersen FH, Artigas A, Bertolini G, et al. The impact of frailty on ICU and 30-day mortality and the level of care in very elderly patients (≥ 80 years). Intensive Care Med. 2017;43(12):1820–8.
40. Montamat SC, Cusack BJ, Vestal RE. Management of drug therapy in the elderly. N Engl J Med. 1989;321(5):303–9.
41. Greenblatt DJ, Sellers EM, Shader RI. Drug therapy: drug disposition in old age. N Engl J Med. 1982;306(18):1081–8.
42. Tosato M, Landi F, Martone AM, Cherubini A, Corsonello A, Volpato S, et al. Potentially inappropriate drug use among hospitalised older adults: results from the CRIME study. Age Ageing. 2014;43(6):767–73.
43. Morandi A, Vasilevskis E, Pandharipande PP, Girard TD, Solberg LM, Neal EB, et al. Inappropriate medication prescriptions in elderly adults surviving an intensive care unit hospitalization. J Am Geriatr Soc. 2013;61(7):1128–34.
44. Lau DT, Kasper JD, Potter DEB, Lyles A, Bennett RG. Hospitalization and death associated with potentially inappropriate medication prescriptions among elderly nursing home residents. Arch Intern Med. 2005;165(1):68–74.
45. Wright RM, Roumani YF, Boudreau R, Newman AB, Ruby CM, Studenski SA, et al. Effect of central nervous system medication use on decline in cognition in community-dwelling older adults: findings from the Health, Aging And Body Composition Study. J Am Geriatr Soc. 2009;57(2):243–50.
46. Page RL, Linnebur SA, Bryant LL, Ruscin JM. Inappropriate prescribing in the hospitalized elderly patient: defining the problem, evaluation tools, and possible solutions. Clin Interv Aging. 2010;5:75–87.
47. Scales DC, Fischer HD, Li P, Bierman AS, Fernandes O, Mamdani M, et al. Unintentional continuation of medications intended for acute illness after hospital discharge: a population-based cohort study. J Gen Intern Med. 2016;31(2):196–202.
48. Morandi A, Vasilevskis EE, Pandharipande PP, Girard TD, Solberg LM, Neal EB, et al. Inappropriate medications in elderly ICU survivors: where to intervene? Arch Intern Med. 2011;171(11):1032–4.
49. Ehlenbach WJ, Hough CL, Crane PK, Haneuse SJPA, Carson SS, Curtis JR, et al. Association between acute care and critical illness hospitalization and cognitive function in older adults. JAMA. 2010;303(8):763–70.

50. Pandharipande P, Shintani A, Peterson J, Pun BT, Wilkinson GR, Dittus RS, et al. Lorazepam is an independent risk factor for transitioning to delirium in intensive care unit patients. Anesthesiology. 2006;104(1):21–6.
51. Swan JT, Fitousis K, Hall JB, Todd SR, Turner KL. Antipsychotic use and diagnosis of delirium in the intensive care unit. Crit Care. 2012;16(3):R84.
52. Tomichek JE, Stollings JL, Pandharipande PP, Chandrasekhar R, Ely EW, Girard TD. Antipsychotic prescribing patterns during and after critical illness: a prospective cohort study. Crit Care. 2016;20(1):378.
53. Jasiak KD, Middleton EA, Camamo JM, Erstad BL, Snyder LS, Huckleberry YC. Evaluation of discontinuation of atypical antipsychotics prescribed for ICU delirium. J Pharm Pract. 2013;26(3):253–6.
54. Kram BL, Kram SJ, Brooks KR. Implications of atypical antipsychotic prescribing in the intensive care unit. J Crit Care. 2015;30(4):814–8.
55. van Eijk MMJ, Roes KCB, Honing MLH, Kuiper MA, Karakus A, van der Jagt M, et al. Effect of rivastigmine as an adjunct to usual care with haloperidol on duration of delirium and mortality in critically ill patients: a multicentre, double-blind, placebo-controlled randomised trial. Lancet. 2010;376(9755):1829–37.
56. AGS Choosing Wisely Workgroup. American Geriatrics Society identifies five things that healthcare providers and patients should question. J Am Geriatr Soc. 2013;61(4):622–31.
57. Zaal IJ, Devlin JW, Hazelbag M, Klein Klouwenberg PMC, van der Kooi AW, Ong DSY, et al. Benzodiazepine-associated delirium in critically ill adults. Intensive Care Med. 2015;41(12):2130–7.
58. Barr J, Fraser GL, Puntillo K, Ely EW, Gélinas C, Dasta JF, et al. Clinical practice guidelines for the management of pain, agitation, and delirium in adult patients in the intensive care unit. Crit Care Med. 2013;41(1):263–306.
59. Riker RR, Shehabi Y, Bokesch PM, Ceraso D, Wisemandle W, Koura F, et al. Dexmedetomidine vs midazolam for sedation of critically ill patients: a randomized trial. JAMA. 2009;301(5):489–99.
60. Garfinkel D, Mangin D. Feasibility study of a systematic approach for discontinuation of multiple medications in older adults: addressing polypharmacy. Arch Intern Med. 2010;170(18):1648–54.
61. O'Mahony D, Gallagher PF. Inappropriate prescribing in the older population: need for new criteria. Age Ageing. 2008;37(2):138–41.
62. Blanco-Reina E, Ariza-Zafra G, Ocaña-Riola R, León-Ortiz M. 2012 American Geriatrics Society Beers criteria: enhanced applicability for detecting potentially inappropriate medications in European older adults? A comparison with the Screening Tool of Older Person's Potentially Inappropriate Prescriptions. J Am Geriatr Soc. 2014;62(7):1217–23.
63. Hill-Taylor B, Sketris I, Hayden J, Byrne S, O'Sullivan D, Christie R. Application of the STOPP/START criteria: a systematic review of the prevalence of potentially inappropriate prescribing in older adults, and evidence of clinical, humanistic and economic impact. J Clin Pharm Ther. 2013;38(5):360–72.
64. Philippart F, Vesin A, Bruel C, Kpodji A, Durand-Gasselin B, Garçon P, et al. The ETHICA study (part I): elderly's thoughts about intensive care unit admission for life-sustaining treatments. Intensive Care Med. 2013;39(9):1565–73.
65. Van den Bulcke B, Piers R, Jensen HI, Malmgren J, Metaxa V, Reyners AK, et al. Ethical decision-making climate in the ICU: theoretical framework and validation of a self-assessment tool. BMJ Qual Saf. 2018;27(10):781–9.
66. Garrouste-Orgeas M, Boumendil A, Pateron D, Aergerter P, Somme D, Simon T, et al. Selection of intensive care unit admission criteria for patients aged 80 years and over and compliance of emer gency and intensive care unit physicians with the selected criteria: an observational, multicenter, prospective study. Crit Care Med. 2009;37(11):2919–28.
67. Garrouste-Orgeas M, Timsit J-F, Montuclard L, Colvez A, Gattolliat O, Philippart F, et al. Decision-making process, outcome, and 1-year quality of life of octogenarians referred for intensive care unit admission. Intensive Care Med. 2006;32(7):1045–51.
68. Andersen FH, Flaatten H, Klepstad P, Follestad T, Strand K, Krüger AJ, et al. Long-term outcomes after ICU admission triage in octogenarians. Crit Care Med. 2017;45(4):e363–71.
69. Sprung CL, Artigas A, Kesecioglu J, Pezzi A, Wiis J, Pirracchio R, et al. The Eldicus prospective, observational study of triage decision making in European intensive care units. Part II: intensive care benefit for the elderly. Crit Care Med. 2012;40(1):132–8.
70. Guidet B, Flaatten H, Boumendil A, Morandi A, Andersen FH, Artigas A, et al. Withholding or withdrawing of life-sustaining therapy in older adults (≥ 80 years) admitted to the intensive care unit. Intensive Care Med. 2018;44(7):1027–38.
71. Benoit DD, Jensen HI, Malmgren J, Metaxa V, Reyners AK, Darmon M, et al. Outcome in patients perceived as receiving excessive care across different ethical climates: a prospective study in 68 intensive care units in Europe and the USA. Intensive Care Med. 2018;44(7):1039–49.
72. Ball IM, Bagshaw SM, Burns KEA, Cook DJ, Day AG, Dodek PM, et al. A clinical prediction tool for hospital mortality in critically ill elderly patients. J Crit Care. 2016;35:206–12.
73. Brandberg C, Blomqvist H, Jirwe M. What is the importance of age on treatment of the elderly in the intensive care unit? Acta Anaesthesiol Scand. 2013;57(6):698–703.
74. Hamel MB, Henderson WG, Khuri SF, Daley J. Surgical outcomes for patients aged 80 and older: morbidity and mortality from major noncardiac surgery. J Am Geriatr Soc. 2005;53(3):424–9.
75. Roger C, Morel J, Molinari N, Orban JC, Jung B, Futier E, et al. Practices of end-of-life decisions in 66 southern French ICUs 4 years after an official legal framework: a 1-day audit. Anaesth Crit Care Pain Med. 2015;34(2):73–7.
76. Azoulay E, Metnitz B, Sprung CL, Timsit J-F, Lemaire F, Bauer P, et al. End-of-life practices in 282 intensive care units: data from the SAPS 3 database. Intensive Care Med. 2009;35(4):623–30.
77. Lecuyer L, Chevret S, Thiery G, Darmon M, Schlemmer B, Azoulay E. The ICU trial: a new admission policy for cancer patients requiring mechanical ventilation. Crit Care Med. 2007;35(3):808–14.
78. Lobo SM, De Simoni FHB, Jakob SM, Estella A, Vadi S, Bluethgen A, et al. Decision-making on withholding or withdrawing life support in the ICU: a worldwide perspective. Chest. 2017;152(2):321–9.
79. Heyland DK, Dodek P, Mehta S, Cook D, Garland A, Stelfox HT, et al. Admission of the very elderly to the intensive care unit: family members' perspectives on clinical decision-making from a multicenter cohort study. Palliat Med. 2015;29(4):324–35.
80. Hua M, Halpern SD, Gabler NB, Wunsch H. Effect of ICU strain on timing of limitations in life-sustaining therapy and on death. Intensive Care Med. 2016;42(6):987–94.
81. Milbrandt EB, Eldadah B, Nayfield S, Hadley E, Angus DC. Toward an integrated research agenda for critical illness in aging. Am J Respir Crit Care Med. 2010;182(8):995–1003.
82. Nin N, Lorente JA, De Paula M, Fernández-Segoviano P, Peñuelas O, Sánchez-Ferrer A, et al. Aging increases the susceptibility to injurious mechanical ventilation. Intensive Care Med. 2008;34(5):923–31.
83. Ray P, Birolleau S, Lefort Y, Becquemin M-H, Beigelman C, Isnard R, et al. Acute respiratory failure in the elderly: etiology, emergency diagnosis and prognosis. Crit Care. 2006;10(3):R82.
84. Rubenfeld GD, Caldwell E, Peabody E, Weaver J, Martin DP, Neff M, et al. Incidence and outcomes of acute lung injury. N Engl J Med. 2005;353(16):1685–93.
85. Bellani G, Laffey JG, Pham T, Fan E, Brochard L, Esteban A, et al. Epidemiology, patterns of care, and mortality for patients with acute respiratory distress syndrome in intensive care units in 50 countries. JAMA. 2016;315(8):788–800.
86. Esteban A, Anzueto A, Frutos F, Alía I, Brochard L, Stewart TE, et al. Characteristics and outcomes in adult patients receiving mechanical ventilation: a 28-day international study. JAMA. 2002;287(3):345–55.
87. Ely EW, Wheeler AP, Thompson BT, Ancukiewicz M, Steinberg KP, Bernard GR. Recovery rate and prognosis in older persons who develop acute lung injury and the acute respiratory distress syndrome. Ann Intern Med. 2002;136(1):25–36.
88. Angus DC, Linde-Zwirble WT, Lidicker J, Clermont G, Carcillo J, Pinsky MR. Epidemiology of severe sepsis in the United States: analysis of incidence, outcome, and associated costs of care. Crit Care Med. 2001;29(7):1303–10.
89. Karakus A, Haas LEM, Brinkman S, de Lange DW, de Keizer NF. Trends in

short-term and 1-year mortality in very elderly intensive care patients in the Netherlands: a retrospective study from 2008 to 2014. Intensive Care Med. 2017;43(10):1476–84.

90. de Rooij SE, Govers A, Korevaar JC, Abu-Hanna A, Levi M, de Jonge E. Short-term and long-term mortality in very elderly patients admitted to an intensive care unit. Intensive Care Med. 2006;32(7):1039–44.

91. Kim S, Han H-S, Jung H, Kim K, Hwang DW, Kang S-B, et al. Multidimensional frailty score for the prediction of postoperative mortality risk. JAMA Surg. 2014;149(7):633–40.

92. Choi J, Tate JA, Donahoe MP, Ren D, Hoffman LA, Chasens ER. Sleep in family caregivers of ICU survivors for two months post-ICU discharge. Intensive Crit Care Nurs. 2016;37:11–8.

93. Lin F, Chaboyer W, Wallis M. A literature review of organisational, individual and teamwork factors contributing to the ICU discharge process. Aust Crit Care. 2009;22(1):29–43.

94. Town JA, Churpek MM, Yuen TC, Huber MT, Kress JP, Edelson DP. Relationship between ICU bed availability, ICU readmission, and cardiac arrest in the general wards. Crit Care Med. 2014;42(9):2037–41.

95. Niven DJ, Bastos JF, Stelfox HT. Critical care transition programs and the risk of readmission or death after discharge from an ICU: a systematic review and meta-analysis. Crit Care Med. 2014;42(1):179–87.

96. van Sluisveld N, Bakhshi-Raiez F, de Keizer N, Holman R, Wester G, Wollersheim H, et al. Variation in rates of ICU readmissions and post-ICU in-hospital mortality and their association with ICU discharge practices. BMC Health Serv Res. 2017;17(1):281.

97. Guidet B, De Lange DW, Christensen S, Moreno R, Fjølner J, Dumas G, Flaatten H. Attitudes of physicians towards the care of critically ill elderly patients—a European survey. Acta Anaesthesiol Scand. 2018;62:207–19.

98. Somme D, Lazarovici C, Dramé M, Blanc P, Lang PO, Gauvain JB, et al. The geriatric patient: use of acute geriatrics units in the emergency care of elderly patients in France. Arch Gerontol Geriatr. 2011;52(1):40–5.

99. Somme D, Andrieux N, Guérot E, Lahjibi-Paulet H, Lazarovici C, Gisselbrecht M, et al. Loss of autonomy among elderly patients after a stay in a medical intensive care unit (ICU): a randomized study of the benefit of transfer to a geriatric ward. Arch Gerontol Geriatr. 2010;50(3):e36–40.

100. Boddaert J, Raux M, Khiami F, Riou B. Perioperative management of elderly patients with hip fracture. Anesthesiology. 2014;121(6):1336–41.

101. Boddaert J, Cohen-Bittan J, Khiami F, Le Manach Y, Raux M, Beinis J-Y, et al. Postoperative admission to a dedicated geriatric unit decreases mortality in elderly patients with hip fracture. PLoS ONE. 2014;9(1):e83795.

102. Soliman IW, Cremer OL, de Lange DW, Slooter AJC, van Delden JHJM, van Dijk D, et al. The ability of intensive care unit physicians to estimate long-term prognosis in survivors of critical illness. J Crit Care. 2018;43:148–55.

103. Herridge MS, Chu LM, Matte A, Tomlinson G, Chan L, Thomas C, et al. The RECOVER program: disability risk groups and 1-year outcome after 7 or more days of mechanical ventilation. Am J Respir Crit Care Med. 2016;194(7):831–44.

104. Heyland DK, Garland A, Bagshaw SM, Cook D, Rockwood K, Stelfox HT, et al. Recovery after critical illness in patients aged 80 years or older: a multi-center prospective observational cohort study. Intensive Care Med. 2015;41(11):1911–20.

105. Khouli H, Astua A, Dombrowski W, Ahmad F, Homel P, Shapiro J, et al. Changes in health-related quality of life and factors predicting long-term outcomes in older adults admitted to intensive care units. Crit Care Med. 2011;39(4):731–7.

106. Iwashyna TJ, Ely EW, Smith DM, Langa KM. Long-term cognitive impairment and functional disability among survivors of severe sepsis. JAMA. 2010;304(16):1787–94.

107. Wassenaar A, de Reus J, Donders ART, Schoonhoven L, Cremer OL, de Lange DW, et al. Development and validation of an abbreviated questionnaire to easily measure cognitive failure in ICU survivors: a multicenter study. Crit Care Med. 2018;46(1):79–84.

108. Wolters AE, Peelen LM, Veldhuijzen DS, Zaal IJ, de Lange DW, Pasma W, et al. Long-term self-reported cognitive problems after delirium in the intensive care unit and the effect of systemic inflammation. J Am Geriatr Soc. 2017;65(4):786–91.

109. Boumendil A, Angus DC, Guitonneau A-L, Menn A-M, Ginsburg C, Takun K, et al. Variability of intensive care admission decisions for the very elderly. PLoS ONE. 2012;7(4):e34387.

110. Guidet B, Leblanc G, Simon T, Woimant M, Quenot J-P, Ganansia O, et al. Effect of systematic intensive care unit triage on long-term mortality among critically ill elderly patients in France: a randomized clinical trial. JAMA. 2017;318(15):1450–9.

111. Sacanella E, Pérez-Castejón JM, Nicolás JM, Masanés F, Navarro M, Castro P, et al. Functional status and quality of life 12 months after discharge from a medical ICU in healthy elderly patients: a prospective observational study. Crit Care. 2011;15(2):R105.

112. Villa P, Pintado M-C, Luján J, González-García N, Trascasa M, Molina R, et al. Functional status and quality of life in elderly intensive care unit survivors. J Am Geriatr Soc. 2016;64(3):536–42.

113. Ferrante LE, Pisani MA, Murphy TE, Gahbauer EA, Leo-Summers LS, Gill TM. Functional trajectories among older persons before and after critical illness. JAMA Intern Med. 2015;175(4):523–9.

114. de Rooij SEJA, Govers AC, Korevaar JC, Giesbers AW, Levi M, de Jonge E. Cognitive, functional, and quality-of-life outcomes of patients aged 80 and older who survived at least 1 year after planned or unplanned surgery or medical intensive care treatment. J Am Geriatr Soc. 2008;56(5):816–22.

115. van der Schaaf M, Beelen A, Dongelmans DA, Vroom MB, Nollet F. Functional status after intensive care: a challenge for rehabilitation professionals to improve outcome. J Rehabil Med. 2009;41(5):360–6.

116. Griffiths J, Hatch RA, Bishop J, Morgan K, Jenkinson C, Cuthbertson BH, et al. An exploration of social and economic outcome and associated health-related quality of life after critical illness in general intensive care unit survivors: a 12-month follow-up study. Crit Care. 2013;17(3):R100.

117. Kaarlola A, Tallgren M, Pettilä V. Long-term survival, quality of life, and quality-adjusted life-years among critically ill elderly patients. Crit Care Med. 2006;34(8):2120–6.

118. Hoffman KR, Loong B, Haren FV. Very old patients urgently referred to the intensive care unit: long-term outcomes for admitted and declined patients. Crit Care Resusc. 2016;18(3):157–64.

119. Cameron JI, Chu LM, Matte A, Tomlinson G, Chan L, Thomas C, et al. One-year outcomes in caregivers of critically ill patients. N Engl J Med. 2016;374(19):1831–41.

120. van den Born-van Zanten SA, Dongelmans DA, Dettling-Ihnenfeldt D, Vink R, van der Schaaf M. Caregiver strain and posttraumatic stress symptoms of informal caregivers of intensive care unit survivors. Rehabil Psychol. 2016;61(2):173–8.

121. Comini L, Rocchi S, Bruletti G, Paneroni M, Bertolotti G, Vitacca M. Impact of clinical and quality of life outcomes of long-stay ICU survivors recovering from rehabilitation on caregivers' burden. Respir Care. 2016;61(4):405–15.

122. Vitacca M, Barbano L, Vanoglio F, Luisa A, Bernocchi P, Giordano A, et al. Does 6-month home caregiver-supervised physiotherapy improve post-critical care outcomes?: a randomized controlled trial. Am J Phys Med Rehabil. 2016;95(8):571–9.

123. Kass JE, Castriotta RJ, Malakoff F. Intensive care unit outcome in the very elderly. Crit Care Med. 1992;20:1666–71.

124. Chelluri L, Pinsky MR, Donahoe MP, Grenvik A. Long-term outcome of critically ill elderly patients requiring intensive care. JAMA. 1993;269:3119–23.

125. Broslawski GE, Elkins M, Algus M. Functional abilities of elderly survivors of intensive care. J Am Osteopath Assoc. 1995;95:712–7.
126. Montuclard L, Garrouste-Orgeas M, Timsit JF, Misset B, De Jonghe B, Carlet J. Outcome, functional autonomy, and quality of life of elderly patients with a long-term intensive care unit stay. Crit Care Med. 2000;28:3389–95.
127. Udekwu P, Gurkin B, Oller D, Lapio L, Bourbina J. Quality of life and functional level in elderly patients surviving surgical intensive care. J Am Coll Surg. 2001;193:245–9.
128. Tabah A, Philippart F, Timsit JF, Willems V, Français A, Leplège A, Carlet J, Bruel C, Misset B, Garrouste-Orgeas M. Quality of life in patients aged 80 or over after ICU discharge. Crit Care. 2010;14(1):R2.
129. Andersen FH, Flaatten H, Klepstad P, Romild U, Kvåle R. Long-term survival and quality of life after intensive care for patients 80 years of age or older. Ann Intensive Care. 2015;5:53.
130. Level C, Tellier E, Dezou P, Chaoui K, Kherchache A, Sejourné P, et al. Outcome of older persons admitted to intensive care unit, mortality, prognosis factors, dependency scores and ability trajectory within 1 year: a prospective cohort study. Aging Clin Exp Res. 2018;30(9):1041–51.

6

Inflammatory and coagulatory parameters linked to survival in critically ill children with sepsis

Christian Niederwanger[1], Mirjam Bachler[2*], Tobias Hell[3], Caroline Linhart[4], Andreas Entenmann[1], Agnes Balog[1], Katharina Auer[5] and Petra Innerhofer[6]

Abstract

Background: Sepsis is associated with a deflection of inflammatory and coagulative parameters, since some clotting factors are known to be involved in the host's defense against infection and inflammation. These parameters could play a crucial role in the course of sepsis and be used as prognostic markers in critically ill children.

Methods: A total of 250 critically ill pediatric patients diagnosed with sepsis were retrospectively analyzed to identify routinely measured predictors for in-hospital mortality at the peak level of C-reactive protein. Those parameters entered multivariate logistic regression analysis as well as a decision tree for survival.

Results: Multivariate logistic regression analysis revealed fibrinogen, platelets and activated partial thromboplastin time (aPTT) at the peak level of C-reactive protein to be predictors for survival ($p=0.03$, $p=0.01$ and $p=0.02$, respectively). An increase in fibrinogen and platelets is linked to survival, whereas an aPTT prolongation is associated with higher mortality; adjusted odds ratios (95% CI) for an increase of 100 mg/dl in fibrinogen are 1.35 (1.04–1.82) per 50 G/l platelets 1.94 (1.3–3.29) and 0.83 (0.69–0.96) for an aPTT prolongation of 10 s. Decision tree analysis shows that a fibrinogen level below 192 mg/dl (90.9% vs. 13% mortality) is most distinctive in non-survivors.

Conclusions: High levels of fibrinogen and platelets as well as a non-overshooting aPTT are associated with a higher survival rate in pediatric patients with diagnosed sepsis. In particular, hypofibrinogenemia is distinctive for a high mortality rate in septic critically ill children.

Keywords: Fibrinogen, Sepsis, Children, Survival, Inflammation, Coagulation, Platelets

Introduction

Although the number of deaths caused by sepsis has drastically decreased in the last couple of decades [1], sepsis remains one of the main causes of mortality in infants and toddlers worldwide [1–3]. Sepsis in children peaks in the neonatal period and symptoms may be nonspecific in those patients [4], while older children may show hyperthermia, tachycardia, tachypnea, hypotension and disorders in hemostasis up to the clinical picture of disseminated intravascular coagulation (DIC).

Sepsis is initially characterized by excessive production of pro-inflammatory cytokines, leukocyte activation and tissue damage, followed by release of anti-inflammatory cytokines, leukocyte deactivation and immunosuppression [5]. In the later phase of sepsis, compensatory release of anti-inflammatory molecules is thought to mediate a state of immunosuppression associated with significant impairment of immune cell function (immunoparalysis) [6].

The systemic inflammation during sepsis is observed by measuring leukocytes, procalcitonin, C-reactive protein and others. Leukocyte count is part of the definition of sepsis, but only at extreme levels are leukocytes

*Correspondence: mirjam.bachler@tirol-kliniken.at
[2] Institute for Sports Medicine, Alpine Medicine and Health Tourism, UMIT - University for Health Sciences, Medical Informatics and Technology, Eduard Wallnöfer Zentrum 1, 6060 Hall in Tirol, Austria
Full list of author information is available at the end of the article

associated with the progression of sepsis [7]. Data confirm that procalcitonin, which specifically increases in bacterial processes [8], is suitable as a diagnostic parameter in many cases in adults due to its high specificity [9, 10]. However, limited data are available for use in pediatric patients [11]. C-reactive protein reflects the inflammatory process and is widely used in clinical routine. Many studies have described an interrelation between an elevated C-reactive protein level and sepsis [12–15]. Thus, in clinical routine, daily C-reactive protein measurements might be used to assess the efficacy of treatment [16]. C-reactive protein can also be an indicator of organ failure [17–21] and therefore has potential for the surveillance of sepsis severity.

Systemic inflammation is followed by activation of the coagulation system, and conversely, components of the coagulation system significantly affect the inflammatory response [22]. This cross-link occurs on several levels: Pro-inflammatory cytokines stimulate the production of coagulation factors and coagulation factors mediate inflammation via binding to receptors of endothelium and immune cells [23]. The coagulation factors also play a direct role in host defense. For example, fibrinogen modulates the immune system [24, 25] and acts as a chemotactical factor for monocytes and neutrophils [26]. Furthermore, as part of the innate immune system, it limits bacterial spreading by forming fiber nets in which the pathogens become immobilized [24].

With few exceptions, such as antithrombin or platelets, the role of coagulation parameters in sepsis is largely ignored. New diagnostic, prognostic and therapeutic strategies can be deduced by observing coagulating laboratory data and, where appropriate, modifying them in the event of excessive activation or dysregulation of the system [27, 28]. An increase in the pro-coagulatory parameters to high level is seen rather negatively in the inflammatory process because of their pro-thrombotic potential [29], although elevation of the pro-coagulatory parameters might be beneficial during sepsis due to their role in host defense.

Therefore, it is worthwhile to examine the behavior and influence of coagulation parameters in combination with the typical inflammatory parameters during sepsis. Correct interpretation of these could facilitate assessment of the course of sepsis in critically ill children.

Methods

This retrospective analysis comprises clinical data and routine laboratory parameters from 250 pediatric patients at the Pediatric Intensive Care Unit of Innsbruck Medical University Hospital.

Inclusion of patients

All medical files of patients younger than 18 years of age who were treated at the pediatric intensive care unit (PICU) between January 1, 2000, and December 31, 2014, with the diagnosis of sepsis or systemic infection were reviewed. A total of 250 patients met the sepsis criteria of Goldstein [1]. There was no need to obtain oral and written informed consent from the study participants since the data were processed anonymously. The study protocol was approved by the institutional review board of the Medical University of Innsbruck (AN2013-0044).

Data collection

We collected the demographic variables age, sex and the diagnosed underlying disease that triggered hospitalization. Septic shock was defined as the need for a vasoactive drug to maintain blood pressure in the normal range during the septic episode [1]. The C-reactive protein level was used to objectify the progression of sepsis, because it is an established parameter of sepsis [12–16] and is used in our clinic in children of all ages as opposed to IL-6 and procalcitonin.

The day on which C-reactive protein peaked was defined as day 0 in the report. The available routine parameters (fibrinogen, platelets, antithrombin, PT, aPTT, leukocytes) were observed from 3 days before until 3 days after day 0. In-hospital mortality was chosen as the outcome parameter.

To evaluate changes in therapy and outcome due to the protracted study period, we grouped patients into four time cohorts (2000–2004, 2005–2007, 2008–2010 and 2011–2014).

Statistical analysis

A mathematician not involved in the study procedures or patient assessment (TH) was responsible for the statistical analyses using R, version 3.4.1. All statistical assessments were two sided, and a significance level of 5% was used. The hypothesis of a normal distribution was not reasonable for most of the continuous variables (Shapiro–Wilk normality test). The Wilcoxon rank sum test and Fisher's exact test were applied to assess differences between survivors and non-survivors. We present continuous data as medians (25th–75th percentile) and binary variables as no./total no. (%). We show effect size and precision with estimated median differences between survivors and non-survivors for continuous data and odds ratios (OR) for binary variables, with 95% CIs.

Stratified by survival, the progression of inflammation- and coagulation-related parameters from 3 days prior to 3 days after the peak of C-reactive protein is illustrated by the sequence of the median with corresponding 95% CIs in a purely descriptive manner.

In the univariate analysis, significant predictors at the peak of C-reactive protein as well as the respective patient's characteristics for survival were identified. Those variables entered a forward–backward stepwise selection by Akaike information criterion (AIC) to fit a logistic regression model for survival [30]. We provide adjusted odds ratios for the remaining predictors with 95% CIs. Receiver operating characteristic (ROC curves) analysis was performed, and ROC AUC is provided with 95% CIs. In addition, with the variables that entered the stepwise model selection, a recursive partitioning tree for survival was fitted using the R package rpart (version 4.1-11). All analyses were performed in a purely exploratory fashion.

Results

Patient characteristics

In total, 250 patients met the eligibility criteria for study inclusion and final analysis. Of those septic children, 41 (16.4%) did not survive while in hospital. Of the critically ill children, 53.2% suffered from sepsis and 26.4% from severe sepsis. Septic shock was reported in 51/250 (20.4%) children, of whom 21/51 (41.2%) died. Patients' baseline characteristics stratified for survival and non-survival are presented in Table 1.

The population consisted of 134/250 (53.6%) male patients, and median (25th–75th percentile) age was 35 (6–109) months. The 22/249 (8.8%) neonates showed a significantly higher ($p = 0.02$) mortality rate, because 8/22 (36.4%) neonates as compared to 33/227 (14.5%) children older than 1 month did not survive the septic episode. The most commonly affected organ systems resulting in ICU admission were the respiratory system in 51/250 (20.4%) and the central nervous system in 46/250 (18.4%) children.

To rule out possible confounding due to the protracted study period (2000–2014), we grouped patients into four time cohorts: 80 patients were included in 2000–2004, 56 in 2005–2007, 68 in 2008–2010 and 46 in 2011–2014. Mortality was 12.5%, 28.6%, 13.2% and 13%, respectively, and was not significantly associated with the time periods (Fisher's exact test: $p = 0.07$).

Univariate analysis of parameters at the peak level of C-reactive protein

As presented in Table 2, no significant difference was observed in C-reactive protein or leukocyte levels between survivors and non-survivors at the peak level of C-reactive protein. There was a difference in the timing between hospital admission and C-reactive protein peak between survivors and non-survivors ($p < 0.0001$) with non-survivors having a longer time period to reach the C-reactive protein peak. In contrast, fibrinogen, platelets and antithrombin significantly differ. This is also the case for aPTT and PT.

Table 1 Characteristics of patients stratified for survival and non-survival

Characteristics[a]	Total ($n = 250$)	Survivors ($n = 209$)	Non-survivors ($n = 41$)	Estimate with 95% CI[b]	p value[c]
Female gender	116/250 (46.4%)	97/209 (46.4%)	19/41 (46.3%)	1 (0.48 to 2.06)	1
Age[d] (months)	34.83 (6.47–108.63)	35.5 (7.16–111.45)	23.8 (1.43–81.97)	3.33 (− 6.55 to 18.07)	0.2725
Neonates < 1 month	22/249 (8.8%)	14/208 (6.7%)	8/41 (19.5%)	3.34 (1.12 to 9.34)	0.0149
Infants 1–3 months	24/249 (9.6%)	20/208 (9.6%)	4/41 (9.8%)	1.02 (0.24 to 3.28)	1
Diagnosed underlying disease					
Central nervous system	46/250 (18.4%)	34/209 (16.3%)	12/41 (29.3%)	2.12 (0.89 to 4.82)	0.075
Cardiovascular	39/250 (15.6%)	31/209 (14.8%)	8/41 (19.5%)	1.39 (0.51 to 3.45)	0.4808
Digestive tract	41/250 (16.4%)	32/209 (15.3%)	9/41 (22%)	1.55 (0.59 to 3.74)	0.3546
Respiratory system	51/250 (20.4%)	41/209 (19.6%)	10/41 (24.4%)	1.32 (0.53 to 3.05)	0.5258
Oncologic	37/250 (14.8%)	31/209 (14.8%)	6/41 (14.6%)	0.98 (0.31 to 2.64)	1
Kidney	30/250 (12%)	22/209 (10.5%)	8/41 (19.5%)	2.05 (0.73 to 5.31)	0.1169
Liver	18/250 (7.2%)	15/209 (7.2%)	3/41 (7.3%)	1.02 (0.18 to 3.87)	1
Skin	11/250 (4.4%)	10/209 (4.8%)	1/41 (2.4%)	0.5 (0.01 to 3.68)	1
Other diagnosis	30/250 (12%)	25/209 (12%)	5/41 (12.2%)	1.02 (0.29 to 2.97)	1

[a] Binary data are presented as no./total no. (%) and continuous data as medians (25th–75th percentile)

[b] Odds ratio for binary variables and estimated median difference for continuous variables

[c] Differences between survivors and non-survivors assessed with Fisher's exact test for binary variables and Wilcoxon rank sum test for continuous variables

[d] For one survivor, the exact age in months is not known

Table 2 Parameters at the peak level of C-reactive protein stratified for survival and non-survival

Parameters[a]	Total ($n=250$)	Survivors ($n=209$)	Non-survivors ($n=41$)	Estimate with 95% CI[b]	p value[c]	Not known[d]
C-reactive protein (mg/dl)	18.5 (9.8–28.4)	18.6 (10–28)	17.6 (7.9–31.9)	−0.13 (−5.3 to 4.55)	0.9491	0/0
Fibrinogen (mg/dl)	506 (329–675)	518 (383–685)	279 (173–514)	206 (118 to 289)	<0.0001	56/9
Platelets (G/l)	124 (50–232)	147 (62.5–247)	63 (29–98)	74 (37 to 111)	<0.0001	5/0
aPTT (s)	47 (38–56)	46 (36–53)	64 (53.5–83)	−20 (−28 to −13)	<0.0001	59/15
PT (%)	71 (51–84)	74 (55–85)	49 (36–71.5)	20 (10 to 30)	0.0001	59/14
Antithrombin (%)	63 (47–81)	65.5 (50–82)	51 (40–66)	14 (5 to 23)	0.0045	75/10
Leukocytes (G/l)	10.4 (4.6–17.8)	11.1 (5.3–17.5)	8.2 (3–20)	1.4 (−1.6 to 5.1)	0.3342	4/5

[a] Data are presented as medians (25th–75th percentile)

[b] Estimated median difference

[c] Differences between survivors and non-survivors assessed with Wilcoxon rank sum test for continuous variables

[d] Number of missing measurements in survivors/non-survivors

Progression of parameters around the peak level of C-reactive protein

The course of fibrinogen and antithrombin seems to be associated with the progression of C-reactive protein (Figs. 1, 2). Fibrinogen concentration followed the progression of C-reactive protein in survivors, but not in non-survivors. Note that for the main portion of the survivors, fibrinogen levels increased distinctly above the norm values around day 0.

Antithrombin levels were constantly higher in survivors than in non-survivors, but, in contrast to fibrinogen, irrespective of the progression of C-reactive protein. In survivors, platelets decreased slightly over time, while patients who did not survive showed a sharp decline in platelets already 2 days before the peak level of C-reactive protein was reached. Survivors showed significantly higher PT levels and shorter aPTT around the peak of C-reactive protein. Progression of leukocytes between survivors and non-survivors is comparable up to day 2.

CRP, fibrinogen, platelets, aPTT, PT and antithrombin levels were comparable between time cohorts (Kruskal–Wallis test: $p=0.40$, $p=0.32$, $p=0.58$, $p=0.90$, $p=0.17$ and $p=0.22$, respectively). Leukocyte count significantly differed between time cohorts (Kruskal–Wallis test: $p=0.04$). Median leukocyte counts in G/l were 12.3 (6.13–20) in 2000–2004, 12.1 (6.8–17.1) in 2005–2007, 10.3 (3.1–16.4) in 2008–2010 and 7.7 (2.8–12) in 2011–2014.

Multivariate logistic regression analysis for survival

The following significant univariate predictors for survival entered a stepwise model selection: fibrinogen, platelets, antithrombin, aPTT, PT and age. The resulting logistic regression model for survival includes fibrinogen, platelets and aPTT as variables, all of them being significant predictors for survival ($p=0.03$, $p=0.01$ and $p=0.02$, respectively).

Figure 3 shows the adjusted odds ratios (95% CI) retrieved from logistic regression. An increase in fibrinogen and platelets is linked to survival, whereas aPTT prolongation is associated with higher mortality. An increase of 100 mg/dl in fibrinogen increases the survival chance by 26%, per 50 G/l platelets by 48.4%, and aPTT prolongation of 10 s increases the mortality risk by 20.8%.

Adding the time cohort or the year of CRP peak as input variables resulted in the identical logistic regression model after stepwise model selection.

The ROC analysis (Additional file 1) for survival predicted by fibrinogen, platelets and aPTT resulted in an AUC of 0.74 (0.63–0.85), 0.71 (0.63–0.79) and 0.81 (0.73–0.90), respectively.

Decision tree for survival

To gain a deeper insight into the interplay of coagulation parameters leading to death in septic children, a decision tree was fitted using the univariate predictors at the peak level of C-reactive protein and age to explore these interrelations.

The obtained classification tree (see Fig. 4) shows that most distinctive in non-survivors is a fibrinogen level below 192 mg/dl [90.9% (58.7–99.8%) vs. 13% (8.1–18.5%) mortality]. For patients presenting with a fibrinogen level of at least 192 mg/dl, an aPTT of less than 58 s is associated with better outcome [8.4% (5.0–13.1%) vs. 37.8% (22.5–55.2%) mortality]. If, in addition, patients show a platelet count of at least 80 G/l, a low mortality rate is observed [4.1% (1.5–8.7%) vs. 20% (10.4–33.0%) mortality]. Patients with a platelet count below 80 G/l and younger than 1.2 months show high mortality as compared to older [57.1% (18.4–90.1%) vs. 14.6% (6.1–27.8%)].

In the case of a fibrinogen level of at least 192 mg/dl and an aPTT prolongation of 58 s or more, antithrombin levels below 58% led to lower mortality [25% (9.8–46.7%)

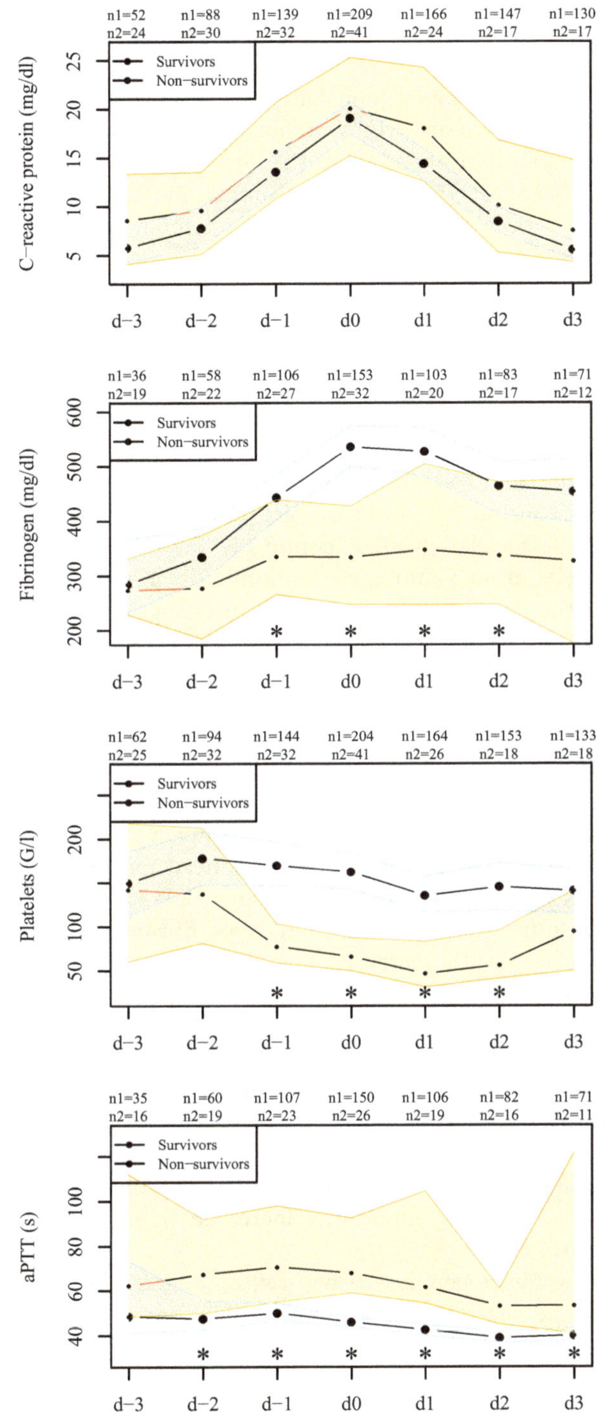

Fig. 1 Progression of C-reactive protein and measured coagulation parameters. Depicted are medians with 95% CIs of the measured parameters for survivors (blue) and non-survivors (red) from 3 days prior to (d-3 to d-1) until 3 days after (d1 to d3) C-reactive protein peaked (d0). Asterisks indicate significant differences between survivors and non-survivors at the respective time point; *n*1 is the number of available measurements for survivors and *n*2 for non-survivors

vs. 61.5% (31.6–86.1%)], especially in patients exceeding an aPTT of 66 s [0% (0.0–24.7%) vs. 54.5% (23.4–83.3%) mortality].

The identical decision tree was obtained when the time cohort or the year of C-reactive protein peak was added as predictors for survival, indicating that there was no confounding due to the protracted study period (2000–2014).

In order to predict mortality with fibrinogen < 192 mg/dl, platelets < 80 G/l and aPTT > 58 s, sensitivity and specificity were calculated (Additional file 2).

Age-adjusted hypofibrinogenemia

The fibrinogen level of each child was classified as hypo-, normo- or hyperfibrinogenemia according to the age-dependent norm value ranges. For normal fibrinogen values, please see the table in Additional file 3.

Patients presenting with hypofibrinogenemia have a significantly higher mortality rate than do patients with normo- or hyperfibrinogenemia: OR 28.42 (5.42–284.81), $p < 0.0001$. As depicted in Fig. 5, 82% of the patients with low fibrinogen levels died, whereas the mortality rate in patients with fibrinogen levels within the normal range was 22% and 10% in children with an elevated fibrinogen level.

No significant difference in the occurrence of a diagnosed thromboembolic event was observed for the 5/128 (3.9%) children with hyperfibrinogenemia as compared to the 4/56 (7.1%) patients with fibrinogen within the normal values or below: OR 0.53 (0.11–2.78), $p = 0.46$.

Discussion

In this study, we investigated the impact of routinely measured coagulation and inflammation parameters on in-hospital survival in pediatric patients diagnosed with sepsis. The main result is that C-reactive protein at its peak level does not significantly differ between survivors and non-survivors, whereas fibrinogen, platelets and aPTT are predictors of survival. An increase in fibrinogen and platelets is linked to survival, whereas aPTT prolongation is associated with higher mortality. Most distinctive for mortality are fibrinogen levels below 192 mg/dl. Especially in children younger than 1.2 months, isolated thrombocytopenia is associated with poor outcome. In general, age-adjusted hypofibrinogenemia is significantly associated with a poor chance of survival.

In some points, these results stand in contrast to findings reported in the literature. Several studies claim that C-reactive protein is of prognostic value in sepsis [12–15]. However, in our study focusing on mortality, C-reactive protein levels did not allow any differentiation between survivors and non-survivors during the observation period of 7 days. Most likely, in children as

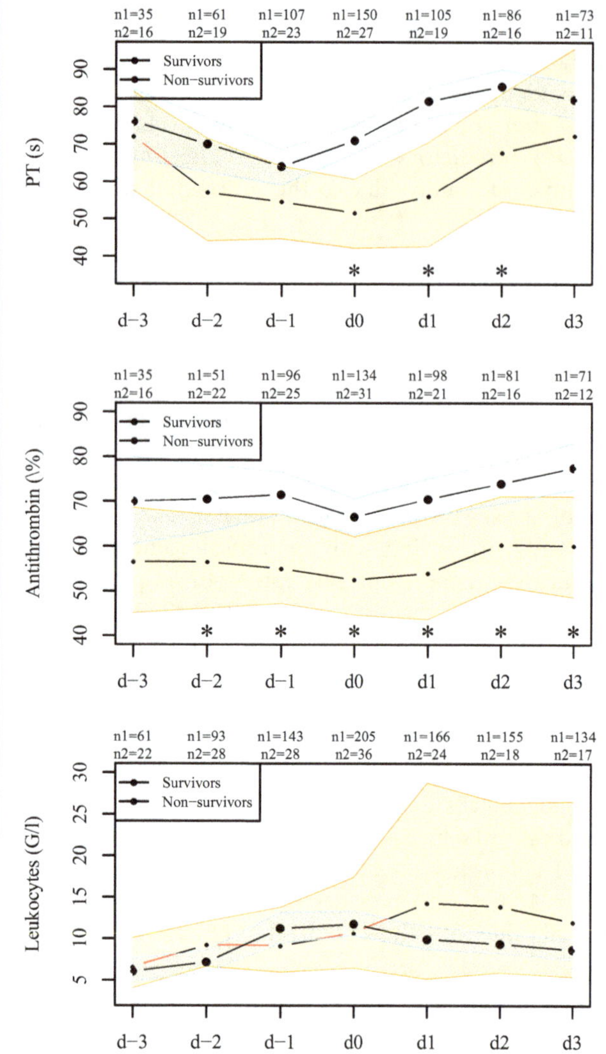

Fig. 2 Progression of measured coagulation parameters. Depicted are medians with 95% CIs of the measured parameters for survivors (blue) and non-survivors (red) from 3 days prior to (d-3 to d-1) until 3 days after (d1 to d3) C-reactive protein peaked (d0). Asterisks indicate significant differences between survivors and non-survivors at the respective time point; *n*1 is the number of available measurements for survivors and *n*2 for non-survivors

well as in adults with diagnosed sepsis C-reactive protein levels are highly elevated without predicting final outcome.

Among the variables routinely measured in our study at the peak level of C-reactive protein, multivariate analysis revealed that only three of these coagulation parameters are essential for the prediction of survival in septic children: An increase in fibrinogen and platelets lowers the mortality risk, while a prolongation of aPTT increases the risk.

We found that hypofibrinogenemia is associated with very high mortality. This is in accordance with Esroy et al., who also confirm in their study that deceased patients exhibited significantly lower fibrinogen levels than did survivors [31]. Moreover, in baboons, survivors had higher fibrinogen levels than did non-survivors after induced sepsis [32]. This was also found in several earlier studies with fibrinogen-deficient mice following induced sepsis [33, 34].

The reason why fibrinogen is associated with survival in sepsis could be that it helps the immune system limit bacterial growth and enhance bacterial clearance [35]. The fibrin net captures and immobilizes invasive bacteria [24], thus restricting local spreading [24, 36]. Once the fibrinolysis sets in, plasminogen releases fibrinogen-derived so-called antimicrobial peptides (AMPs), thus causing an antimicrobial environment to arise within the clot. Such a peptide is the Bß15–42 fragment, and an unambiguous antimicrobial effect of this protein was already proven by S. aureus, group A Streptococcus (GAS) and group B Streptococcus (GBS) [25]. Besides that, this peptide binds to the VE cadherin of the endothelial cells and thus reinforces the tight junctions, which has a positive effect on organ failure and survival during sepsis [37, 38]. The importance of fibrinogen, fibrinolysis and the consequently released peptides during sepsis and their beneficial impact on infection, multiple-organ dysfunction and reduced mortality have already been proven in several studies [39–41].

In our study, age-adjusted hyperfibrinogenemia is associated with increased survival in sepsis. In studies of adult patients, this connection between acute and transient fibrinogen levels in the context of sepsis and survival was also observed [42]. In this context of high levels of pro-thrombotic factors, the fear of a hypercoagulatory state during sepsis is present and justified, since this could contribute to the development of thrombosis. In our study, the incidence rate of thromboembolic events was not significantly increased in patients with hyperfibrinogenemia.

Low fibrinogen levels may reflect ongoing consumption and deposition, development of DIC and MODS [43, 44]. Sepsis itself also causes severe damage to the liver, via hemodynamic changes as well as the direct or indirect destruction of hepatocytes or both [45]. The destroyed hepatocytes are no longer able to synthesize a sufficient amount of fibrinogen, which might be another reason for the low fibrinogen levels in non-survivors.

High concentrations of fibrinogen before the C-reactive protein peak in our study rarely coincided with platelet concentrations below the critical limit of 100 G/l. Low platelets in addition to low fibrinogen levels result in weak clot firmness, which is known to lead

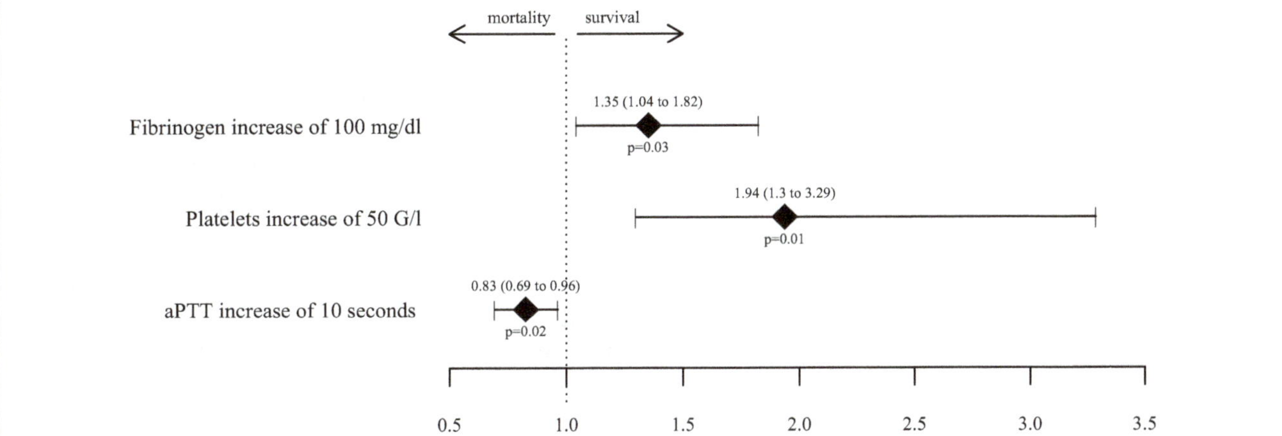

Fig. 3 Adjusted odds ratios (95% CI) for survival retrieved from logistic regression. For an odds ratio greater than 1, an increase in the parameter decreases the mortality risk

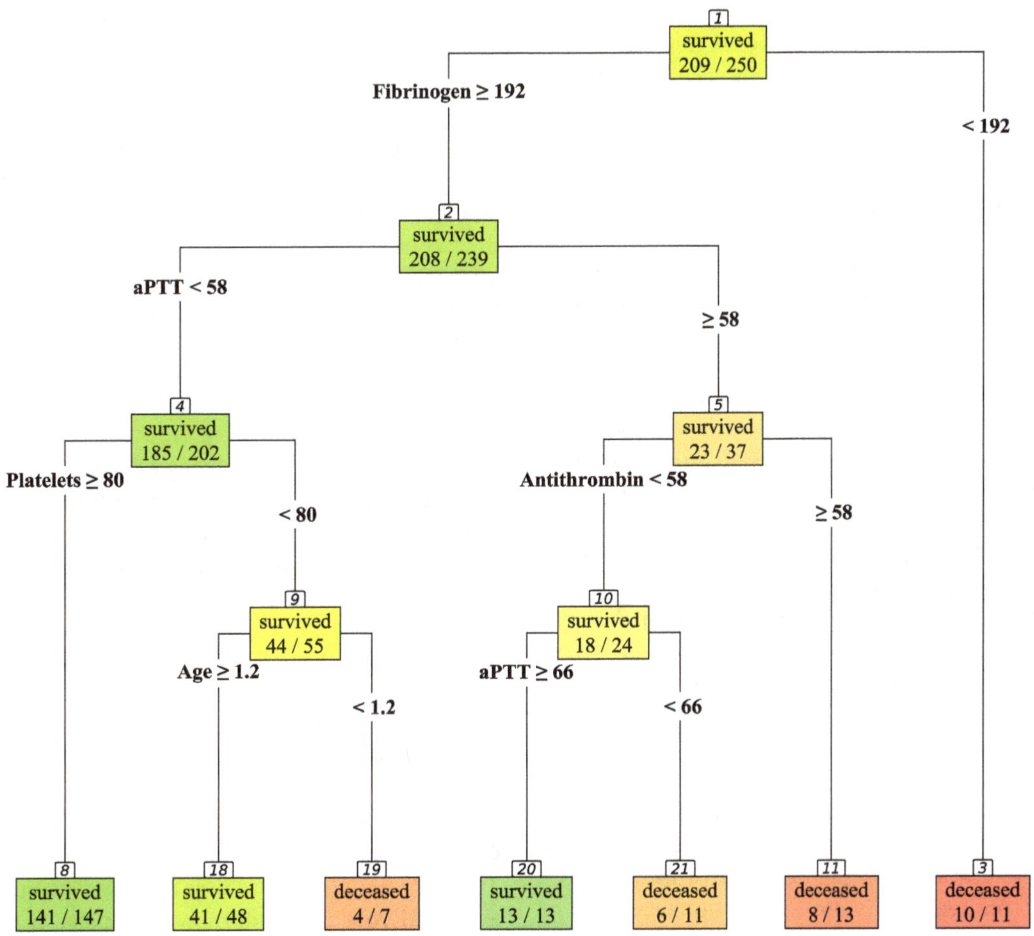

Fig. 4 Decision tree for survival. The classification tree was fitted with univariate predictors at the peak of C-reactive protein and age

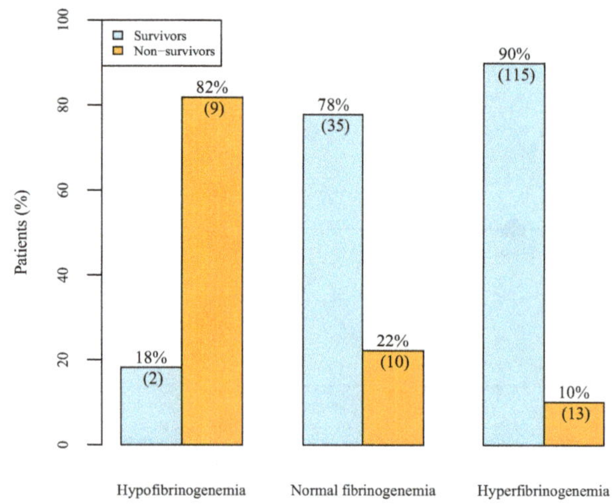

Fig. 5 Survival by age-adjusted hypofibrinogenemia, normal fibrinogenemia and hyperfibrinogenemia. The classification is based on the age-adjusted norm value ranges

to poor outcome [4, 46]. Especially in neonates, isolated thrombocytopenia leads to increased mortality. This may be explained by the fact that during the first 6 weeks after birth, the plasmatic coagulation cascade is not fully developed and therefore hemostatic competence heavily relies on platelet function [47].

Overall, a decreased platelet count is associated with mortality. This might be due to the fact that thrombocytes are also an important part of the innate immune system. Whenever pathogens are present, platelets bind to them via the glycoprotein receptor IIb/IIIa and Toll-like receptors. That either happens directly, or it is mediated by plasma proteins like fibrinogen [48]. The activated platelets release antimicrobial peptides like defensins, kinocidins and thrombocidins to kill bacteria. In addition, they release members of the chemokine family like platelet factor 4 (PF4, CXCL-4) in order to attract other immune cells [49, 50].

The third coagulation parameter essential for the prediction of mortality in septic children in our study was aPTT. Prolongation leads to poorer outcome. A long aPTT might reflect the most severe cases of sepsis due to consumption of coagulation factors or high-dose heparin therapy, but may also be caused by a FXII deficiency. In septic patients, FXII deficiency can be protective via attenuation of the FXII-dependent bradykinin generation, complement activation and further contact pathway activation. This consequence of low FXII levels might explain why 13/13 children with fibrinogen levels above 192 mg/dl and an aPTT above 66 s survived, despite an antithrombin level below 58.

Compared with developed countries, at 16.4% the overall mortality of our children was in the upper frame [51, 52]. Due to the tertiary care status of our university hospital, the study included a large number of seriously ill children. Of them, 20.4% developed septic shock with a mortality rate of 41.2%. The literature reports a mortality rate of 20–30% in the presence of septic shock [53, 54], which increases to 52% in the case of additional MODS.

The limitations of our study have to be mentioned. The retrospective design of the study precludes assessment of causal relationships. Nevertheless, the main finding that high fibrinogen levels are beneficial in sepsis can be well explained by recently reported pathophysiological mechanisms. Further, not all the considered parameters were available throughout the observation period of 7 days. Especially for children who died rapidly or were transferred to another hospital soon after C-reactive protein peaked, data are lacking and a bias could be present in the consecutive days due to the smaller sample size. Therefore, the main analyses were performed solely on the day of C-reactive protein peak. The number of 250 sepsis cases diagnosed in children over a period of 14 years could be considered low. A deeper insight might be gained in a prospective setting.

Interpretation of the results of the multivariate logistic regression analysis for survival and decision tree analysis should be done carefully, since it cannot be concluded that these coagulation parameters are independently associated with survival because major well-known risk factors for death such as organ dysfunction or lactate were not taken into account. These analyses were used solely in an explorative fashion to describe the relation of the inflammatory and coagulatory parameters to survival. Therefore, this study is mainly descriptive and cannot determine the predictive value of coagulation parameters for outcome after sepsis. Another limitation is the fact that some values, such as low fibrinogen or low platelets, might have led to interventions that were not captured by this retrospective study. This could have influenced the magnitude of the associations. Despite all limitations, this study gives new insight into the course of sepsis and provides a good basis for a prospective study using these parameters as proxy for mortality, like organ dysfunction resolution or new and progressive MODS.

Conclusion

The link between inflammation and coagulation plays a crucial role in children with sepsis. C-reactive protein does not allow discrimination between survivors and non-survivors. In contrast, increased levels of fibrinogen and platelets are linked to survival and distinctively reflect the inflammatory process. Prolonged aPTT is associated with lower survival, which might reflect therapy-related measures needed due to disease severity.

Additional files

Additional file 1. Receiver operating characteristic (ROC) curves and area under the ROC curve (AUC) values for survival. The ROC curves showing the predictive value of fibrinogen. (A) Platelets (B) and aPTT (C). ROC AUC is provided with 95% CIs.

Additional file 2. Sensitivity and specificity analysis for mortality of fibrinogen, platelets and aPTT.

Additional file 3. Fibrinogen (Clauss method) norm value ranges for female and male children.

Abbreviations
AIC: Akaike information criterion; AMP: antimicrobial peptides; aPTT: activated partial thromboplastin time; CRP: C-reactive protein; DIC: disseminated intravascular coagulopathy; FXII: coagulation factor XII; GAS: group A Streptococci; GBS: group B Streptococci; ICD: International Statistical Classification of Diseases and Related Health Problems; MODS: multiple organ dysfunction syndrome; OR: odds ratio; PF4: platelet factor 4; PICU: pediatric intensive care unit; PT: prothrombin time.

Authors' contributions
CN conceived the study, developed the study design, contributed to the acquisition and interpretation of data and drafted and edited the manuscript. MB conceived the study, developed the study design and contributed to the acquisition and interpretation of data. She also drafted and edited the manuscript. She was responsible for ensuring that this study was reported honestly, accurately and transparently and also for the overall work by ensuring that questions pertaining to the accuracy or integrity of any portion of the work were appropriately investigated and resolved (corresponding author). TH performed the statistical analysis and gave support in interpretation of the data. He also contributed significantly to the drafting and editing the manuscript. CL gave support in development of the study design and contributed to the statistical analysis. She contributed to the drafting and editing the manuscript. AE contributed to the interpretation of data. He also gave support in drafting and editing the manuscript. AB helped with the English translation and assisted with drafting and editing the manuscript. KA contributed to the acquisition and interpretation of data. She also assisted with drafting and editing the manuscript. KA contributed to the acquisition and interpretation of data. She also assisted with drafting and editing the manuscript. PI contributed to the interpretation of data and gave major support in drafting and editing the manuscript. All authors read and approved the final manuscript.

Author details
[1] Department of Pediatrics, Pediatrics I, Medical University of Innsbruck, Anichstrasse 35, 6020 Innsbruck, Austria. [2] Institute for Sports Medicine, Alpine Medicine and Health Tourism, UMIT - University for Health Sciences, Medical Informatics and Technology, Eduard Wallnöfer Zentrum 1, 6060 Hall in Tirol, Austria. [3] Department of Mathematics, Faculty of Mathematics, Computer Science and Physics, University of Innsbruck, Technikerstraße 13, 6020 Innsbruck, Austria. [4] Department of Medical Statistics, Informatics and Health Economics, Medical University of Innsbruck, Anichstrasse 35, 6020 Innsbruck, Austria. [5] Department of General and Surgical Critical Care Medicine, Medical University of Innsbruck, Anichstrasse 35, 6020 Innsbruck, Austria. [6] Department of Anaesthesiology and Critical Care Medicine, Medical University of Innsbruck, Anichstrasse 35, 6020 Innsbruck, Austria.

Acknowledgements
We thank Dr. Sophie Hofer, Dr. Christina Schoner, Dr. Daniela Hainz, Dr. Ahmed Fideh, Martin Wagner, Dr. Thomas Varga and Dr. Dietmar Fries for their assistance in executing this project.

Competing interests
The authors state that they have no competing interests in regard to this study. MB has received personal fees from LFB Biomedicaments, Baxter GmbH, CSL Behring GmbH and Mitsubishi Tanabe and non-financial support from TEM International outside the submitted work. PI has received personal fees from Baxter GmbH, personal fees from CSL Behring GmbH, personal fees from Fresenius Kabi GmbH Austria, personal fees from Bayer GmbH Austria and personal fees from LFB and non-financial support from TEM International outside the submitted work.

Funding
There is no funding to declare.

References
1. Goldstein B, Giroir B, Randolph A. International pediatric sepsis consensus conference: definitions for sepsis and organ dysfunction in pediatrics. Pediatr Crit Care Med. 2005;6(1):2–8.
2. Randolph AG, McCulloh RJ. Pediatric sepsis: important considerations for diagnosing and managing severe infections in infants, children, and adolescents. Virulence. 2014;5(1):179–89.
3. Hartman ME, Linde-Zwirble WT, Angus DC, Watson RS. Trends in the epidemiology of pediatric severe sepsis*. Pediatr Crit Care Med. 2013;14(7):686–93.
4. Sokou R, Giallouros G, Konstantinidi A, Pantavou K, Nikolopoulos G, Bonovas S, et al. Thromboelastometry for diagnosis of neonatal sepsis-associated coagulopathy: an observational study. Eur J Pediatr. 2018;177(3):355–62.
5. van der Poll T, van Deventer SJ. Cytokines and anticytokines in the pathogenesis of sepsis. Infect Dis Clin North Am. 1999;13(2):413–26.
6. Reddy RC, Chen GH, Tekchandani PK, Standiford TJ. Sepsis-induced immunosuppression. Immunol Res. 2001;24(3):273–87.
7. Levy MM, Fink MP, Marshall JC, Abraham E, Angus D, Cook D, et al. 2001 SCCM/ESICM/ACCP/ATS/SIS international sepsis definitions conference. Crit Care Med. 2003;31(4):1250–6.
8. Schneider HG, Lam QT. Procalcitonin for the clinical laboratory: a review. Pathology. 2007;39(4):383–90.
9. Castelli GP, Pognani C, Meisner M, Stuani A, Bellomi D, Sgarbi L. Procalcitonin and C-reactive protein during systemic inflammatory response syndrome, sepsis and organ dysfunction. Crit Care. 2004;8(4):R234–42.
10. Clec'h C, Ferriere F, Karoubi P, Fosse JP, Cupa M, Hoang P, et al. Diagnostic and prognostic value of procalcitonin in patients with septic shock. Crit Care Med. 2004;32(5):1166–9.
11. Chiesa C, Natale F, Pascone R, Osborn JF, Pacifico L, Bonci E, et al. C reactive protein and procalcitonin: reference intervals for preterm and term newborns during the early neonatal period. Clin Chim Acta. 2011;412(11):1053–9.
12. Schentag JJ, O'Keeffe D, Marmion M, Wels PB. C-reactive protein as an indicator of infection relapse in patients with abdominal sepsis. Arch Surg. 1984;119(3):300–4.
13. Maury CP. Monitoring the acute phase response: comparison of tumour necrosis factor (cachectin) and C-reactive protein responses in inflammatory and infectious diseases. J Clin Pathol. 1989;42(10):1078–82.
14. Povoa P, Almeida E, Moreira P, Fernandes A, Mealha R, Aragao A, et al. C-reactive protein as an indicator of sepsis. Intensive Care Med. 1998;24(10):1052–6.
15. Presterl E, Staudinger T, Pettermann M, Lassnigg A, Burgmann H, Winkler S, et al. Cytokine profile and correlation to the APACHE III and MPM II scores in patients with sepsis. Am J Respir Crit Care Med. 1997;156(3 Pt 1):825–32.
16. Yentis SM, Soni N, Sheldon J. C-reactive protein as an indicator of resolution of sepsis in the intensive care unit. Intensive Care Med. 1995;21(7):602–5.
17. Pinilla JC, Hayes P, Laverty W, Arnold C, Laxdal V. The C-reactive protein to prealbumin ratio correlates with the severity of multiple organ dysfunction. Surgery. 1998;124(4):799–805 **(discussion-6)**.

18. Waydhas C, Nast-Kolb D, Trupka A, Zettl R, Kick M, Wiesholler J, et al. Posttraumatic inflammatory response, secondary operations, and late multiple organ failure. J Trauma. 1996;40(4):624–30 **(discussion 630-1)**.
19. Ikei S, Ogawa M, Yamaguchi Y. Blood concentrations of polymorphonuclear leucocyte elastase and interleukin-6 are indicators for the occurrence of multiple organ failures at the early stage of acute pancreatitis. J Gastroenterol Hepatol. 1998;13(12):1274–83.
20. de Beaux AC, Goldie AS, Ross JA, Carter DC, Fearon KC. Serum concentrations of inflammatory mediators related to organ failure in patients with acute pancreatitis. Br J Surg. 1996;83(3):349–53.
21. Rau B, Steinbach G, Baumgart K, Gansauge F, Grunert A, Beger HG. Serum amyloid A versus C-reactive protein in acute pancreatitis: clinical value of an alternative acute-phase reactant. Crit Care Med. 2000;28(3):736–42.
22. Levi M, van der Poll T. Inflammation and coagulation. Crit Care Med. 2010;38(2 Suppl):S26–34.
23. van der Poll T, Levi M. Crosstalk between inflammation and coagulation: the lessons of sepsis. Curr Vasc Pharmacol. 2012;10(5):632–8.
24. Berends ET, Kuipers A, Ravesloot MM, Urbanus RT, Rooijakkers SH. Bacteria under stress by complement and coagulation. FEMS Microbiol Rev. 2014;38(6):1146–71.
25. Pahlman LI, Morgelin M, Kasetty G, Olin AI, Schmidtchen A, Herwald H. Antimicrobial activity of fibrinogen and fibrinogen-derived peptides—a novel link between coagulation and innate immunity. Thromb Haemost. 2013;109(5):930–9.
26. Senior RM, Skogen WF, Griffin GL, Wilner GD. Effects of fibrinogen derivatives upon the inflammatory response. Studies with human fibrinopeptide B. J Clin Invest. 1986;77(3):1014–9.
27. Lauterbach R, Pawlik D, Radziszewska R, Wozniak J, Rytlewski K. Plasma antithrombin III and protein C levels in early recognition of late-onset sepsis in newborns. Eur J Pediatr. 2006;165(9):585–9.
28. Semeraro F, Colucci M, Caironi P, Masson S, Ammollo CT, Teli R, et al. Platelet drop and fibrinolytic shutdown in patients with sepsis. Crit Care Med. 2018;46(3):e221–8.
29. Esmon CT. The interactions between inflammation and coagulation. Br J Haematol. 2005;131(4):417–30.
30. Akaike H. A new look at the statistical model identification. IEEE Trans Autom Control. 1974;19(6):716–23.
31. Ersoy B, Nehir H, Altinoz S, Yilmaz O, Dundar PE, Aydogan A. Prognostic value of initial antithrombin levels in neonatal sepsis. Indian Pediatr. 2007;44(8):581–4.
32. Taylor FB Jr, Kinasewitz GT, Lupu F. Pathophysiology, staging and therapy of severe sepsis in baboon models. J Cell Mol Med. 2012;16(4):672–82.
33. Luo D, Szaba FM, Kummer LW, Plow EF, Mackman N, Gailani D, et al. Protective roles for fibrin, tissue factor, plasminogen activator inhibitor-1, and thrombin activatable fibrinolysis inhibitor, but not factor XI, during defense against the gram-negative bacterium *Yersinia enterocolitica*. J Immunol. 2011;187(4):1866–76.
34. Mullarky IK, Szaba FM, Berggren KN, Parent MA, Kummer LW, Chen W, et al. Infection-stimulated fibrin deposition controls hemorrhage and limits hepatic bacterial growth during listeriosis. Infect Immun. 2005;73(7):3888–95.
35. Davalos D, Akassoglou K. Fibrinogen as a key regulator of inflammation in disease. Semin Immunopathol. 2012;34(1):43–62.
36. McAdow M, Missiakas DM, Schneewind O. *Staphylococcus aureus* secretes coagulase and von Willebrand factor binding protein to modify the coagulation cascade and establish host infections. J Innate Immun. 2012;4(2):141–8.
37. Jennewein C, Mehring M, Tran N, Paulus P, Ockelmann PA, Habeck K, et al. The fibrinopeptide bbeta15–42 reduces inflammation in mice subjected to polymicrobial sepsis. Shock. 2012;38(3):275–80.
38. Wolf T, Kann G, Becker S, Stephan C, Brodt HR, de Leuw P, et al. Severe Ebola virus disease with vascular leakage and multiorgan failure: treatment of a patient in intensive care. Lancet. 2015;385(9976):1428–35.
39. Wada H, Mori Y, Okabayashi K, Gabazza EC, Kushiya F, Watanabe M, et al. High plasma fibrinogen level is associated with poor clinical outcome in DIC patients. Am J Hematol. 2003;72(1):1–7.
40. Renckens R, Roelofs JJ, Stegenga ME, Florquin S, Levi M, Carmeliet P, et al. Transgenic tissue-type plasminogen activator expression improves host defense during Klebsiella pneumonia. J Thromb Haemost. 2008;6(4):660–8.
41. Asakura H, Ontachi Y, Mizutani T, Kato M, Saito M, Kumabashiri I, et al. An enhanced fibrinolysis prevents the development of multiple organ failure in disseminated intravascular coagulation in spite of much activation of blood coagulation. Crit Care Med. 2001;29(6):1164–8.
42. Mihajlovic D, Lendak D, Mitic G, Cebovic T, Draskovic B, Novakov A, et al. Prognostic value of hemostasis-related parameters for prediction of organ dysfunction and mortality in sepsis. Turk J Med Sci. 2015;45(1):93–8.
43. Semeraro N, Ammollo CT, Semeraro F, Colucci M. Coagulopathy of acute sepsis. Semin Thromb Hemost. 2015;41(6):650–8.
44. Parker RI. Coagulopathies in the PICU: DIC and liver disease. Crit Care Clin. 2013;29(2):319–33.
45. Nesseler N, Launey Y, Aninat C, Morel F, Malledant Y, Seguin P. Clinical review: the liver in sepsis. Crit Care. 2012;16(5):235.
46. Ostrowski SR, Haase N, Muller RB, Moller MH, Pott FC, Perner A, et al. Association between biomarkers of endothelial injury and hypocoagulability in patients with severe sepsis: a prospective study. Crit Care. 2015;19(191):015–0918.
47. Andrew M, Vegh P, Johnston M, Bowker J, Ofosu F, Mitchell L. Maturation of the hemostatic system during childhood. Blood. 1992;80(8):1998–2005.
48. Yeaman MR. Platelets in defense against bacterial pathogens. Cell Mol Life Sci. 2010;67(4):525–44.
49. Clemetson KJ. The role of platelets in defence against pathogens. Hamostaseologie. 2011;31(4):264–8.
50. Saloga J, Klimek L, Buhl R, Mann W, Knop J, Grabbe S. Allergologie-Handbuch: Grundlagen und klinische Praxis. Stuttgart: Schattauer Verlag; 2012.
51. Taori RN, Lahiri KR, Tullu MS. Performance of PRISM (pediatric risk of mortality) score and PIM (pediatric index of mortality) score in a tertiary care pediatric ICU. Indian J Pediatr. 2010;77(3):267–71.
52. Kutko MC, Calarco MP, Flaherty MB, Helmrich RF, Ushay HM, Pon S, et al. Mortality rates in pediatric septic shock with and without multiple organ system failure. Pediatr Crit Care Med. 2003;4(3):333–7.
53. Hatherill M, Tibby SM, Turner C, Ratnavel N, Murdoch IA. Procalcitonin and cytokine levels: relationship to organ failure and mortality in pediatric septic shock. Crit Care Med. 2000;28(7):2591–4.
54. Wilkinson JD, Pollack MM, Ruttimann UE, Glass NL, Yeh TS. Outcome of pediatric patients with multiple organ system failure. Crit Care Med. 1986;14(4):271–4.

7

Large-volume paracentesis effects plasma disappearance rate of indo-cyanine green in critically ill patients with decompensated liver cirrhosis and intraabdominal hypertension

Ulrich Mayr*, Leonie Fahrenkrog-Petersen, Gonzalo Batres-Baires, Alexander Herner, Sebastian Rasch, Roland M. Schmid, Wolfgang Huber and Tobias Lahmer

Abstract

Background: Ascites is a major complication of decompensated liver cirrhosis. Intraabdominal hypertension and structural alterations of parenchyma involve decisive changes in hepatosplanchnic blood flow. Clearance of indo-cyanine green (ICG) is mainly dependent on hepatic perfusion and hepatocellular function. As a consequence, plasma disappearance rate of ICG (ICG-PDR) is rated as a useful dynamic parameter of liver function. This study primarily evaluates the impact of large-volume paracentesis (LVP) on ICG-PDR in critically ill patients with decompensated cirrhosis. Additionally, it describes influences on intraabdominal pressure (IAP), abdominal perfusion pressure (APP), hepatic blood flow, hemodynamic and respiratory function.

Methods: We analyzed LVP in 22 patients with decompensated liver cirrhosis. ICG-PDR was assessed by using noninvasive LiMON technology (Pulsion® Medical Systems; Maquet Getinge Group), and hepatic blood flow was analyzed by color-coded duplex sonography.

Results: Paracentesis of a median volume of 3450 mL ascites evoked significant increases of ICG-PDR from 3.6 (2.8–4.6) to 5.1 (3.9–6.2)%/min ($p<0.001$). Concomitantly, we observed a raise in "ICG-Clearance" from 99 (73.5–124.5) to 104 (91–143.5) mL/min/m^2 ($p=0.005$), while circulating blood volume index was unchanged [2412 (1983–3025) before paracentesis vs. 2409 (1997–2805) mL/m^2, $p=0.734$]. Sonography revealed a significant impact of paracentesis on hepatic blood flow: Hepatic artery resistance index dropped from 0.74 (0.68–0.75) to 0.68 (0.65–0.71) ($p<0.001$) and maximum flow velocity in hepatic vein increased from 24 (17–30) to 30 (22–36) cm/s ($p<0.001$). Consistent with previous studies, paracentesis caused significant decreases in IAP from 19.0 (15.0–20.3) to 11.0 (8.8–12.3) mmHg ($p<0.001$) and central venous pressure from 22.5 (17.8–29.0) to 17.5 (12.8–24.0) mmHg ($p<0.001$) with inverse increases in APP from 63.0 (56.8–69.5) to 71.0 (65.5–78.5) mmHg ($p<0.001$). Changes in ICG-PDR were concomitant with changes in IAP ($r=-0.602$) and APP ($r=0.576$). Moreover, we found a substantial improvement in respiratory function. By contrast, hemodynamic parameters assessed by transpulmonary thermodilution, serum bilirubin and international normalized ratio did not change after paracentesis.

Conclusion: Critically ill patients with decompensated cirrhosis and elevated IAP showed dramatically impaired ICG-PDR. Paracentesis evoked an improvement in ICG-PDR in parallel with a decreased IAP and an increased APP, while conventional parameters of liver function did not change. This effect on ICG-PDR is mainly referable to a relief of intraabdominal hypertension and changes in hepatosplanchnic blood flow.

*Correspondence: mayr.ulrich@gmx.net
Klinik und Poliklinik für Innere Medizin II, Klinikum rechts der Isar, Technische Universität München, Ismaninger Strasse 22, 81675 Munich, Germany

Keywords: Indo-cyanine green (ICG), Plasma disappearance rate (PDR), Large-volume paracentesis (LVP), Intraabdominal hypertension (IAH), Intraabdominal pressure (IAP), Decompensated liver cirrhosis, Hepatosplanchnic blood flow, Transpulmonary thermodilution, Color-coded duplex sonography, Hepatic artery resistance index

Background

Decompensated liver cirrhosis implies serious consequences for affected patients. Ascites is one major and highly frequently emerging complication [1, 2]. Intraabdominal hypertension (IAH) is associated with poor prognosis and high mortality [3, 4]. Increased intraabdominal pressure (IAP) involves multiple organ dysfunction regarding cardiovascular, respiratory, renal and abdominal impairment [5–8]. In particular, IAH interferes with proper abdominal perfusion, including hepatosplanchnic blood flow [9, 10].

Furthermore, advanced cirrhosis is accompanied by structural alterations leading to increased intrahepatic vascular resistance [11, 12]. Restrictions of intrahepatic blood flow cause portal hypertension, further aggravated by compensatory splanchnic arterial vasodilation [13]. Moreover, cirrhosis provokes impairment of blood flow in hepatic veins as well as increases in hepatic artery resistance index [14, 15]. Color-coded duplex sonography provides a subjective, but noninvasive diagnostic approach regarding vascular disorders in advanced liver disease [16].

Finally, end-stage liver disease is associated with progressive loss of functional liver capacity. Conventional laboratory assessment of liver function is mainly based on liver enzymes, bilirubin and the coagulation parameter international normalized ratio (INR) [17]. Dynamic tests of liver function at bedside might be more precise and objective relating to actual, short-term functional status [18]. Promising experiences were achieved with noninvasive measurement of plasma disappearance rate of indo-cyanine green (ICG-PDR). ICG is injected intravenously, distributed via blood circulation and excreted hepatobiliary [19]. ICG-PDR reflects both hepatosplanchnic blood flow and hepatocellular and excretory function [20, 21]. Some previous data described an interaction of ICG-PDR with intraabdominal pressure level [22–24]. Recently, one of these studies affirmed that ICG-PDR correlates inversely with IAP, suggesting that IAH restrains hepatosplanchnic and sinusoidal perfusion [25]. The abdominal perfusion pressure (APP), defined as difference between mean arterial pressure (MAP) and IAP, was positively correlated with ICG-PDR.

The accumulation of ascites is a typical complication of decompensated cirrhosis with elevated IAP and restricted organ perfusion [2, 10]. The evacuation of ascites by large-volume paracentesis (LVP) is one of the few nonsurgical treatment options [26]. ICG-PDR was already labeled as an accurate test for prediction of survival in advanced cirrhosis [27]. So far, none of the previous studies focused on the impact of LVP on dynamic liver assessment by ICG-PDR in this patient population. Consequently, the aim of our study was to investigate the effect of LVP on ICG-PDR in critically ill patients with decompensated liver cirrhosis (primary endpoint). This evaluation was supplemented by analyses of IAP, APP, hepatic blood flow by sonography, respiratory function as well as hemodynamic monitoring by using transpulmonary thermodilution.

Methods

Study design

This observational study was approved by the institutional review board (Ethikkommission Technische Universität München; Fakultät für Medizin; Project Number 5384/12), and informed consent was obtained by all patients.

Between April 2016 and July 2017, a total of 29 critically ill patients with decompensated liver cirrhosis on our university hospital general ICU were screened for the feasibility of LVP, analyses of ICG-PDR, IAP and hemodynamic monitoring via transpulmonary thermodilution. LVP was performed irrespective of the study based on the indication made by the treating ICU physician. We released a maximum of mobilizable ascites in each individual case of LVP; laboratory analyses of ascites revealed a cell count $< 500/\mu L$ and polymorphonuclear neutrophils $< 250/\mu L$ in every single patient. Due to potential influences on hepatosplanchnic blood flow, analysis was considered feasible only in patients without terlipressin treatment, portal vein thrombosis or transjugular intrahepatic portosystemic stent shunt. Therefore, 6 patients with terlipressin-treatment, 1 patient with portal vein thrombosis and 2 patients with portosystemic stent were restrained from the study. Finally, we analyzed a total of 22 critically ill patients with decompensated liver cirrhosis and tense ascites.

Techniques

Assessment of ICG-PDR, BVI, CBI and laboratory tests

ICG-PDR, circulating blood volume index (BVI) and "ICG-Clearance" (CBI) were analyzed immediately before and after paracentesis by using noninvasive LiMON technology (Pulsion® Medical Systems; Maquet

Getinge Group) via a disposable finger color sensor as previously described [28]. We used ICG solubilized in distilled water and injected via a central venous catheter at a dose of 0.5 mg/kg of ICG-solution for measurement of ICG-PDR and additional assessment of BVI and CBI. Normally, ICG-PDR amounts to 18–25%/min [20]. Measurements of BVI and CBI were performed in parallel with ICG-PDR after manual input of current cardiac output and automatically indexed according to manufacturer's recommendations.

Main laboratory tests of excretory liver function and synthesis (Bilirubin, INR) were analyzed once a day—corresponding to current standard in our intensive care unit. Overall time interval between blood sampling was 24 h.

LVP, IAP, abdominal compliance, APP and CVP

LVP was performed ultrasound guided after bringing the patient in supine position [29]. IAP was determined by intravesical measurement using a home-made technique according to The Abdominal Compartment Society (WSACS), and IAH was defined as IAP $\geq$ 12 mmHg [30, 31]. Abdominal compliance was expressed as the change of ascites volume per change in IAP (delta IAP) before and after paracentesis [32]. APP was calculated as MAP minus IAP by using concomitantly obtained values as explained previously [25, 31]. Substitution of albumin followed current guidelines and was performed after the final analyses [33]. Central venous pressure (CVP) was measured via jugular central venous catheters at end-expiration.

Ventilator setting and respiratory function

Patients with spontaneous breathing received a demand-based application of oxygen. Mechanical ventilation was performed using the routine ventilator device EVITA XL of our ICU (Dräger, Lübeck, Germany). Parameters were set according to current ARDSNet recommendations, especially regarding positive end-expiratory pressure (PEEP) [34]. Ventilator setting was based on medical assessment by the treating ICU physician irrespective of the study. The EVITA XL ventilator continuously monitored levels of airway pressures and corresponding volumes. Routine ventilatory parameters such as PEEP, tidal volume (TV), mean airway pressure, dynamic respiratory system compliance (C_{dyn}) and fraction of inspired oxygen (F_iO_2) were recorded at baseline and at the end of LVP. P_aO_2 and P_aCO_2 were derived from a fully automatic blood gas analysis device (Rapid Point 400, Siemens Healthcare Diagnostic GmbH, Eschborn, Germany). Blood gas analysis and ventilatory parameters were used for calculation of Horowitz-index (P_aO_2/F_iO_2) and oxygenation index ($OI = F_iO_2$ * mean airway pressure * $100/P_aO_2$) [35].

Hemodynamic monitoring

With the exception of only a single subject, all patients were under hemodynamic monitoring irrespective of the study, by using transpulmonary thermodilution with the PiCCO-2-device (Pulsion Medical Systems SE, Maquet Getinge Group) as described previously [36]: A 5 Fr thermistor-tipped arterial line (Pulsiocath, Pulsion® Medical Systems; Maquet Getinge Group) inserted through a femoral artery and a hemodynamic monitor (PiCCO-2, Pulsion® Medical Systems, Maquet Getinge Group) served to derive and analyze the thermodilution curve after injection of a cold indicator bolus (15 ml of saline cooled down to 4 °C) through a jugular central venous catheter. Measurements were done in triplicate, averaged and automatically indexed according to manufacturer's recommendations.

Color-coded duplex sonography

Transabdominal ultrasound examination was accomplished noninvasively at the bedside in a supine position of the patients. All analyses were performed by a single physician with 6 years of institutional experience in the field of abdominal ultrasound. We used the mobile ultrasound scanner ACUSON X300 (Siemens Healthcare GmbH, Erlangen, Germany) and a convex 3.5 MHz transducer with color Doppler capacity. The transducer was placed in the right intercostal space due to the intraabdominal fluid accumulation. Doppler-analyses of blood flow were performed of the portal vein, hepatic artery and right hepatic vein; middle hepatic vein was chosen only when analysis of right hepatic vein was insufficient [14].

Data collection

Clinical and laboratory parameters for the calculation of APACHE II-, SOFA-, MELD- and Child–Pugh scores were recorded on the day of paracentesis. Measurements of ICG-PDR, BVI and CBI were done immediately before and after LVP, with a median time interval of 210 (180–255) min. Ventilatory parameters, hemodynamic profiles as well as IAP-assessment and ultrasound examinations were performed immediately before as well as after the maximal mobilizable release of ascites.

Statistical analysis and primary endpoint

For primary outcome analysis, we investigated ICG-PDR at the end of LVP compared to baseline. All analyses and graphs were generated using GraphPad Prism 7.0 (GraphPad Software, La Jolla, CA, USA). Correlations were calculated using Pearson`s correlation coefficient r and linear regressions using the coefficient R^2. Continuous variables are expressed as median and interquartile range (IQR). Categorical variables are expressed as percentages. To compare continuous variables, we used nonparametric Wilcoxon test for paired samples. Significance was assumed at a p value < 0.05.

Results

Patients' baseline characteristics

Patients' baseline characteristics and clinical scores are presented in Table 1.

We performed LVP procedures in a total of 22 patients (7 female, 15 male) with decompensated liver cirrhosis and tense ascites. APACHE-, SOFA-, MELD- and Child–Pugh scores are explainable by advanced hepatic impairment and critical illness. The etiology of cirrhosis was predominantly alcoholic-toxic. About 75% of patients were mechanically ventilated and about 25% were spontaneously breathing. Regarding mechanically ventilated patients, PEEP-setting was unchanged during LVP and study measurements.

LVP, ICG-PDR, BVI, CBI and laboratory tests

Twenty-two LVP procedures with a median volume of 3450 (3075–4700) mL removed ascites (≥3000 mL for every paracentesis) were analyzed. We noticed a median ascitic cell count of 180 (100–310)/μL (≤500/μL in all patients), with polymorphonuclear neutrophils < 250/μL in each patient to exclude spontaneous bacterial peritonitis and to justify a release of a maximum of mobilizable ascites volume.

ICG-PDR at baseline was decreased substantially to 3.6 (2.8–4.6)%/min compatible with dramatic hepatic impairment of advanced liver cirrhosis. LVP provoked a significant increase of ICG-PDR to 5.1 (3.9–6.2)%/min ($p < 0.001$) (Fig. 1). Median change of ICG-PDR (delta ICG-PDR) induced by LVP was 1.2 (1.0–2.1)%/min.

Circulating blood volume index (BVI) was unchanged after LVP [2412 (1983–3025) before paracentesis vs. 2409 (1997–2805) mL/m^2, $p = 0.734$], while "ICG-Clearance" (CBI) increased from 99 (73.5–124.5) to 104 (91–143.5) mL/min/m^2 ($p = 0.005$) (Fig. 2).

In comparison, main laboratory tests of liver function showed no significant changes after an overall time interval of 24 h: Parameter of liver excretion function bilirubin as well as plasmatic coagulation parameter INR remained stable (Table 2).

IAP, abdominal compliance, APP and CVP

Paracentesis caused a distinct relief of IAH: At the end of LVP, pressure levels of IAP had lowered from 19.0 (15.0–20.3) to 11.0 (8.8–12.3) mmHg ($p < 0.001$). Grading of IAH before and after LVP is listed in Table 3, according to the definition established by the WSACS [31]. Median abdominal compliance based on paracentesis of 3450 (3075–4700) mL was 461 (383–659) mL/mmHg.

Consecutively, we noticed a marked improvement of APP from 63.0 (56.8–69.5) to 71.0 (65.5–78.5)

Table 1 Patients baseline characteristics and clinical scores

Patients characteristics	
Male sex [*n*/total (%)]	15/22 (68%)
Age (years)	55 (52–69.3)
Body weight (kg)	82.5 (70–100)
Body height (cm)	180 (170–183)
APACHE II	24 (19–29.3)
SOFA	12 (9.8–16)
MELD	27.5 (23.8–36.3)
Child–Pugh	12 (10–13)
Child C [*n*/total (%)]	19/22 (86%)
Etiology of cirrhosis [*n*/total (%)]	Alcoholic 16/22 (72%)
	Viral 3/22 (14%)
	Cryptogenic 3/22 (14%)
Admission diagnoses [*n*/total (%)]	Sepsis/Pneumonia 10/22 (45%)
	Acute kidney failure 7/22 (32%)
	Hepatic encephalopathy 5/22 (23%)
Mode of ventilation [*n*/total (%)]	Spontaneous breathing 6/22 (27%)
	Pressure-supported 6/22 (27%)
	Pressure-controlled 10/22 (46%)
Ascites volume (mL)	3450 (3075–4700)
Total cell count (*n*/μL)	180 (100–310)
PEEP-level (cmH$_2$O)	8 (8–10)
Baseline F$_i$O$_2$ (%)	45 (35–60)

APACHE acute physiology and chronic health evaluation, *SOFA* sequential organ failure assessment, *MELD* model of end-stage liver disease, *PEEP* positive end-expiratory pressure, F_iO_2 fraction of inspired oxygen

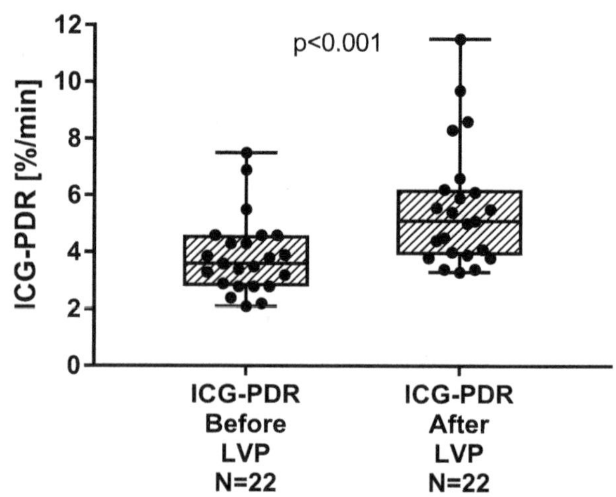

Fig. 1 ICG-PDR at baseline and after large-volume paracentesis (LVP), depicted as box plots (median and IQR, min to max) and showing all individual points

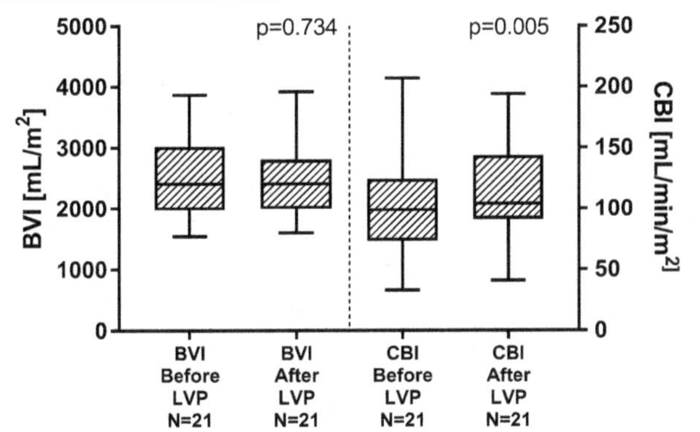

Fig. 2 Circulating blood volume index (BVI) and "ICG-Clearance" (CBI) before and after large-volume paracentesis (LVP), depicted as box plots (median and IQR, min to max)

Table 2 Main conventional laboratory parameters of liver function before and after paracentesis (overall time interval of 24 h)

Conventional laboratory tests of hepatic function			
	Before paracentesis Median (IQR)	After paracentesis Median (IQR)	*p* value
Bilirubin (mg/dL)	7.8 (3.3–19.0)	7.6 (2.5–21.4)	0.868
INR	1.8 (1.4–2.2)	1.8 (1.4–2.5)	0.094

INR international normalized ratio

Table 3 Grading of intraabdominal hypertension before and after paracentesis

Grading of IAH according to WSACS definition		
	Before LVP *n*/total (%)	After LVP *n*/total (%)
No IAH, IAP ≤ 11 mmHg	1/22 (5%)	13/22 (59%)
IAH Grade I, IAP 12–15 mmHg	5/22 (23%)	6/22 (27%)
IAH Grade II, IAP 16–20 mmHg	11/22 (50%)	2/22 (9%)
IAH Grade III, IAP 21–25 mmHg	3/22 (13%)	1/22 (5%)
IAH Grade IV, IAP > 25 mmHg	2/22 (9%)	0/22 (0%)

IAH intraabdominal hypertension, *WSACS* The Abdominal Compartment Society, *LVP* large-volume paracentesis, *IAP* Intraabdominal pressure

mmHg ($p < 0.001$). Pressure levels of IAP and APP are depicted in Fig. 3. In parallel with the decline of IAP, LVP induced a significant decrease of CVP from 22.5 (17.8–29.0) to 17.5 (12.8–24.0) mmHg ($p = 0.001$).

Median changes in IAP (delta IAP) and APP (delta APP) caused by paracentesis were -8.0 (− 5.0 to − 10.0) mmHg and 8.5 (5.8–10.3) mmHg, respectively. Furthermore, LVP provoked a median change in CVP (delta CVP) of − 5.0 (− 3.0 to − 7.0) mmHg.

Correlations and regression plots

Analyses according to Pearson as well as linear regressions are illustrated in Fig. 4. Paracentesis of a median volume of 3450 (3075–4700) mL in a total of 22 patients provoked concomitant changes of ICG-PDR (delta ICG-PDR) with changes in IAP (panel A, $r = -0.602$, $p = 0.003$). In parallel, delta ICG-PDR correlated significantly with delta APP (panel B, $r = 0.576$, $p = 0.005$). In contrast, delta ICG-PDR was not significantly associated with evacuated ascites volume (panel C, $r = 0.281$, $p = 0.205$). Concerning concomitant changes of IAP and CVP after LVP, correlation analyses outlined an association of delta IAP and delta CVP (panel D, $r = 0.637$, $p = 0.001$).

Color-coded duplex sonography

By sonographic examination, we registered a significant impact of LVP on hepatic blood flow: Hepatic artery resistance index dropped from 0.74 (0.68–0.75) to 0.68 (0.65–0.71) ($p < 0.001$). This reduction was mainly reflected in an increase of diastolic hepatic arterial flow velocity, while systolic arterial flow velocity was steady. Furthermore, LVP provoked an increase of maximum hepatic vein flow velocity. In contrast, maximum flow velocity in portal vein was mainly unaffected by paracentesis (Table 4).

Respiratory and ventilatory parameters

Respiratory function improved by paracentesis without changes of PEEP-level, outlined in Table 5. Horowitz-index (P_aO_2/F_iO_2) increased and oxygenation index (OI) improved. Furthermore, we registered a significant raise in TV and C_{dyn}. We also recorded a decrease in respiratory rate and P_aCO_2, but results were not statistically significant.

Hemodynamic parameters

Hemodynamic assessment by transpulmonary thermodilution and pulse contour analysis revealed overall unchanged parameters of hemodynamic function after LVP: Mean arterial pressure MAP, cardiac Index CI, cardiac output CO, global end-diastolic volume index GEDVI, extravascular lung water index EVLWI and systemic vascular resistance index SVRI did not change significantly (Table 6).

Discussion

The present study shows that large-volume paracentesis (LVP) induced an improvement in ICG-PDR in critically ill patients with decompensated liver cirrhosis. This effect comes along with a relief of intraabdominal hypertension

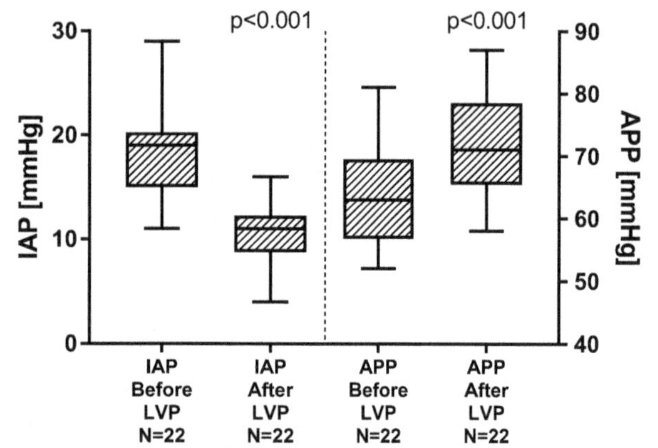

Fig. 3 Intraabdominal pressure (IAP) and abdominal perfusion pressure (APP) before and after large-volume paracentesis (LVP), depicted as box plots (median and IQR, min to max)

(IAH) reflected in a decrease in intraabdominal pressure (IAP) and an inverse raise of abdominal perfusion pressure (APP).

ICG-PDR represents a useful dynamic liver test in addition to conventional laboratory parameters [17]. On the one hand, ICG-PDR is dependent on hepatocellular function [18–20, 37, 38]. On the other hand, it is highly influenced by sufficient hepatosplanchnic blood flow and sinusoidal perfusion [18, 21, 39]. Normal range of ICG-PDR is between 18 and 25%/min. Advanced liver cirrhosis involves severe decreases of ICG-PDR with consecutively grave consequences on patients outcome [20].

This dramatic impairment of ICG-PDR in case of end-stage liver disease is confirmed in our study. Median baseline ICG-PDR was reduced markedly to 3.6%/min. Large-volume paracentesis (LVP) provoked a significant increase in ICG-PDR. Additionally, we noticed an increase in "ICG-Clearance" in contrast to unchanged circulating blood volume index, but data on the relevance of these parameters are rare so far. As opposed to this, paracentesis had no influence on main laboratory parameters of hepatic function. In this context, it should be pointed out that an earlier study found no correlation

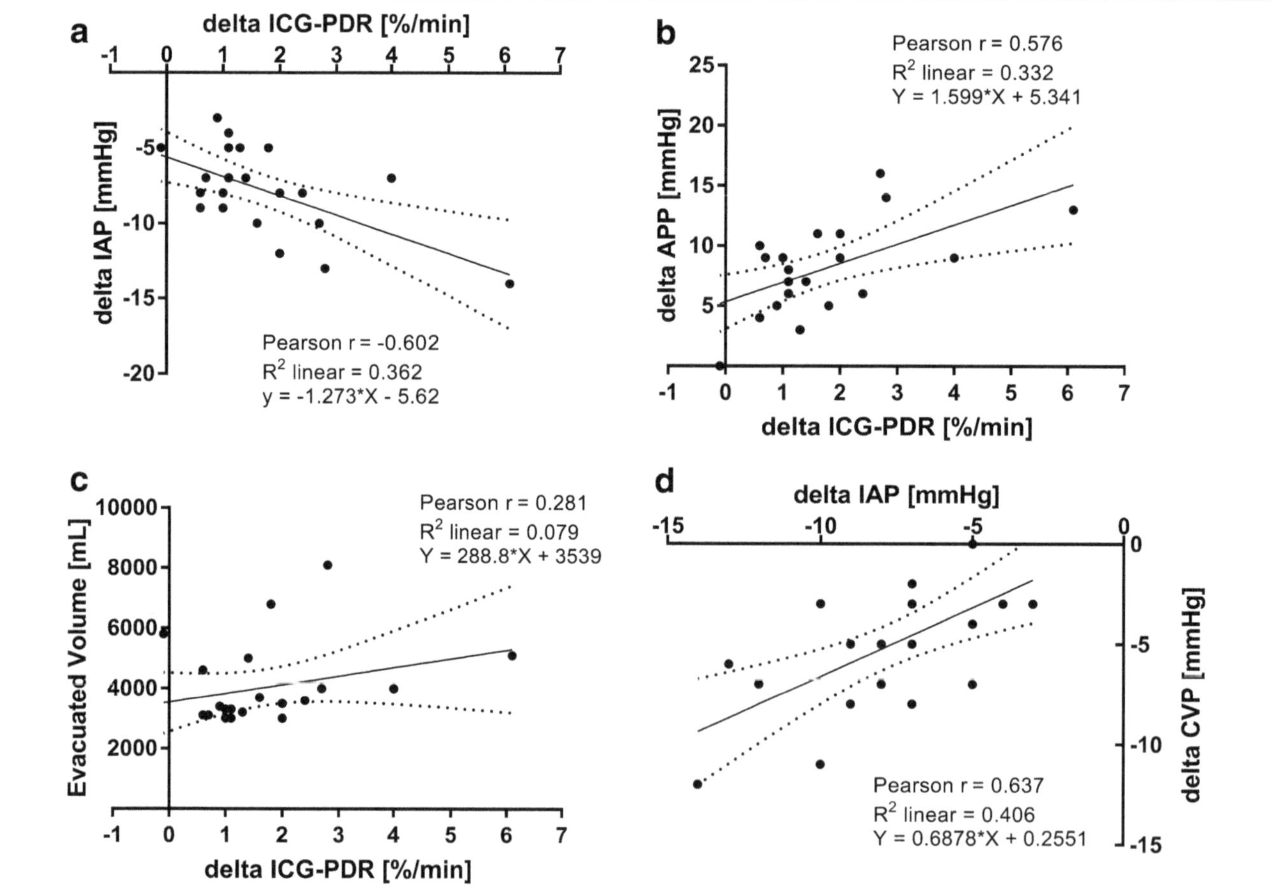

Fig. 4 Pearson correlations and regression plots of changes caused by paracentesis per patient ($n = 22$). **a** delta ICG-PDR correlated with delta IAP. **b** delta ICG-PDR correlated with delta APP. **c** delta ICG-PDR correlated with evacuated volume. **d** delta IAP correlated with delta CVP

Table 4 Ultrasound examination of hepatic blood flow by color-coded duplex sonography of hepatic artery, portal vein and hepatic vein before and after paracentesis

Color-coded duplex sonography of hepatic blood flow			
	Before paracentesis	After paracentesis	*p* value
	Median (IQR)	Median (IQR)	
HARI	0.74 (0.68–0.75)	0.68 (0.65–0.71)	< 0.001
Systolic HAF (cm/s)	129 (115–145)	123 (114–140)	0.100
Diastolic HAF (cm/s)	35 (24–48)	40 (31–50)	0.009
PVF (cm/s)	20 (16–28)	21 (15–32)	0.753
HVF (cm/s)	24 (17–30)	30 (22–36)	< 0.001

HARI hepatic artery resistance index, *HAF* maximum hepatic arterial flow velocity, *PVF* maximum portal vein flow velocity, HVF: Maximum hepatic vein flow velocity

Table 5 Respiratory and ventilatory parameters before and after paracentesis

Respiratory and ventilatory parameters			
	Before paracentesis	After paracentesis	*p* value
	Median (IQR)	Median (IQR)	
P_aO_2/F_iO_2	220 (126–271)	247 (138–321)	< 0.001
OI (cmH_2O/mmHg)	8.0 (4.8–12.3)	5.8 (3.8–11.1)	< 0.001
TV (mL)	491 (337–542)	530 (414–590)	0.001
C_{dyn} (mL/cmH_2O)	41 (21–46)	49 (24–65)	< 0.001
Respiratory rate (min^{-1})	24 (18–26)	22 (16–26)	0.062
P_aCO_2	36.7 (32.6–46.4)	37.0 (32.7–41.2)	0.115

OI oxygenation index, *TV* tidal volume, C_{dyn} dynamic respiratory system compliance, P_aCO_2 arterial partial pressure of carbon dioxide

Table 6 Parameters of hemodynamic monitoring before and after paracentesis

Hemodynamic parameters assessed by transpulmonary thermodilution			
	Before paracentesis	After paracentesis	*p* value
	Median (IQR)	Median (IQR)	
MAP (mmHg)	82 (76–91)	79 (74–91)	0.134
CI (L/min/m^2)	4.5 (3.8–6.5)	5.0 (3.8–6.6)	0.522
CO (L/min)	8.9 (7.5–13.1)	10.3 (7.3–13.4)	0.579
GEDVI (mL/m^2)	880 (788–1021)	902 (758–1021)	0.437
EVLWI (mL/kg)	12 (9.5–15)	12 (9.5–14.5)	0.918
SVRI (dyn * s * cm^{-5} * m^{-2})	978 (725–1254)	1064 (713–1236)	0.772
CVP (mmHg)	22.5 (17.8–29.0)	17.5 (12.8–24)	0.001

CI cardiac index, *CO* cardiac output, *GEDVI* global end-diastolic volume index, *EVLWI* extravascular lung water index, *SVRI* systemic vascular resistance index, *CVP* central venous pressure

between ICG-PDR and standard laboratory liver tests [25].

The improvement in ICG-PDR is in parallel with a decline of IAP after evacuation of ascites. Correlation analyses revealed a statistically significant association of changes in ICG-PDR with changes in IAP. Previously, a few studies described a relationship between ICG-PDR and IAP. Some of them focused on the effect of prone positioning on IAP and ICG-PDR in patients with respiratory failure [22, 40, 41]. Two studies characterized the inverse correlation of ICG-PDR with the dimension of IAP in critically ill patients [24, 25]. Sakka presented a case of abdominal compartment syndrome with impaired ICG-PDR and a significant increase after surgical relief [42]. Not less interesting is another report from the same author describing the beneficial effect of paracentesis on ICG-PDR in a woman with ascites due to chronic heart failure; while IAP dropped from 18 to 12 mmHg, ICG-PDR rose from 11.6 to 15.6%/min [23]. The basic rationale behind all these findings seems to be that IAH compromises APP and consecutively restrains hepatosplanchnic blood flow and sinusoidal perfusion [25]. According to this, decompression of abdomen with a decrease in IAP improves hepatic blood flow and increases ICG-PDR [23].

The results of our study reaffirmed previous trials concerning a significant and immediate drop of IAP after LVP in patients with decompensated cirrhosis and tense ascites [27, 30, 43]. The relief of IAH is paralleled by a significant raise of APP, suggesting a substantial effect on hepatic perfusion. In the present study, we used color-coded duplex sonography for analyses of liver blood flow. At baseline, we found an elevated hepatic artery resistance index. This observation is in line with former ultrasound examinations showing increased resistance index in case of advanced liver fibrosis and cirrhosis [15, 44–46]. The alterations of intrahepatic circulation in cirrhosis with endothelial dysfunction and increased vasoconstrictor activity are well established [13, 47]. We recognized a significant decrease in hepatic artery resistance index after LVP, mainly referable to a change in diastolic blood flow. The hypothesis behind this finding is that LVP reduces hepatic vascular resistance and enhances sinusoidal perfusion. Moreover, sonography revealed a raise in maximum blood flow velocity in hepatic vein after LVP. Damping of hepatic venous waveform is a frequent observation in advanced cirrhosis, but the significance of blood flow velocity in hepatic vein alone is not investigated so far [14, 48]. In contrast, there was no relevant change of portal vein flow after paracentesis, indicating an obvious portal hypertension in the studied population with advanced liver cirrhosis.

Considered as secondary endpoints of this study, we analyzed the impact of LVP on respiratory and circulatory function in case of decompensated cirrhosis. We registered an overall beneficial effect on parameters of oxygenation and ventilation. Several studies underlined that respiratory improvement was particularly attributable to decreases in IAP, enhanced ventilatory mechanics with increased compliance as well as alveolar recruitment with increased end-expiratory lung volume [43, 49–51]. Concerning hemodynamic function, previous studies yielded diverging results about the existing threat of paracentesis-induced cardiocirculatory dysfunction [52–54]. Nevertheless, a recent study demonstrated that LVP did not impair hemodynamic parameters assessed by transpulmonary thermodilution [43]. Our analyses via transpulmonary thermodilution reconfirmed this favorable situation with steady parameters of hemodynamic function after LVP. However, we noticed a significant decrease in central venous pressure after LVP, most probably due to the decrease in IAP and therefore extra-thoracic pressure level. In line with this, we found a significant association of changes in IAP with changes in central venous pressure.

Altogether, the present study emphasizes the inverse correlation of ICG-PDR with IAP and the far-reaching effects of IAH in critically ill patients with decompensated cirrhosis. Hydropic decompensation evokes harmful increases of IAP with negative effects on abdominal perfusion and liver blood flow. LVP immediately lowers IAP in combination with an increase in ICG-PDR. According to ultrasound examination, this beneficial effect on ICG-PDR is mainly referable to improved arterial liver perfusion and decreased hepatic vascular resistance. By implication, our study to some extent questions the significance of ICG-PDR for an exclusive evaluation of hepatocellular function in case of IAH.

Strengths and limitations

To our knowledge, this is the first study evaluating the effects of LVP on ICG-PDR in a characterized population of critically ill patients with decompensated cirrhosis and tense ascites. The study combines ICG-PDR with assessments of IAP and APP, ultrasound examinations as well as respiratory and advanced hemodynamic monitoring. Despite the overall modest beneficial effect of paracentesis on ICG-PDR, the results are conclusive with high levels of statistical significance.

However, this is a single-center study with consecutively a very limited number of patients. Paracentesis was performed with a maximum release of mobilizable ascites instead of a stepwise release of predefined fluid amounts. Therefore, our data allowed only the calculation of an "overall" abdominal compliance with limited validity considering its evolution during progressive, stepwise evacuation of ascites [32]. Moreover, this study provides no further information about a possible influence of LVP on kidney function. In light of highly frequently occurring hepatorenal syndrome in case of decompensated liver cirrhosis, further studies would be interesting to investigate the impact of paracentesis on renal perfusion. In consideration of a relatively high baseline EVLWI in our patients, hemodynamic monitoring via transpulmonary thermodilution would have been even more accurate when performed with a higher saline bolus [55]. Ultrasound examinations via color-coded duplex sonography are operator-dependent and were performed only by one physician. Beside ICG-PDR, reliable data on additional parameters CBI and BVI provided by LiMON technology are rare.

Conclusion

Decompensated cirrhosis is associated with a marked decrease of dynamic liver test ICG-PDR, reflecting reduced hepatocellular capacity as well as impaired hepatosplanchnic blood flow. LVP evokes a modest but significant improvement in ICG-PDR, primarily referable to a decline in IAP and an inverse increase in APP. While conventional laboratory parameters of liver function did not change, the increase in ICG-PDR is mainly attributable to changes in hepatic perfusion.

Moreover, LVP induced substantial improvement in respiratory parameters, while hemodynamic profiles remained stable.

Abbreviations

IAH: intraabdominal hypertension; IAP: intraabdominal pressure; INR: international normalized ratio; ICG: indo-cyanine green; PDR: plasma disappearance rate; APP: abdominal perfusion pressure; MAP: mean arterial pressure; LVP: large-volume paracentesis; ICU: intensive care unit; BVI: circulating blood volume index; CBI: "ICG-Clearance"; WSACS: The Abdominal Compartment Society; CVP: central venous pressure; ARDS: acute respiratory distress syndrome; PEEP: positive end-expiratory pressure; TV: tidal volume; C_{dyn}: dynamic respiratory system compliance; F_iO_2: fraction of inspired oxygen; P_aO_2: arterial partial pressure of oxygen; P_aCO_2: arterial partial pressure of carbon dioxide; OI: oxygenation Index; APACHE: acute and physiology chronic health evaluation; SOFA: sequential organ failure assessment; MELD: model of end-stage liver disease; IQR: interquartile range; HARI: hepatic artery resistance index; HAF: maximum hepatic arterial flow; PVF: maximum portal vein flow; HVF: maximum hepatic vein flow; CI: cardiac index; CO: cardiac output; GEDVI: global end-diastolic volume index; EVLWI: extravascular lung water index; SVRI: systemic vascular resistance index.

Authors' contributions

UM, WH and TL designed the study. UM, LF and TL collected data, performed statistical analysis and drafted the manuscript. GB, AH, SR and RS also collected data, participated in the analysis of the data and helped to draft the manuscript. All authors read and approved the final manuscript.

Acknowledgements
None.

Competing interests
Wolfgang Huber collaborates with Pulsion Medical Systems SE, Feldkirchen, Germany, as member of the Medical Advisory Board. All other authors have no competing interests to disclose.

Funding
Funding was provided by Pulsion Medical Systems SE, Feldkirchen, Germany.

References

1. Gines P, Quintero E, Arroyo V, Teres J, Bruguera M, Rimola A, et al. Compensated cirrhosis: natural history and prognostic factors. Hepatology. 1987;7(1):122–8.
2. Bernardi M, Moreau R, Angeli P, Schnabl B, Arroyo V. Mechanisms of decompensation and organ failure in cirrhosis: from peripheral arterial vasodilation to systemic inflammation hypothesis. J Hepatol. 2015;63(5):1272–84. https://doi.org/10.1016/j.jhep.2015.07.004.
3. Malbrain ML, Chiumello D, Pelosi P, Bihari D, Innes R, Ranieri VM, et al. Incidence and prognosis of intraabdominal hypertension in a mixed population of critically ill patients: a multiple-center epidemiological study. Crit Care Med. 2005;33(2):315–22.
4. Malbrain ML, Chiumello D, Pelosi P, Wilmer A, Brienza N, Malcangi V, et al. Prevalence of intra-abdominal hypertension in critically ill patients: a multicentre epidemiological study. Intensive Care Med. 2004;30(5):822–9. https://doi.org/10.1007/s00134-004-2169-9.
5. Rouby JJ, Constantin JM, De Roberto AGC, Zhang M, Lu Q. Mechanical ventilation in patients with acute respiratory distress syndrome. Anesthesiology. 2004;101(1):228–34.
6. Barnes GE, Laine GA, Giam PY, Smith EE, Granger HJ. Cardiovascular responses to elevation of intra-abdominal hydrostatic pressure. Am J Physiol. 1985;248(2 Pt 2):R208–13.
7. Malbrain ML, Cheatham ML, Kirkpatrick A, Sugrue M, Parr M, De Waele J, et al. Results from the international conference of experts on intra-abdominal hypertension and abdominal compartment syndrome. I. Definitions. Intensive Care Med. 2006;32(11):1722–32. https://doi.org/10.1007/s00134-006-0349-5.
8. von Delius S, Karagianni A, Henke J, Preissel A, Meining A, Frimberger E, et al. Changes in intra-abdominal pressure, hemodynamics, and peak inspiratory pressure during gastroscopy in a porcine model. Endoscopy. 2007;39(11):962–8. https://doi.org/10.1055/s-2007-966973.
9. Malbrain ML, Deeren D, De Potter TJ. Intra-abdominal hypertension in the critically ill: it is time to pay attention. Curr Opin Crit Care. 2005;11(2):156–71.
10. Cresswell AB, Wendon JA. Hepatic function and non-invasive hepatosplanchnic monitoring in patients with abdominal hypertension. Acta Clin Belg. 2007;62(Suppl 1):113–8.
11. Bosch J. Vascular deterioration in cirrhosis: the big picture. J Clin Gastroenterol. 2007;41(Suppl 3):S247–53. https://doi.org/10.1097/MCG.0b013e3181572357.
12. Iwakiri Y, Groszmann RJ. The hyperdynamic circulation of chronic liver diseases: from the patient to the molecule. Hepatology. 2006;43(2 Suppl 1):S121–31. https://doi.org/10.1002/hep.20993.
13. Iwakiri Y. Pathophysiology of portal hypertension. Clin Liver Dis. 2014;18(2):281–91. https://doi.org/10.1016/j.cld.2013.12.001.
14. Scheinfeld MH, Bilali A, Koenigsberg M. Understanding the spectral Doppler waveform of the hepatic veins in health and disease. Radiographics. 2009;29(7):2081–98. https://doi.org/10.1148/rg.297095715.
15. Zekanovic D, Ljubicic N, Boban M, Nikolic M, Delic-Brkljacic D, Gacina P, et al. Doppler ultrasound of hepatic and system hemodynamics in patients with alcoholic liver cirrhosis. Dig Dis Sci. 2010;55(2):458–66. https://doi.org/10.1007/s10620-009-0760-1.
16. Zwiebel WJ. Sonographic diagnosis of hepatic vascular disorders. Semin Ultrasound CT MRI. 1995;16(1):34–48.
17. Sakka SG. Assessing liver function. Curr Opin Crit Care. 2007;13(2):207–14. https://doi.org/10.1097/MCC.0b013e328012b268.
18. Sakka SG, Klein M, Reinhart K, Meier-Hellmann A. Prognostic value of extravascular lung water in critically ill patients. Chest. 2002;122(6):2080–6.
19. Stehr A, Ploner F, Traeger K, Theisen M, Zuelke C, Radermacher P, et al. Plasma disappearance of indocyanine green: a marker for excretory liver function? Intensive Care Med. 2005;31(12):1719–22. https://doi.org/10.1007/s00134-005-2826-7.
20. Faybik P, Hetz H. Plasma disappearance rate of indocyanine green in liver dysfunction. Transplant Proc. 2006;38(3):801–2. https://doi.org/10.1016/j.transproceed.2006.01.049.
21. Seibel A, Muller A, Sakka SG. Indocyanine green plasma disappearance rate for monitoring hepatosplanchnic blood flow. Intensive Care Med. 2011;37(2):357–9. https://doi.org/10.1007/s00134-010-2063-6.
22. Michelet P, Roch A, Gainnier M, Sainty JM, Auffray JP, Papazian L. Influence of support on intra-abdominal pressure, hepatic kinetics of indocyanine green and extravascular lung water during prone positioning in patients with ARDS: a randomized crossover study. Crit Care. 2005;9(3):R251–7. https://doi.org/10.1186/cc3513.
23. Sakka SG. Indocyanine green plasma disappearance rate during relief of increased abdominal pressure. Intensive Care Med. 2006;32(12):2090–1. https://doi.org/10.1007/s00134-006-0411-3.
24. Inal MT, Memis D, Sezer YA, Atalay M, Karakoc A, Sut N. Effects of intra-abdominal pressure on liver function assessed with the LiMON in critically ill patients. Can J Surg. 2011;54(3):161–6. https://doi.org/10.1503/cjs.042709.
25. Malbrain ML, Viaene D, Kortgen A, De Laet I, Dits H, Van Regenmortel N, et al. Relationship between intra-abdominal pressure and indocyanine green plasma disappearance rate: hepatic perfusion may be impaired in critically ill patients with intra-abdominal hypertension. Ann Intensive Care. 2012;2(Suppl 1):S19. https://doi.org/10.1186/2110-5820-2-S1-S19.
26. Zipprich A, Kuss O, Rogowski S, Kleber G, Lotterer E, Seufferlein T, et al. Incorporating indocyanin green clearance into the Model for End Stage Liver Disease (MELD-ICG) improves prognostic accuracy in intermediate to advanced cirrhosis. Gut. 2010;59(7):963–8. https://doi.org/10.1136/gut.2010.208595.
27. Cheatham ML. Nonoperative management of intraabdominal hypertension and abdominal compartment syndrome. World J Surg. 2009;33(6):1116–22. https://doi.org/10.1007/s00268-009-0003-9.
28. Sakka SG, Reinhart K, Meier-Hellmann A. Comparison of invasive and noninvasive measurements of indocyanine green plasma disappearance rate in critically ill patients with mechanical ventilation and stable hemodynamics. Intensive Care Med. 2000;26(10):1553–6.
29. Umgelter A, Reindl W, Wagner KS, Franzen M, Stock K, Schmid RM, et al. Effects of plasma expansion with albumin and paracentesis on haemodynamics and kidney function in critically ill cirrhotic patients with tense ascites and hepatorenal syndrome: a prospective uncontrolled trial. Crit Care. 2008;12(1):R4. https://doi.org/10.1186/cc6765.
30. Malbrain ML. Different techniques to measure intra-abdominal pressure (IAP): time for a critical re-appraisal. Intensive Care Med. 2004;30(3):357–71. https://doi.org/10.1007/s00134-003-2107-2.
31. Kirkpatrick AW, Roberts DJ, De Waele J, Jaeschke R, Malbrain ML, De Keulenaer B, et al. Intra-abdominal hypertension and the abdominal compartment syndrome: updated consensus definitions and clinical practice guidelines from the World Society of the Abdominal Compartment Syndrome. Intensive Care Med. 2013;39(7):1190–206. https://doi.org/10.1007/s00134-013-2906-z.
32. Malbrain ML, Peeters Y, Wise R. The neglected role of abdominal compliance in organ–organ interactions. Crit Care. 2016;20:67. https://doi.org/10.1186/s13054-016-1220-x
33. Gines A, Fernandez-Esparrach G, Monescillo A, Vila C, Domenech E, Abecasis R, et al. Randomized trial comparing albumin, dextran 70, and polygeline in cirrhotic patients with ascites treated by paracentesis. Gastroenterology. 1996;111(4):1002–10.
34. Bein T, Grasso S, Moerer O, Quintel M, Guerin C, Deja M, et al. The standard of care of patients with ARDS: ventilatory settings and rescue therapies for refractory hypoxemia. Intensive Care Med. 2016;42(5):699–711. https://doi.org/10.1007/s00134-016-4325-4.
35. Bone RC, Maunder R, Slotman G, Silverman H, Hyers TM, Kerstein MD, et al. An early test of survival in patients with the adult respiratory distress syndrome. The P_aO_2/F_iO_2 ratio and its differential response to conventional therapy. Prostaglandin E1 Study Group. Chest. 1989;96(4):849–51.

36. Huber W, Umgelter A, Reindl W, Franzen M, Schmidt C, von Delius S, et al. Volume assessment in patients with necrotizing pancreatitis: a comparison of intrathoracic blood volume index, central venous pressure, and hematocrit, and their correlation to cardiac index and extravascular lung water index. Crit Care Med. 2008;36(8):2348–54. https://doi.org/10.1097/CCM.0b013e3181809928.
37. Hemming AW, Scudamore CH, Shackleton CR, Pudek M, Erb SR. Indocyanine green clearance as a predictor of successful hepatic resection in cirrhotic patients. Am J Surg. 1992;163(5):515–8.
38. Scheingraber S, Richter S, Igna D, Flesch S, Kopp B, Schilling MK. Indocyanine green disappearance rate is the most useful marker for liver resection. Hepatogastroenterology. 2008;55(85):1394–9.
39. Inal MT, Memis D, Kargi M, Sut N. Prognostic value of indocyanine green elimination assessed with LiMON in septic patients. J Crit Care. 2009;24(3):329–34. https://doi.org/10.1016/j.jcrc.2008.11.012.
40. Hering R, Vorwerk R, Wrigge H, Zinserling J, Schroder S, von Spiegel T, et al. Prone positioning, systemic hemodynamics, hepatic indocyanine green kinetics, and gastric intramucosal energy balance in patients with acute lung injury. Intensive Care Med. 2002;28(1):53–8. https://doi.org/10.1007/s00134-001-1166-5.
41. Kirkpatrick AW, Pelosi P, De Waele JJ, Malbrain ML, Ball CG, Meade MO, et al. Clinical review: intra-abdominal hypertension: does it influence the physiology of prone ventilation? Crit Care. 2010;14(4):232. https://doi.org/10.1186/cc9099.
42. Sakka SG. Indocyanine green plasma disappearance rate as an indicator of hepato-splanchnic ischemia during abdominal compartment syndrome. Anesth Analg. 2007;104(4):1003–4. https://doi.org/10.1213/01.ane.0000256097.61730.cc.
43. Phillip V, Saugel B, Ernesti C, Hapfelmeier A, Schultheiss C, Thies P, et al. Effects of paracentesis on hemodynamic parameters and respiratory function in critically ill patients. BMC Gastroenterol. 2014;14:18. https://doi.org/10.1186/1471-230X-14-18.
44. Sacerdoti D, Merkel C, Bolognesi M, Amodio P, Angeli P, Gatta A. Hepatic arterial resistance in cirrhosis with and without portal vein thrombosis: relationships with portal hemodynamics. Gastroenterology. 1995;108(4):1152–8.
45. Lutz HH, Gassler N, Tischendorf FW, Trautwein C, Tischendorf JJ. Doppler ultrasound of hepatic blood flow for noninvasive evaluation of liver fibrosis compared with liver biopsy and transient elastography. Dig Dis Sci. 2012;57(8):2222–30. https://doi.org/10.1007/s10620-012-2153-0.
46. Glisic TM, Perisic MD, Dimitrijevic S, Jurisic V. Doppler assessment of splanchnic arterial flow in patients with liver cirrhosis: correlation with ammonia plasma levels and MELD score. J Clin Ultrasound. 2014;42(5):264–9. https://doi.org/10.1002/jcu.22135.
47. Gracia-Sancho J, Lavina B, Rodriguez-Vilarrupla A, Garcia-Caldero H, Bosch J, Garcia-Pagan JC. Enhanced vasoconstrictor prostanoid production by sinusoidal endothelial cells increases portal perfusion pressure in cirrhotic rat livers. J Hepatol. 2007;47(2):220–7. https://doi.org/10.1016/j.jhep.2007.03.014.
48. Kim MY, Baik SK, Park DH, Lim DW, Kim JW, Kim HS, et al. Damping index of Doppler hepatic vein waveform to assess the severity of portal hypertension and response to propranolol in liver cirrhosis: a prospective nonrandomized study. Liver Int. 2007;27(8):1103–10. https://doi.org/10.1111/j.1478-3231.2007.01526.x.
49. Levesque E, Hoti E, Jiabin J, Dellamonica J, Ichai P, Saliba F, et al. Respiratory impact of paracentesis in cirrhotic patients with acute lung injury. J Crit Care. 2011;26(3):257–61. https://doi.org/10.1016/j.jcrc.2010.08.020.
50. Byrd RP Jr, Roy TM, Simons M. Improvement in oxygenation after large volume paracentesis. South Med J. 1996;89(7):689–92.
51. Wauters J, Claus P, Brosens N, McLaughlin M, Hermans G, Malbrain M, et al. Relationship between abdominal pressure, pulmonary compliance, and cardiac preload in a porcine model. Crit Care Res Pract. 2012;2012:763181. https://doi.org/10.1155/2012/763181.
52. Cabrera J, Falcon L, Gorriz E, Pardo MD, Granados R, Quinones A, et al. Abdominal decompression plays a major role in early postparacentesis haemodynamic changes in cirrhotic patients with tense ascites. Gut. 2001;48(3):384–9.
53. Nasr G, Hassan A, Ahmed S, Serwah A. Predictors of large volume paracantesis induced circulatory dysfunction in patients with massive hepatic ascites. J Cardiovasc Dis Res. 2010;1(3):136–44. https://doi.org/10.4103/0975-3583.70914
54. Peltekian KM, Wong F, Liu PP, Logan AG, Sherman M, Blendis LM. Cardiovascular, renal, and neurohumoral responses to single large-volume paracentesis in patients with cirrhosis and diuretic-resistant ascites. Am J Gastroenterol. 1997;92(3):394–9.
55. Hofkens PJ, Verrijcken A, Merveille K, Neirynck S, Van Regenmortel N, De Laet I, et al. Common pitfalls and tips and tricks to get the most out of your transpulmonary thermodilution device: results of a survey and state-of-the-art review. Anaesthesiol Intensive Ther. 2015;47(2):89–116. https://doi.org/10.5603/AIT.a2014.0068.

8

Renal failure in critically ill patients, beware of applying (central venous) pressure on the kidney

Xiukai Chen[1*], Xiaoting Wang[2], Patrick M. Honore[3], Herbert D. Spapen[4] and Dawei Liu[2*]

Abstract

The central venous pressure (CVP) is traditionally used as a surrogate of intravascular volume. CVP measurements therefore are often applied at the bedside to guide fluid administration in postoperative and critically ill patients. Pursuing high CVP levels has recently been challenged. A high CVP might impede venous return to the heart and disturb microcirculatory blood flow which may cause tissue congestion and organ failure. By imposing an increased "afterload" on the kidney, an elevated CVP will particularly harm kidney hemodynamics and promote acute kidney injury (AKI) even in the absence of volume overload. Maintaining the lowest possible CVP should become routine to prevent and treat AKI, especially when associated with septic shock, cardiac surgery, mechanical ventilation, and intra-abdominal hypertension.

Keywords: Acute kidney injury, Central venous pressure, Afterload

Background

Acute kidney injury (AKI) is a common complication in critically ill patients with high attributable morbidity and mortality [1, 2]. Systemic and renal perfusion considerably determines the development and course of AKI. Yet, optimal hemodynamic targets to minimize the risk of AKI are not precisely defined [3, 4]. In critical care, hypotension and shock are the "rogue enemies." Resuscitation primarily focuses on optimizing mean arterial pressure (MAP) to improve renal perfusion [5]. However, there is little evidence that MAP correctly reflects organ perfusion. Moreover, aggressive fluid loading may contribute to an increased central venous pressure (CVP). By accepting high CVP levels [6–10], clinicians neglect that volume treatment and AKI are closely intertwined.

CVP is traditionally used for assessing volume status and volume responsiveness at the bedside [11]. However, CVP measurements to direct volume management in critically ill patients have repeatedly been found unreliable [12]. Whether and how CVP monitoring should be adapted to a particular patient (e.g., postsurgical, cardiac, septic) population is topic of controversy and debate [13, 14]. Monitoring CVP also does not guarantee preservation of renal function. A recent study reported a higher incidence of AKI in patients undergoing CVP monitoring as compared with unmonitored subjects. A 1 cm H_2O higher CVP was associated with a 1.02 (95% CI 1.00–1.03, $p=0.02$) risk of AKI. No association was found between pulmonary edema and AKI [13]. Till recently, the innate pressure character of CVP and its pathophysiological impact have been largely underestimated. What follows is a thorough discussion about the role of CVP, beyond its value as volume indicator, in various diseases.

Main text

CVP is a pressure used to estimate volume

The CVP is the pressure recorded from the superior vena cava or right atrium which, in the absence of tricuspid stenosis, equals right ventricular end-diastolic pressure. CVP is determined by the interaction between cardiac function and venous return which both depend

*Correspondence: xic91@pitt.edu; dwliu98@163.com
[1] Pittsburgh Heart, Lung, Blood and Vascular Medicine Institute, University of Pittsburgh, 200 Lothrop Street, BST E1240, Pittsburgh, PA 15261, USA
[2] Department of Critical Care Medicine, Peking Union Medical College Hospital, Peking Union Medical College, Chinese Academy of Medical Sciences, 1 Shuaifuyuan, Dongcheng District, Beijing 100073, China
Full list of author information is available at the end of the article

on changes in total blood volume, vascular tone, cardiac output (CO), right ventricular compliance, intrathoracic and pericardial pressure [15]. CVP measurements are especially useful when followed over time and combined with a CO recording. A properly measured CVP can successfully guide right ventricular filling [16]. Within a certain range, CVP increases with expanding blood volume. However, excessive fluid administration may augment CVP and end-diastolic pressure without increasing end-diastolic or stroke volume. On the other hand, an increased CVP is often associated with decreased right ventricular compliance. Additionally, CVP is the downstream pressure for venous return and close to the minimum pressure in the global circulation [17].

CVP and kidney "afterload"

CVP must be lower than renal venous pressure (RVP) in order to allow an adequate venous renal blood flow (RBF) to the heart. Accordingly, the presence of a high CVP requires a much higher RVP to ensure this flow. Renal perfusion pressure (RPP) approximates the difference between renal arterial pressure and RVP. As such, a higher RVP lowers RPP. In analogy with cardiac physiology, this forms the basis for the renal "afterload" concept [18]. Recent studies focusing on kidney "afterload" have revived interest in older studies which suggested that kidney dysfunction resulted from venous congestion transmitted to the renal venous compartment. Almost a century ago, it was indeed demonstrated that an hypervolemia-induced increase in RVP caused AKI independently of CO or RBF [19].

Effect of CVP on pressure and flow in the kidney

Kidney perfusion is pressure and flow dependent. If intravascular volume augments without excessive CVP elevation, the unstressed volume (i.e., the fluid volume to fill the vascular bed to the point where it exerts force on the vessel walls) may incrementally follow a CO increase and RBF will rise. When CVP is already high, however, any additional volume load may increase CVP without a subsequent increase in CO and RBF. Right ventricular function then may deteriorate and evolve into acute cor pulmonale [17]. The difference between mean system filling pressure (MSFP) and CVP is the driving force behind venous return. Thus, with increasing CVP, a venous return will drop [20, 21]. With the heart functioning on the steep portion of the Starling curve, volume expansion will increase MSFP more than CVP. In contrast, changes in MSFP are approximately similar to CVP changes on the flat part of the Starling curve with no or minimal effects on CO [22, 23]. If fluid administration fails to obtain a higher MSFP, CVP must be kept low to enhance venous return, cardiac preload and CO. In isolated kidneys of healthy dogs, renal venous and tissue pressures were unaffected over a large range of increased venous pressures. However, RBF fell when RVP approached or exceeded renal venous and tissue pressure [24]. Critically ill patients even have a more narrow pressure autoregulation range [25]. In the cardiorenal syndrome, an elevated CVP causes lowering of RPP below the kidney autoregulation threshold, resulting in pressure-dependent renal perfusion [26]. The rise in CVP is transmitted to the renal veins, sustains the cardiorenal syndrome, and induces a detrimental feedback loop via the renin–angiotensin–aldosterone and neuroendocrine pathways that leads to refractory heart failure. Worsening congestion also enhances sodium retention which exacerbates heart failure.

CVP can be more than a volume "indicator"

Many studies report a weak relationship between CVP and blood volume. CVP itself or changes in CVP evolution over time also failed to predict the hemodynamic response to a fluid challenge or to correctly estimate cardiac filling. As a result, it was suggested to abandon CVP to guide fluid resuscitation in critically ill patients [11, 27]. However, a more thorough understanding of various parameters and variables (i.e., preload, measurements in fluid-filled systems, impact of respiration, physiological determinants of CVP, and the point on the tracing that best estimates cardiac preload) may revalue CVP as a reproducible indicator of cardiac preload [16]. This is best illustrated by looking at the relationship between CVP and AKI in cardiac disease and sepsis.

Heart failure and cardiorenal syndrome

Since pressure/volume relationships are largely determined by heart compliance, a high CVP indicates volume overload, cardiac dysfunction, or both [28, 29]. Traditionally, AKI in congestive heart failure or cardiorenal syndrome is attributed to a reduction in CO and MAP which elicits a series of neurohumoral events resulting in increased renal vascular resistance and decreased renal function [30]. The degree of AKI is closely associated with congestive venous "backward failure." In 2557 patients who underwent right heart catheterization, Damman et al. found that an increased CVP was not only associated with impaired renal function but also independently related to all-cause mortality [31]. A study in patients with advanced decompensated heart failure showed that those with worsening renal function had a higher CVP on admission and after intensive medical therapy [32]. Worsening renal function occurred less frequently in patients in whom CVP was kept below 8 mmHg. An apparent potential of CVP for AKI risk stratification was noted across the spectrum of systemic blood pressure, pulmonary capillary wedge pressure, cardiac index, and estimated glomerular filtration rate [32]. In adults with chronic heart disease after biventricular repair, Ohuchi et al. found that a high CVP predicted kidney enlargement and abnormal intrarenal flow dynamics that were closely associated with severity of heart failure and with cardiovascular events [33]. Right ventricular dysfunction and increased CVP are frequently observed in cardiac surgery patients and may lead to congestive renal dysfunction [34]. Studies in patients with acute right ventricular failure suggest that a high CVP is associated with a marked reduction in RBF by increasing renal backward pressure [35, 36]. A strong relationship was observed between CVP and RBF in both acute and chronic heart failure. Reducing CVP markedly improved renal function [35]. Cardiovascular surgery patients with progressive AKI had greater diastolic perfusion pressure deficits as compared to patients without AKI progression. Almost 25% of the diastolic perfusion pressure deficit was due to an increase in CVP [36]. This underscores the strong relationship between back (renal venous) pressure and CVP in the development of AKI.

Taken together, more attention must be paid to the pressure effect of CVP in heart failure/cardiorenal syndrome, regardless of whether fluid overload is present or not.

Sepsis and septic shock

Based on the landmark article of Rivers et al. which highlighted a striking mortality benefit of early goal-directed therapy (EGDT) in severe sepsis and septic shock [37], the Surviving Sepsis Campaign guidelines endorsed a CVP of 8–12 mmHg (12–15 mmHg in mechanically ventilated patients) as a key resuscitation target [38]. However, fluid load after 72 h in the Rivers study was equally high (approximately 13.5 L) in the EGDT and control arm. A major drawback of the study was the lack of data on occurrence and incidence of AKI. Recently, EGDT was assessed in the multicenter ProCESS [39, 40], ARISE [41], and ProMISE [42] trials which all used a CVP target ≥ 8 mmHg for guiding fluid resuscitation. The results of these trials, while reporting an all-time low sepsis mortality, question the need to use all elements of EGDT or the need for protocolized care in general. Limited data suggest that EGDT does not improve incidence of AKI and outcome of patients with AKI [43]. A CVP >8 mmHg decreased microcirculatory and renal blood flow and increased AKI and mortality risk [44]. After adjustment for fluid balance and positive end-expiratory pressure ventilation, a lower diastolic arterial pressure and an elevated CVP were found to correlate with a high AKI incidence in septic patients [45–48].

Overzealous fluid treatment may result in interstitial edema which may worsen AKI or hamper renal recovery [49]. This underscores the potential role of venous congestion as one of the factors potentially implicated in the pathogenesis of septic AKI. CVP-directed fluid resuscitation in septic shock might harm the kidney if the target point is not correctly determined. Consequently, conservative fluid management [44] and permissive hypofiltration ("unburdening" the kidney by providing early renal replacement therapy, avoiding new injurious events such as fluid overload, and initiating therapies to improve survival and avoid ongoing loss of kidney function) [50, 51] are emerging treatment options in septic AKI. CVP should play a "limiting" rather than a target role within fluid resuscitation protocols [52]. Chen et al. found that early goal-directed diuretic therapy can improve the prognosis of sepsis [53]. In 105 patients with septic shock, Wang et al. showed that CVP was associated with kidney, liver, and lung function, sequential organ failure assessment scores, and lactate. Patients whose CVP remained below 8 mmHg during 7 days had a higher survival rate [54]. However, hypovolemia and renal hypoperfusion may occur in AKI patients if a too excessive fluid removal is pursued with diuretics or extracorporeal therapy [55].

Taken together, CVP plays an important role in the development of septic AKI by actively sustaining renal venous congestion and enhancing sepsis-related tissue edema.

A high CVP should be avoided

Healthy persons have a low CVP [56]. A high CVP does not always signify fluid overload, yet may impede RBF return to the right atrium and increase the risk of AKI. Ventricular preload is determined by transmural pressure, which is the difference between intracardiac and extracardiac intrathoracic pressure. Changes in right or left ventricular compliance, pulmonary hypertension, pulmonary venous disease, chronic airway disease, positive pressure ventilation, cardiac tamponade, pleural effusion, and increased intra-abdominal pressure all can increase intrathoracic or pericardial pressure [57] and thus augment CVP, decrease venous return, and potentially injure the kidney. Any elevation or significant change in CVP may refer to either presence or severity of a particular disease process and its response to treatment (Fig. 1).

Intra-abdominal hypertension

Intra-abdominal hypertension is defined as an intra-abdominal pressure exceeding 1.6 kPa. Abdominal compartment syndrome is diagnosed when the intra-abdominal pressure persists above 2.7 kPa in association with new organ dysfunction or failure. Various diseases

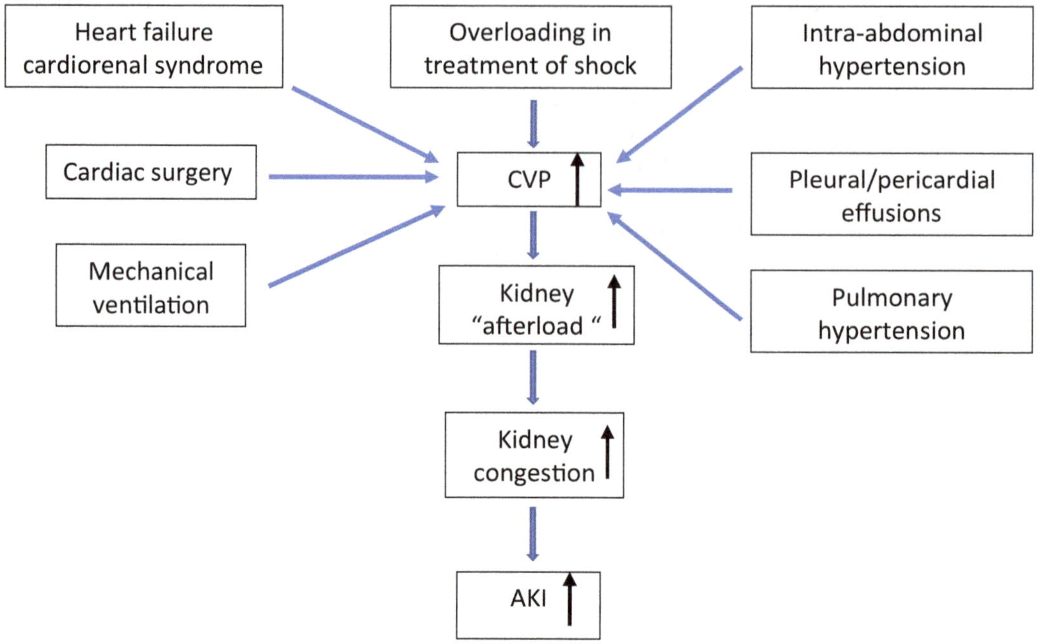

Fig. 1 Relationship of all-caused high CVP and AKI. *CVP* central venous pressure, *AKI* acute kidney injury

or conditions (e.g., pancreatitis, bile peritonitis, intra-abdominal hemorrhage, large abdominal masses, blunt abdominal trauma, recent abdominal surgery, ...) but also ample fluid resuscitation may cause abdominal hypertension and abdominal compartment syndrome [58–61]. Sepsis is an important trigger of AKI in postoperative and trauma patients with intra-abdominal hypertension [62]. AKI related to high intra-abdominal pressure is mainly due to an increase in inferior vena cava and intrathoracic pressure resulting in CVP elevation. A close relationship exists between an increased intra-abdominal pressure and the presence of oliguria and a high serum creatinine. The impact of diuretics on CVP and recovery of renal function is limited. However, lowering intra-abdominal pressure decreased CVP, restored diuresis, and normalized serum creatinine levels [61]. In a swine model, elevated intra-abdominal pressure increased renal venous, pleural, wedge, and pulmonary artery pressures, whereas cardiac index and urine output decreased. Intravascular volume expansion significantly increased urine output [63]. Decreasing intra-abdominal pressure to offer more space for volume expansion may be the best option to lower CVP.

Cardiac surgery

The CVP recorded 6 h after elective or urgent coronary artery bypass grafting was a strong and independent predictor of mortality and AKI [64]. The risk-adjusted OR for AKI was 5.5 (95% CI 1.93, 15.5; $p=0.001$) with every 5 mmHg rise in CVP for patients with a CVP < 9 mmHg. For patients with a CVP ≥ 9 mmHg at 6 h, risk-adjusted OR was 1.3 (95% CI 1.01, 1.65; $p=0.045$) with every 5 mmHg rise in CVP [64]. Guinot et al. observed that renal dysfunction in cardiac surgery patients was associated with early postoperative vena cava dilatation and elevated CVP, secondary to an increase in right heart filling pressure due to impaired right ventricular diastolic function [65].

Mechanical ventilation

Mechanical ventilation, especially when combined with high positive end-expiratory pressure (PEEP), prone positioning, and lung recruitment maneuvers, induces a high CVP [57, 66, 67]. Lung recruitment decreased renal arterial blood flow and perfusion of renal cortex and medulla in both healthy pigs and in pigs with endotoxin-induced pulmonary arterial hypertension [66, 67]. A balance must be sought between adequate blood volume, lowest CVP, and lowest intrathoracic pressure by carefully titrating PEEP under hemodynamic monitoring [68].

Specific conditions

Pleural and pericardial effusions are often associated with an increase in CVP. Pleural or pericardial puncture and drainage will reduce CVP. An increased CVP is a hallmark of diseases accompanied by pulmonary hypertension. Specific treatments (e.g., inhaled nitric oxide) can decrease pulmonary pressure and CVP, yet may increase

AKI risk [69]. The intrinsic response of renal vessels must thus always be weighed against the potential benefit of decreasing CVP when treating the primary disease.

The "optimal" CVP should be personalized and kept as low as possible

Currently, no exact definition of "lowest possible CVP" can be given except that it should be a CVP that assures adequate cardiac output and preserves organ perfusion. It becomes evident that a personalized approach is needed to aim at the most optimal CVP. In different patient populations or cohorts of similar patients with different disease stages, this optimal CVP level also will be different. A retrospective analysis of more than 500,000 CVP recordings in more than 9000 patients showed that the highest quartile of mean CVP during the first 3 days [mean (SD); 17.4 (4.1) mmHg] was associated with a 33.6% higher adjusted risk of death as compared with the lowest quartile [7.4 (1.9) mmHg]. Poor secondary outcomes (i.e., prolonged mechanical ventilation or vasopressor use, longer ICU and hospital stay) were also associated with higher quartiles of elevated mean CVP. Prolonged duration of CVP > 10 mmHg was significantly higher in non-survivors [70]. Keeping CVP and fluid in balance is more challenging in patients exhibiting a high CVP but no volume overload. In addition, extracting volume is not always the best way to decrease CVP. Overzealous use of diuretics or excessive ultrafiltration may indeed cause unwarranted volume loss resulting in lower cardiac preload, CO, and RBF. Strict and continuous monitoring of cardiac output, CVP, and kidney perfusion is imperative to avoid under- or over-treatment [71, 72]. Patients with acute heart failure and a CVP < 10 cm H2O were more likely to develop worsening renal function within the first 24 h than those presenting with a CVP > 15 cm H2O [73]. This does not imply that a higher CVP must be targeted in this population but rather that a volume "deficit" due to excessive fluid restriction or elimination should absolutely be avoided. Any decision to lower CVP should be individualized. Improving lung–right heart interactions that sustain an elevated CVP in heart failure and cardiorenal syndrome appears to be more efficacious than reducing intravascular volume [26, 30].

Conclusions

CVP is an innate pressure that is not only affected by manipulation of intravascular volume (fluid administration, restriction, or elimination) but also determined by various disease processes (intra-abdominal hypertension, pulmonary hypertension,...) or treatment (mechanical ventilation). Irrespective of volume status, an elevated CVP may harm the kidney by impeding renal venous return and causing renal interstitial edema. Individualizing CVP measurements and keeping CVP as low as possible should be encouraged to preserve kidney function or to avoid unnecessary renal damage.

Abbreviations

AKI: acute kidney injury; CVP: central venous pressure; MAP: mean arterial pressure; RVP: renal venous pressure; RPP: renal perfusion pressure; CO: cardiac output; RBF: renal blood flow; MSFP: mean system filling pressure; EGDT: early goal-directed therapy; PEEP: positive end-expiratory pressure.

Authors' contributions

XC performed the literature search and wrote the first draft of the paper. XW, PMH, HDS, and DL reviewed and contributed to the manuscript. All authors read and approved the final manuscript.

Author details

[1] Pittsburgh Heart, Lung, Blood and Vascular Medicine Institute, University of Pittsburgh, 200 Lothrop Street, BST E1240, Pittsburgh, PA 15261, USA. [2] Department of Critical Care Medicine, Peking Union Medical College Hospital, Peking Union Medical College, Chinese Academy of Medical Sciences, 1 Shuaifuyuan, Dongcheng District, Beijing 100073, China. [3] Department of Intensive Care, Centre Hospitalier Universitaire Brugmann, Brugmann University Hospital, 4 Place Van Gehuchtenplein, 1020 Brussels, Belgium. [4] Department of Intensive Care, University Hospital, Vrije Universiteit Brussel (VUB), 101, Laarbeeklaan, Jette 1090 Brussels, Belgium.

Acknowledgements

Thanks to Dr. Wenzhao Chai, Hongmin Zhang, Rongli Yang, Qing Zhang, and Suwei Li's help in the formatting of the idea. Thanks to Dr. John A. Kellum's comments. Thanks to Seth Morrisroe for draft editing.

Competing interests

The authors declare that they have no competing interests.

Funding

Not applicable.

References

1. Parmar A, Langenberg C, Wan L, May CN, Bellomo R, Bagshaw SM. Epidemiology of septic acute kidney injury. Curr Drug Targets. 2009;10(12):1169–78.
2. Kellum JA. Why are patients still getting and dying from acute kidney injury? Curr Opin Crit Care. 2016;22(6):513–9.
3. Matejovic M, Ince C, Chawla LS, Blantz R, Molitoris BA, Rosner MH, et al. Renal hemodynamics in AKI. In search of new treatment targets. J Am Soc Nephrol JASN. 2016;27(1):49–58.
4. Zhang H, Liu D, Wang X, Chen X, Zhang Q, Tang B, et al. Variations of renal vascular score and resistive indices in septic shock patients. Zhonghua Yi Xue Za Zhi. 2014;94(27):2102–5.
5. Badin J, Boulain T, Ehrmann S, Skarzynski M, Bretagnol A, Buret J, et al. Relation between mean arterial pressure and renal function in the early phase of shock: a prospective, explorative cohort study. Crit Care. 2011;15(3):R135.
6. Gambardella I, Gaudino M, Ronco C, Lau C, Ivascu N, Girardi LN. Congestive kidney failure in cardiac surgery: the relationship between central venous pressure and acute kidney injury. Interact Cardiovasc Thorac Surg. 2016;23(5):800–5.

7. Bagshaw SM, Delaney A, Jones D, Ronco C, Bellomo R. Diuretics in the management of acute kidney injury: a multinational survey. Contrib Nephrol. 2007;156:236–49.
8. Chuasuwan A, Kellum JA. Cardio-renal syndrome type 3: epidemiology, pathophysiology, and treatment. Semin Nephrol. 2012;32(1):31–9.
9. Jones SL, Martensson J, Glassford NJ, Eastwood GM, Bellomo R. Loop diuretic therapy in the critically ill: a survey. Crit Care Resusc. 2015;17(3):223–6.
10. Fiaccadori E. Fluid overload in acute kidney injury: an underestimated toxin? G Ital Nefrol. 2011;28(1):11.
11. Marik PE, Baram M, Vahid B. Does central venous pressure predict fluid responsiveness? A systematic review of the literature and the tale of seven mares. Chest. 2008;134(1):172–8.
12. Ho KM. Pitfalls in haemodynamic monitoring in the postoperative and critical care setting. Anaesth Intensive Care. 2016;44(1):14–9.
13. Chen KP, Cavender S, Lee J, Feng M, Mark RG, Celi LA, et al. Peripheral edema, central venous pressure, and risk of AKI in critical illness. Clin J Am Soc Nephrol. 2016;11(4):602–8.
14. Magder S, Bafaqeeh F. The clinical role of central venous pressure measurements. J Intensive Care Med. 2007;22(1):44–51.
15. Gelman S. Venous function and central venous pressure: a physiologic story. Anesthesiology. 2008;108(4):735–48.
16. Magder S. Understanding central venous pressure: not a preload index? Curr Opin Crit Care. 2015;21(5):369–75.
17. Magder S. Volume and its relationship to cardiac output and venous return. Crit Care. 2016;20:271.
18. Honore PM, Jacobs R, Hendrickx I, Bagshaw SM, Joannes-Boyau O, Boer W, et al. Prevention and treatment of sepsis-induced acute kidney injury: an update. Ann Intensive Care. 2015;5(1):51.
19. Winton FR. The influence of venous pressure on the isolated mammalian kidney. J Physiol. 1931;72(1):49–61.
20. Brengelmann GL. A critical analysis of the view that right atrial pressure determines venous return. J Appl Physiol. 2003;94(3):849–59.
21. Beard DA, Feigl EO. Understanding Guyton's venous return curves. Am J Physiol Heart Circ Physiol. 2011;301(3):H629–33.
22. Den Hartog EA, Versprille A, Jansen JR. Systemic filling pressure in intact circulation determined on basis of aortic vs. central venous pressure relationships. Am J Physiol. 1994;267(6 Pt 2):H2255–8.
23. Gupta K, Sondergaard S, Parkin G, Leaning M, Aneman A. Applying mean systemic filling pressure to assess the response to fluid boluses in cardiac post-surgical patients. Intensive Care Med. 2015;41(2):265–72.
24. Hinshaw LB, Brake CM, Iampietro PF, Emerson TE Jr. Effect of increased venous pressure on renal hemodynamics. Am J Physiol. 1963;204:119–23.
25. Burban M, Hamel JF, Tabka M, de La Bourdonnaye MR, Duveau A, Mercat A, et al. Renal macro- and microcirculation autoregulatory capacity during early sepsis and norepinephrine infusion in rats. Crit Care. 2013;17(4):R139.
26. Guazzi M, Gatto P, Giusti G, Pizzamiglio F, Previtali I, Vignati C, et al. Pathophysiology of cardiorenal syndrome in decompensated heart failure: role of lung-right heart-kidney interaction. Int J Cardiol. 2013;169(6):379–84.
27. Toyoda D, Fukuda M, Iwasaki R, Terada T, Sato N, Ochiai R, et al. The comparison between stroke volume variation and filling pressure as an estimate of right ventricular preload in patients undergoing renal transplantation. J Anesth. 2015;29(1):40–6.
28. Cui K, Wang X, Zhang H, Chai W, Liu D. The application of combined central venous pressure and oxygen metabolism parameters monitoring in diagnosing septic shock-induced left ventricular dysfunction. Zhonghua Nei Ke Za Zhi. 2015;54(10):855–9.
29. Zhang HM, Liu DW, Wang XT, Long Y, Shi Y, Chai WZ, et al. Correlation between pressure and volume parameters of septic shock patients with cardiac depression. Zhonghua Wai Ke Za Zhi [Chin J Surg]. 2010;48(3):201–4.
30. McCullough PA, Kellum JA, Haase M, Muller C, Damman K, Murray PT, et al. Pathophysiology of the cardiorenal syndromes: executive summary from the eleventh consensus conference of the acute dialysis quality initiative (ADQI). Contrib Nephrol. 2013;182:82–98.
31. Damman K, van Deursen VM, Navis G, Voors AA, van Veldhuisen DJ, Hillege HL. Increased central venous pressure is associated with impaired renal function and mortality in a broad spectrum of patients with cardiovascular disease. J Am Coll Cardiol. 2009;53(7):582–8.
32. Mullens W, Abrahams Z, Francis GS, Sokos G, Taylor DO, Starling RC, et al. Importance of venous congestion for worsening of renal function in advanced decompensated heart failure. J Am Coll Cardiol. 2009;53(7):589–96.
33. Ohuchi H, Ikado H, Noritake K, Miyazaki A, Yasuda K, Yamada O. Impact of central venous pressure on cardiorenal interactions in adult patients with congenital heart disease after biventricular repair. Congenit Heart Dis. 2013;8(2):103–10.
34. Romagnoli S, Ricci Z, Ronco C. Therapy of acute kidney injury in the perioperative setting. Curr Opin Anaesthesiol. 2017;30(1):92–9.
35. Mebazaa A. Congestion and cardiorenal syndromes. Contrib Nephrol. 2010;165:140–4.
36. Saito S, Uchino S, Takinami M, Uezono S, Bellomo R. Postoperative blood pressure deficit and acute kidney injury progression in vasopressor-dependent cardiovascular surgery patients. Crit Care. 2016;20:74.
37. Rivers E, Nguyen B, Havstad S, Ressler J, Muzzin A, Knoblich B, et al. Early goal-directed therapy in the treatment of severe sepsis and septic shock. N Engl J Med. 2001;345(19):1368–77.
38. Rhodes A, Evans LE, Alhazzani W, Levy MM, Antonelli M, Ferrer R, et al. Surviving sepsis campaign: international guidelines for management of sepsis and septic shock: 2016. Crit Care Med. 2017;45(3):486–552.
39. Pro CI, Yealy DM, Kellum JA, Huang DT, Barnato AE, Weissfeld LA, et al. A randomized trial of protocol-based care for early septic shock. N Engl J Med. 2014;370(18):1683–93.
40. Angus DC, Yealy DM, Kellum JA, Pro CI. Protocol-based care for early septic shock. N Engl J Med. 2014;371(4):386.
41. Investigators A, Group ACT, Peake SL, Delaney A, Bailey M, Bellomo R, et al. Goal-directed resuscitation for patients with early septic shock. N Engl J Med. 2014;371(16):1496–506.
42. Mouncey PR, Osborn TM, Power GS, Harrison DA, Sadique MZ, Grieve RD, et al. Protocolised Management In Sepsis (ProMISe): a multicentre randomised controlled trial of the clinical effectiveness and cost-effectiveness of early, goal-directed, protocolised resuscitation for emerging septic shock. Health Technol Assess. 2015;19(97):i–xxv, 1–150.
43. Ahmed W, Memon JI, Rehmani R, Al Juhaiman A. Outcome of patients with acute kidney injury in severe sepsis and septic shock treated with early goal-directed therapy in an intensive care unit. Saudi J Kidney Dis Transpl. 2014;25(3):544–51.
44. Schrier RW. Fluid administration in critically ill patients with acute kidney injury. Clin J Am Soc Nephrol. 2010;5(4):733–9.
45. Marik PE. Iatrogenic salt water drowning and the hazards of a high central venous pressure. Ann Intensive Care. 2014;4:21.
46. Legrand M, Dupuis C, Simon C, Gayat E, Mateo J, Lukaszewicz AC, et al. Association between systemic hemodynamics and septic acute kidney injury in critically ill patients: a retrospective observational study. Crit Care. 2013;17(6):R278.
47. Wong BT, Chan MJ, Glassford NJ, Martensson J, Bion V, Chai SY, et al. Mean arterial pressure and mean perfusion pressure deficit in septic acute kidney injury. J Crit Care. 2015;30(5):975–81.
48. Chen XK, Li SW, Liu DW, Yang RL, Zhang HM, Zhang H, et al. Effects of central venous pressure on acute kidney injury in septic shock. Zhonghua Yi Xue Za Zhi. 2011;91(19):1323–7.
49. Prowle JR, Bellomo R. Fluid administration and the kidney. Curr Opin Crit Care. 2010;16(4):332–6.
50. Chawla LS, Kellum JA, Ronco C. Permissive hypofiltration. Crit Care. 2012;16(4):317.
51. Chen X, Yang R, Liu D. Permissive hypohemofiltration and blood purification to salvage acute kidney injury. Zhonghua Nei Ke Za Zhi. 2014;53(6):428–30.
52. Pinsky MR, Kellum JA, Bellomo R. Central venous pressure is a stopping rule, not a target of fluid resuscitation. Crit Care Resusc. 2014;16(4):245–6.
53. Chen XK, Ding Q, Liu DW, Li WX, Huang LF, Sui F, et al. Effects of early goal-directed diuresis therapy on the outcomes of critical ill patients. Zhonghua Yi Xue Za Zhi. 2013;93(23):1815–8.
54. Wang XT, Yao B, Liu DW, Zhang HM. Central venous pressure dropped early is associated with organ function and prognosis in septic shock patients: a retrospective observational study. Shock. 2015;44(5):426–30.
55. Prowle JR, Echeverri JE, Ligabo EV, Ronco C, Bellomo R. Fluid balance and acute kidney injury. Nat Rev Nephrol. 2010;6(2):107–15.
56. Pinsky MR, Payen D. Functional hemodynamic monitoring. Crit Care. 2005;9(6):566–72.
57. Berger D, Moller PW, Weber A, Bloch A, Bloechlinger S, Haenggi M, et al.

Effect of PEEP, blood volume, and inspiratory hold maneuvers on venous return. Am J Physiol Heart Circ Physiol. 2016;311(3):H794–806.
58. Chen XK, Li WX. Intra-abdominal hypertension induced acute kidney injury: pressure overweigh volume. Zhonghua Yi Xue Za Zhi. 2012;92(15):1009–11.
59. Mohmand H, Goldfarb S. Renal dysfunction associated with intra-abdominal hypertension and the abdominal compartment syndrome. J Am Soc Nephrol. 2011;22(4):615–21.
60. Ross EA. Congestive renal failure: the pathophysiology and treatment of renal venous hypertension. J Card Fail. 2012;18(12):930–8.
61. Wu YF, Zheng YP, Zhang N, Liu H, Zheng QX, Yang FT, et al. Study on the correlation between the changes in intra-abdominal pressure and renal functional in the patients with abdominal compartment syndrome. Eur Rev Med Pharmacol Sci. 2015;19(19):3682–7.
62. Honore PM, Jacobs R, Joannes-Boyau O, De Regt J, Boer W, De Waele E, et al. Septic AKI in ICU patients. diagnosis, pathophysiology, and treatment type, dosing, and timing: a comprehensive review of recent and future developments. Ann Intensive Care. 2011;1(1):32.
63. Bloomfield GL, Blocher CR, Fakhry IF, Sica DA, Sugerman HJ. Elevated intra-abdominal pressure increases plasma renin activity and aldosterone levels. J Trauma. 1997;42(6):997–1004 (**discussion-5**).
64. Williams JB, Peterson ED, Wojdyla D, Harskamp R, Southerland KW, Ferguson TB, et al. Central venous pressure after coronary artery bypass surgery: does it predict postoperative mortality or renal failure? J Crit Care. 2014;29(6):1006–10.
65. Guinot PG, Abou-Arab O, Longrois D, Dupont H. Right ventricular systolic dysfunction and vena cava dilatation precede alteration of renal function in adult patients undergoing cardiac surgery: an observational study. Eur J Anaesthesiol. 2015;32(8):535–42.
66. Daudel F, Gorrasi J, Bracht H, Brandt S, Krejci V, Jakob SM, et al. Effects of lung recruitment maneuvers on splanchnic organ perfusion during endotoxin-induced pulmonary arterial hypertension. Shock. 2010;34(5):488–94.
67. Nunes S, Rothen HU, Brander L, Takala J, Jakob SM. Changes in splanchnic circulation during an alveolar recruitment maneuver in healthy porcine lungs. Anesth Analg. 2004;98(5):1432–8.
68. Vieillard-Baron A, Matthay M, Teboul JL, Bein T, Schultz M, Magder S, et al. Experts' opinion on management of hemodynamics in ARDS patients: focus on the effects of mechanical ventilation. Intensive Care Med. 2016;42(5):739–49.
69. Ruan SY, Huang TM, Wu HY, Wu HD, Yu CJ, Lai MS. Inhaled nitric oxide therapy and risk of renal dysfunction: a systematic review and meta-analysis of randomized trials. Crit Care. 2015;19:137.
70. Li DK, Wang XT, Liu DW. Association between elevated central venous pressure and outcomes in critically ill patients. Ann Intensive Care. 2017;7(1):83.
71. Honore PM, Pierrakos C, Spapen HD. Relationship between central venous pressure and acute kidney injury in critically ill patients. Annu Update Intensive Care Emerg Med. 2019.
72. Legrand M, Soussi S, Depret F. Cardiac output and CVP monitoring… to guide fluid removal. Crit Care. 2018;22(1):89.
73. Uthoff H, Breidthardt T, Klima T, Aschwanden M, Arenja N, Socrates T, et al. Central venous pressure and impaired renal function in patients with acute heart failure. Eur J Heart Fail. 2011;13(4):432–9.

9

MicroDAIMON study: Microcirculatory DAIly MONitoring in critically ill patients

Claudia Scorcella[1], Elisa Damiani[1], Roberta Domizi[1], Silvia Pierantozzi[1], Stefania Tondi[1], Andrea Carsetti[1], Silvia Ciucani[1], Valentina Monaldi[1], Mara Rogani[1], Benedetto Marini[1], Erica Adrario[1], Rocco Romano[1], Can Ince[2], E. Christiaan Boerma[3] and Abele Donati[1*]

Abstract

Background: Until now, the prognostic value of microcirculatory alterations in critically ill patients has been mainly evaluated in highly selected subgroups. Aim of this study is to monitor the microcirculation daily in mixed group of Intensive Care Unit (ICU)-patients and to establish the association between (the evolution of) microcirculatory alterations and outcome.

Methods: This is a prospective longitudinal observational single-centre study in adult patients admitted to a 12-bed ICU in an Italian teaching hospital. Sublingual microcirculation was evaluated daily, from admission to discharge/death, using Sidestream Dark Field imaging. Videos were analysed offline to assess flow and density variables. Laboratory and clinical data were recorded simultaneously. A priori, a Microvascular Flow Index (MFI) < 2.6 was defined as abnormal. A binary logistic regression analysis was performed to evaluate the association between microcirculatory variables and outcomes; a Kaplan–Meier survival curve was built. Outcomes were ICU and 90-day mortality.

Results: A total of 97 patients were included. An abnormal MFI was present on day 1 in 20.6%, and in 55.7% of cases during ICU admission. Patients with a baseline MFI < 2.6 had higher ICU, in-hospital and 90-day mortality (45 vs. 15.6%, $p = 0.012$; 55 vs. 28.6%, $p = 0.035$; 55 vs. 26%, $p = 0.017$, respectively). An independent association between baseline MFI < 2.6 and outcome was confirmed in a binary logistic analysis (odds ratio 4.594 [1.340–15.754], $p = 0.015$). A heart rate (HR) ≥ 90 bpm was an adjunctive predictor of mortality. However, a model with stepwise inclusion of mean arterial pressure < 65 mmHg, HR ≥ 90 bpm, lactate > 2 mmol/L and MFI < 2.6 did not detect significant differences in ICU mortality. In case an abnormal MFI was present on day 1, ICU mortality was significantly higher in comparison with patients with an abnormal MFI after day 1 (38 vs. 6%, $p = 0.001$), indicating a time-dependent significant difference in prognostic value.

Conclusions: In a general ICU population, an abnormal microcirculation at baseline is an independent predictor for mortality. In this setting, additional routine daily microcirculatory monitoring did not reveal extra prognostic information. Further research is needed to integrate microcirculatory monitoring in a set of commonly available hemodynamic variables.

Keywords: Microcirculation, Physiologic monitoring, Critical illness, Tachycardia, Video microscopy, Capillaries

*Correspondence: a.donati@univpm.it
[1] Anaesthesia and Intensive Care, Department of Biomedical Sciences and Public Health, Università Politecnica delle Marche, via Tronto 10/a, 60126 Ancona, Italy
Full list of author information is available at the end of the article

Background

The microcirculation is a vast network of small vessels (terminal arterioles, capillaries and venules < 100 μm diameter) in which the exchange of oxygen and nutrients with tissues takes place [1]. Its derangement, defined as "microcirculatory shock" [2], is recognised as an important cause of organ dysfunction in critically ill patients, affected by various disease states, such as sepsis, severe trauma, haemorrhagic shock and post-cardiac arrest [2–5]. Furthermore, microcirculatory abnormalities and its persistence despite adequate macro-hemodynamic resuscitation were independently associated with morbidity and mortality in many critical conditions [6–12].

Today, the development of new technologies of in vivo video microscopy and its integration in easy-to-handle microscopes as in Sidestream Dark Field (SDF) imaging allow us to assess the (sublingual) microcirculation at the bedside, in a non-invasive way [13]. However, until 2015, data on microcirculatory alterations in the Intensive Care Unit (ICU) were restricted to small sample-sized studies in high-risk patients [7, 8, 14].

The MicroSOAP study by Vellinga and colleagues [15] gave a first insight in the *prevalence* of microcirculatory alterations in a large number of ICU patients. However, due to its design with a single time-point observation, the *incidence* in a time-dependent manner remains to be elucidated. Primary aim of the study was to detect a difference in the incidence of microvascular flow abnormalities between ICU survivors and non-survivors. Secondary outcomes were long-term mortality (in-hospital mortality and 90-day mortality) and development of organ dysfunction (described by sequential organ failure assessment, SOFA).

Methods

Patients enrolment and data collection

The MicroDAIMON (Microcirculation DAIly MONitoring in critically ill patients) is a single-centre prospective observational study (clinicaltrials.gov, NCT 02649088 registered on 23 December; retrospectively registered). The recruiting phase was performed in a 9-month period in 2013 (from 1 April to 31 December) in a 12-bed mixed ICU of an Italian teaching hospital with a mean number of yearly-admitted patients of 400. The ICU was structured in three subunits of four beds each, caring for respiratory, traumatology and medical critically ill patients, respectively. For the study purpose, each subunit was subsequently included and monitored during a 3-month period for patients' screening and the recruitment: from 1 April to 30 June 2013, the medical subunit, from 1 July to 30 September 2013, the traumatology subunit and from 1st October to 31st December 2013, the respiratory subunit.

Patients were screened and included in the study within the first 12 h from ICU admission. Exclusion criteria were age < 18 years, lack of informed consent and pathophysiological conditions that may interfere with the sublingual microcirculation videos acquisition (maxillofacial traumas/surgery, oral bleeding, mucositis, etc.). In context to the microcirculatory assessments, demographic, laboratory, microbiologic, hemodynamic and other clinical data were recorded. All patients were followed up for 90 days after the ICU admission.

The study protocol was approved by the Local Ethics Committee and conducted in respect of the principles of Helsinki declaration (last revision, Edinburgh 2000). A written informed consent was obtained from all the included subjects or their next of kin in compliance with national applicable laws.

Microcirculation assessment

The sublingual microcirculation was evaluated at the moment of the inclusion and every 24 h until discharge/death with SDF imaging (Microscan®, Microvision Medical, Amsterdam, The Netherlands) [13].

The video acquisition technique is extensively described in previous papers [16]. For every session, videos from at least five different sites were registered trying to obtain a good video quality and to avoid artefacts that may affect flow or vessels density variables [16].

The three best videos were chosen from each session, in compliance with recommendations from Massey et al. [17] and blindly analysed offline with a dedicated software (Automated Vascular Analysis, AVA Software 3.0, MicroVision Medical, Amsterdam, The Netherlands) by a restricted group of four experienced investigators. Interobserver variability was calculated, based on the simultaneous analysis of ten randomly selected SDF videos by all the investigators. Variables of flow (Microvascular Flow Index, MFI and proportion of perfused vessels, PPV), as well as capillary density (total vessel density, TVD, perfused vessel density, PVD) and flow distribution (Heterogeneity Index, HI) were calculated according to international criteria [18, 19]. Flow was scored per quadrant as 0 (no flow), 1 (intermittent flow), 2 (sluggish flow) and 3 (continuous flow). The MFI is the average over 4 quadrants × 3 areas of interest. Total vessel density (TVD, mm/mm^2) was calculated as the total length of vessels divided by the total area of the image. The percentage of perfused vessels (PPV) was estimated as follows: 100 × [(total number of grid crossings − [no flow + intermittent flow])/total number of grid crossings] and expressed as percentage. The perfused vessel density (PVD, mm/mm^2) was estimated by multiplying TVD by PPV as estimated with the De Backer method. The Flow Heterogeneity Index (FHI, arbitrary units) was calculated as the highest MFI minus the lowest MFI, divided by the mean MFI of all sublingual sites [18].

Analogous to previous data, a threshold for the MFI < 2.6 was a priori established to define an abnormal microcirculation [3, 8, 15, 20].

Statistical analysis

Data analysis was conducted with SPSS Software 17.0 (IBM, New York, NY) and GraphPad Prism 6 (GraphPad Software, La Jolla, CA). All data are presented as mean ± standard deviation (SD) or median [interquartile range, IQR].

Descriptive statistics were performed to obtain patients' baseline characteristics. Quantitative variables distribution was tested with Kolmogorov–Smirnov normality test. Parametric (Student's *t* test with Welch's correction) and nonparametric tests (Mann–Whitney *U* test) were applied to describe the differences between groups for the variables of interest as appropriate. Fisher's exact test was performed for comparisons between categorical variables, and the results are presented as percentage, odds ratio (OR) and 95% confidence interval (CI). Kaplan–Meier 90-day survival curves with Tarone–Ware test for the comparison of the hazard ratio between groups were built for the survival analysis.

Binary logistic regression analysis was performed with a forward stepwise entry method. A p value of less than 0.05 was considered statistically significant.

Results

Population characteristics

During the study period, 40, 37 and 38 patients were admitted, respectively, in the medical, traumatology and respiratory ICU subunits, for a total amount of 115 patients. Hundred patients met the inclusion criteria. All the patients were included in the study within 12 h from ICU admission, with no exceptions due to timing or organizational issues. Three patients were a posteriori excluded because no SDF videos were available for the baseline assessment. Therefore, 97 patients were included in the final analysis. The flow chart for the patients' inclusion process is illustrated in Additional file 1.

Baseline characteristics of the patients are illustrated in Table 1. Patients were predominantly male (66%) with a median age of 67 years [46–75], a mean acute physiology and chronic health evaluation (APACHE) II score of 16 ± 7 and a median SOFA score of 7 [4–10]; the most frequent cause of ICU admission was trauma (38.1%). Patients admitted for sepsis represented the 9.3% of the sample. During the ICU stay, ten more patients developed sepsis: two trauma patients (5.4%), one neurologic patient (4.8%), two respiratory patients (18.2%) and five other patients (26.3%).

Median ICU length of stay was 7 [4–15] days; ICU mortality was 21.6%, in-hospital mortality 34%, 90-day mortality 31.9% (two patients died in the hospital after 90 days from ICU admission).

Microcirculatory abnormalities at baseline and outcome

2455 videos were collected and analysed offline to obtain microcirculatory variables. The coefficient of variation (inter-observer variability) for MFI was 1.4 ± 3% for small vessels. Baseline microcirculatory variables are described in Table 1. The incidence of MFI abnormality at the day of ICU admission was 20.6%.

ICU non-survivors showed a higher baseline APACHE II score and SOFA score, higher age, heart rate (HR), Cumulative Vasopressor Index [21], arterial lactate level, serum creatinine and lower platelets count (Table 1).

Subsequently, patients were divided into two groups based on normal (≥ 2.6) or abnormal (< 2.6) baseline MFI. In comparison with patients with a normal MFI at baseline, patients with an abnormal MFI showed a higher ICU mortality (45 vs. 15.6%, $p = 0.012$) (Table 1), in-hospital mortality (55 vs. 28.6%, $p = 0.035$) and 90-day mortality (55 vs. 26%, $p = 0.017$). (Additional files 2, 3)

Survival analysis, by Kaplan–Meier method, confirmed a significant difference between the two groups for 90-day mortality (Tarone–Ware $\chi^2 = 6.15$, $p = 0.003$) (Fig. 1a). In the binary logistic regression analysis, the presence of an abnormal MFI at baseline was associated with ICU mortality (OR 4.594 [95% CI 1.340–15.754], $p = 0.015$) independently of the APACHE II score (Table 2).

The role of tachycardia in combination with an abnormal microcirculation was additionally tested. Patients were divided into four groups based on the presence of tachycardia (defined as the presence of an HR ≥ 90 beats per minute, bpm) [22–25] and/or MFI abnormality at the baseline. ICU mortality was significantly different between the four groups (overall $\chi^2 = 12.76$, $p = 0.002$). Survival analysis confirmed a significant difference between the groups in terms of 90-day mortality (Tarone–Ware $\chi^2 = 24.98$, $p < 0.0001$) with a survival rate as low as 12.5% among patients with tachycardia plus abnormal MFI (Fig. 1b). The combination of tachycardia and an abnormal MFI on day 1 was associated with an increased risk for ICU mortality (OR 10.732 [95% CI 1.685–68.354], $p = 0.012$) independently of the APACHE II score (Table 2).

Integration of an abnormal microcirculation in a set of common hemodynamic variables

In order to clarify the additional prognostic value of an abnormal microcirculation (MFI < 2.6) at baseline in a set of commonly available hemodynamic variables, i.e. mean arterial blood pressure (MAP), HR and lactate,

Table 1 Baseline characteristics and comparison between ICU survivors versus non-survivors

Patients characteristics	n	All (97)	ICU survivors (76)	ICU non-survivors (21)	p
Male gender (n, %)	97	64 (66)	50 (65.8)	14 (66.7)	1
Age (years, n)	97	67 [46–75]	64 [44–73]	71 [56–81]	0.034
APACHE II (pts)	97	16±7	14±7	22±6	< 0.001
SOFA (pts)	97	7 [4–10]	6 [4–9]	12 [8–15]	< 0.001
ICU admission diagnosis, n (%)	97				0.046
		Trauma 37 (38.1)	34	3(8.1)	
		Neurologic 21 (21.6)	17	4(19)	
		Respiratory 11 (11.3)	8	3(27.3)	
		Sepsis 9 (9.3)	6	3 (33.3)	
		Other 19 (19.7)	11	8(42.1)	
Heart rate (bpm)	97	79 [61–102]	77 [61–95]	96 [69–107]	0.045
Mean arterial pressure (mmHg)	97	84±19	86±17	79±27	0.255
Vasoactive drugs (treated)	54		38(50)	16(76.2)	0.046
Noradrenaline (mcg/kg/min)	52	0.28 [0.14–0.61]			
Dopamine (mcg/kg/min)	5	6.1 [4.8–7.4]			
Dobutamine (mcg/kg/min)	8	2.54 [2–4.5]			
Cumulative Vasopressor Index	54	4 [4]	1 [0–4]	4 [2–4]	0.008
Glasgow Coma Scale (pts)	97	10 [3–15]	10 [4–15]	4 [3–14]	0.074
Mechanical ventilation (n, %)	97	91 (93.8)	71(93.4)	21(100)	0.581
Peep (cmH_2O)	91	7 [6–9]	7 [6–9]	8 [7–10]	0.095
Haemoglobin (g/dL)	97	11±1.78	11.1±1.7	10.8±2.2	0.58
White blood cells ($n \times 10^3$/mmc)	97	12.1 [8.83–14.81]	11.3 [8.8–15.7]	12.7 [9.5–14.6]	0.518
Platelets ($n \times 10^3$/mmc)	97	150 [102–199]	165 [110–201]	115 [56–173]	0.02
Creatinine (mg/dL)	97	1.0 [0.8–1.45]	1 [0.8–1.2]	1.4 [1.1–1.8]	< 0.001
Bilirubine (mg/dL)	97	0.8 [0.5–1.2]	0.75 [0.5–1.1]	0.9 [0.4–1.8]	0.264
PaO_2 (mmHg)	97	146 [104–175]	147 [106–176]	140 [93–172]	0.63
Arterial lactates (mmol/L)	97	1.4 [1.0–2.15]	1.3 [0.9–1.67]	3.1 [1.4–5.6]	< 0.001
$ScvO_2$ (%)	60	77.2 [71–82.3]	77.7 [72.3–82.5]	75.6 [62.7–80.8]	0.24
Microcirculatory variables					
TVD (small) (mm/mm²)	97	20.4±3.7	20.5 [17.2–22.7]	20.9 [17.8–22.7]	0.817
PVD (small) (mm/mm²)	97	19.3±4.4	19.3±4	19.3±6	0.951
De Backer score (small) (n/mm)	97	11.9±2	11.8±2	12.2±2	0.489
PPV (small) (%)	97	98.3 [95.4–100]	98.2 [94.8–100]	98.3 [97–100]	0.688
MFI (small) (AU)	97	3 [2.7–3.0]	3 [2.75–3]	2.93 [2.3–3]	0.155
HI (small)	97	0 [0.0–0.2]	0 [0–0.2]	0 [0–0.3]	0.417
Abnormal MFI (n, %)	97	20 (20.6)	11 (14.5)	9 (42.9)	0.012

Data are presented as mean ± or as median [IQR] unless stated otherwise

APACHE acute physiologic and chronic health evaluation II, calculated over the first 24 h from ICU admission; *SOFA* sequential organ failure assessment, calculated over the first 24 h from ICU admission; *CVI* cumulative vasopressor index; *ICU* Intensive Care Unit; *COPD*, chronic obstructive pulmonary disease. *TVD* total vessel density; *PVD* perfused vessel density; *PPV* proportion of perfused vessel; *HI* Heterogeneity Index; *MFI* Microvascular Flow Index. Abnormal MFI is defined as MFI < 2.6. Cut-off value for small vessels diameter < 20 μm

we divided these variables into normal and abnormal: MAP ≥ 65 mmHg = normal, < 65 mmHg = abnormal; HR < 90 bpm = normal, ≥ 90 bpm = abnormal; and arterial lactate ≤ 2 mmol/L = normal, > 2 mmol/L = abnormal. In the first model, all variables were normal. A stepwise addition of each variable was associated with a non-significant reduction in ICU mortality (Fig. 2). In the second model, all variables were abnormal. A stepwise addition of each variable was associated with a non-significant increment in ICU mortality (Fig. 2). The comparison between the two models revealed in each step a significantly higher ICU mortality in the 'abnormal' model (Fig. 2).

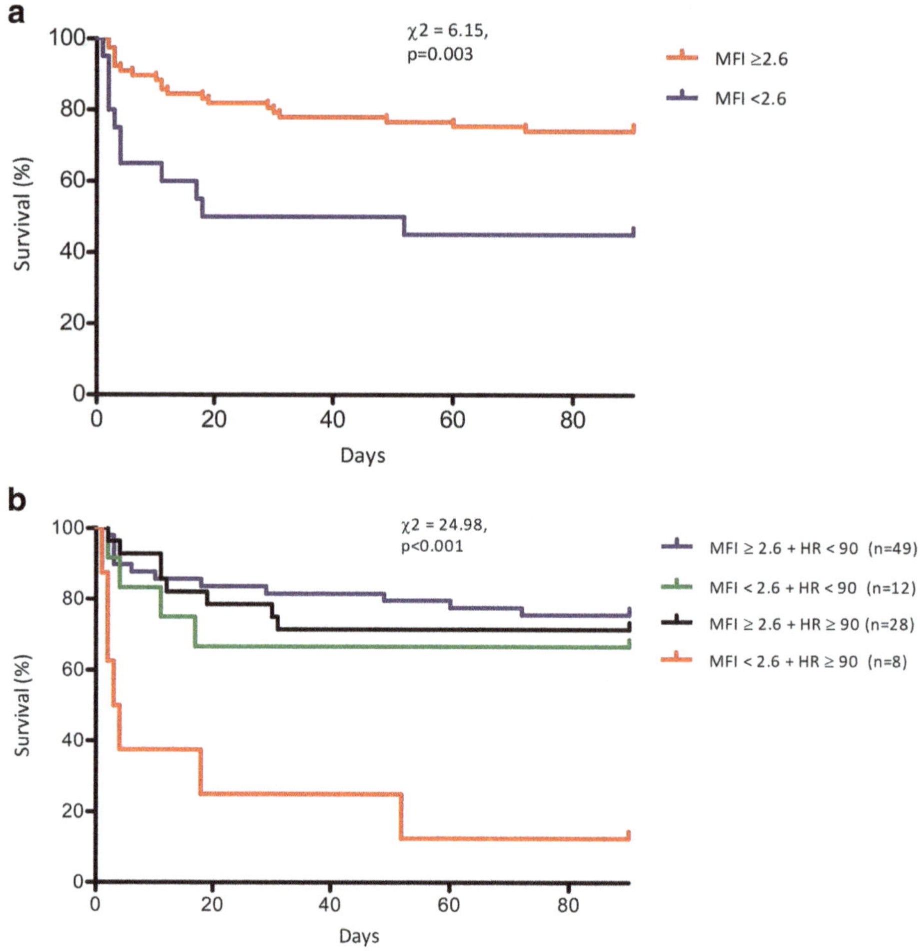

Fig. 1 Kaplan–Meier survival analysis. **a** Represents two subgroups, separated by microvascular blood flow (MFI) < 2.6 versus MFI ≥ 2.6. **b** Represents four subgroups, separated by MFI with identical cut-off value and heart rate (HR) ≥ 90 versus < 90 bpm

Table 2 Binary logistic regression analysis for ICU mortality

Variables	Odds ratio (95% CI)	p value
ICU MORTALITY (abnormal MFI)		
APACHE II score	1.204 (1.089–1.331)	< 0.001
MFI < 2.6	4.594 (1.340–15.754)	0.015
ICU MORTALITY (abnormal MFI + tachycardia)		
APACHE II score	1.191 (1.077–1.316)	0.001
MFI < 2.6 + tachycardia	10.732 (1.685–68.354)	0.012

In the upper model baseline, MFI abnormality was the independent variable. Model AUC 0.836 [0.747–0.904], Nagelkerke R^2 0.359, Hosmer and Lemeshow χ^2 4.733, $p = 0.822$. In the lower model, the presence of abnormal MFI plus tachycardia was the independent variable. Model AUC 0.836 [0.747–0.903], Nagelkerke R^2 0.374, Hosmer and Lemeshow χ^2 2.670, $p = 0.914$

APACHE acute physiologic and chronic health evaluation II, calculated in the first 24 h from ICU admission; *ICU* Intensive Care Unit; *MFI* Microvascular Flow Index. Abnormal MFI is defined as MFI < 2.6 for small vessels (diameter < 20 μm). Tachycardia is defined as a heart rate ≥ 90 bpm

Microcirculatory longitudinal monitoring and outcome

The median duration of follow-up for each patient category was: 6 [3–12] days for trauma, 8 [3–14] days for neurologic, 5 [1–6] days for respiratory, 8 [3–11] days for septic and 4 [2–8] days for other patients.

The total *incidence* of an abnormal microcirculation during the entire ICU stay was 55.7% (20.6% on day 1, 35.1% after day 1). Microcirculatory imaging was restricted to day 1 in ten patients (six died, four were discharged); missing data (SOFA and/or MFI) prevented further analysis in 19 patients. MFI and SOFA score over time are depicted in Fig. 3. Twenty-two patients showed an increment in MFI between days 1 and 2 (ΔMFI (+)), 21 patients showed a reduction in MFI between days 1 and 2 (ΔMFI (−)) and 25 remained indifferent. ΔMFI (+) was not associated with a significant reduction in SOFA score between days 2 and 3 (corresponding with the same time frame of MFI days 1 and 2) or mortality,

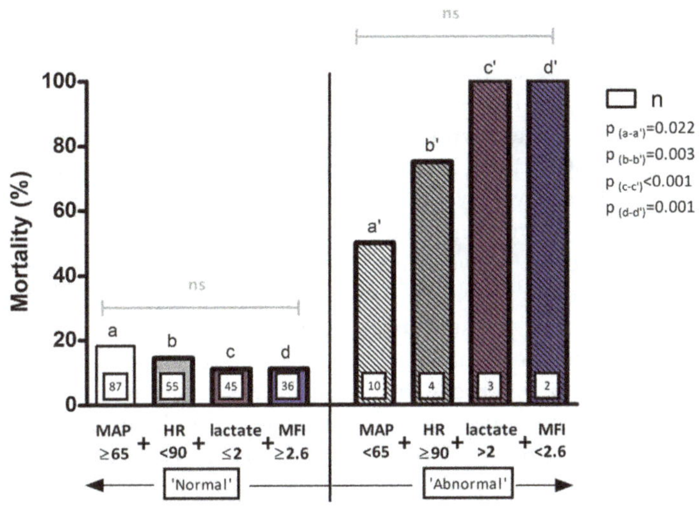

Fig. 2 Prognostic model with stepwise inclusion of consecutive hemodynamic variables: mean arterial pressure (MAP) in mmHg, heart rate (HR) in bpm, (arterial) lactate in mmol/L and Microvascular Flow Index (MFI) in AU

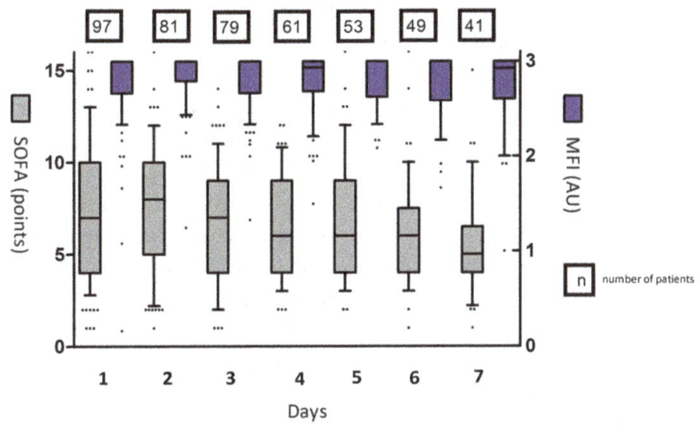

Fig. 3 Evolvement over time of sequential organ failure assessment (SOFA) score and Microvascular Flow Index (MFI) in the first 7 days of ICU admission. Box and 10–90th percentile whisker plots with individual outliers

as compared to patients with a ΔMFI (−). Any increase/decrease in MFI was considered relevant for this analysis.

Post hoc, patients were divided into four groups according to the timing of the presence of an abnormal MFI. Group 1: patients with a normal MFI on day 1 and later on ($n=36$). Group 2: patients with a normal MFI on day 1 but with one or more episodes of an abnormal MFI later on ($n=34$). Group 3: patients with an abnormal MFI on day 1 and a normal MFI later on ($n=6$). Group 4: patients with an abnormal MFI on day 1 and one or more episodes of an abnormal MFI later on ($n=10$). Mortality was significantly different across groups ($p<0.001$). If an abnormal MFI was present on day one (groups 3 and 4), mortality was 6/16 (38%), whereas in patients with an abnormal MFI only after day 1 (group 2), ICU mortality was 2/34 (6%, $p=0.001$), indicating a significant difference in prognostic value of an abnormal MFI on day 1 in comparison with an abnormal MFI after day 1.

Discussion

This MicroDAIMON study is currently the largest prospective longitudinal observational study to describe the incidence of microcirculatory derangements among a mixed group of critically ill patients, offering a day-by-day follow-up. The incidence of baseline microcirculatory flow abnormalities was 20.6%, and more than half (55.7%) of the patients displayed an abnormal MFI in at least one observation during ICU stay. The main finding of this study is that in this mixed ICU population, an abnormal baseline MFI is independently associated with unfavourable outcome in terms of ICU, in-hospital and 90-day mortality. In addition, the contemporary presence of tachycardia showed an additive predictive power towards mortality in the survival analysis. However, the change of MFI over time was not associated with outcome, in terms of both organ failure (SOFA) and mortality. In contrast to an abnormal MFI on day 1, we could not associate an abnormal MFI after day 1 with unfavourable outcome. No associations were found between the other microvascular variables and outcome.

In 2015, the MicroSOAP study provided the first and largest database on the prevalence and the significance of the microcirculatory alterations in a heterogeneous ICU population, with a time-point observation across 36 ICUs worldwide [15]. The authors reported a prevalence of MFI abnormalities of 17%, using the same predefined cut-off value [15, 26]. This difference in reported percentage of MFI abnormalities can be explained by the difference in study design (longitudinal vs. point prevalence). Our data confirm previous observations, showing an important prognostic role of the microcirculation in various subsets of critically ill patients [4–9, 14]. In contrast to the existing literature, these findings extend the predictive value of early microcirculatory alterations towards 90-day mortality. Patients with an abnormal MFI at baseline showed an absolute risk of non-survival almost three times higher in comparison with patients with a normal MFI.

However, in the present study, routine day-by-day microcirculatory monitoring does not confirm previous observations. In 2004, Sakr et al. [11] introduced for the first time the concept of serial observations of microcirculation in a cohort of 49 patients with septic shock. In this highly selected group of patients, the persistence of microcirculatory alterations was associated with persistence of shock, development of multiple organ failure and mortality.

Conversely, ICU survivors showed early improvement of microcirculation. These data were confirmed by others [21]. Duranteau and colleagues observed in another selected cohort of 18 patients with traumatic haemorrhagic shock, early derangements of microcirculatory flow and vessel density, as well as its persistence, were able to predict a worse SOFA score after 96 h from ICU admission [5]. A possible explanation for this discrepancy may lie in the heterogeneous composition of our study population and in considerable differences in microcirculatory baseline abnormalities. Alternatively, microvascular alterations represent differences in underlying pathology between study populations. Careful selection of patients at risk may contribute to the prognostic power of microcirculatory observation. As of now, our data indicate that routine daily monitoring of the microcirculation in an unselected group of ICU patients is of limited prognostic value.

This study has several limitations. Although this study contains the largest reported database on day-by-day monitoring of the microcirculation in critically ill, it appears to have insufficient sample size to correlate differences in the evolution of microcirculatory conditions over time with clinically relevant endpoints (SOFA, mortality) also due to the considerable number of patients lost to follow-up, due to death/discharge. And although the independent predictive value of an abnormal MFI on day 1 was established, the integration of such variable in a model with more commonly used hemodynamic variables was clearly limited by the sample size as well. Further research is needed to establish the additive value of microcirculatory imaging on top of the existing hemodynamic variables. In addition, it is conceivable that other microvascular variables and different cut-off yield different results. We did not found any significant association between the other microcirculatory variables (TVD, PVD, PPV) and the outcome either on day 1 or in the following days. This could be explained by the fact that the MFI, especially if used as a dichotomous variable based on an a priori cut-off of 2,6, could have been the most sensitive variable to detect an association with the outcome in a such heterogeneous population which is expected to cause a "dilution effect" on the microcirculatory alterations. It is also possible that a vessel-by-vessel MFI calculation could have been more precise and provide different results depending on a more accurate evaluation of the capillary blood flow, especially in the presence of marked heterogeneity. In this respect, the burden of time-consuming offline analysis remains a major practical limitation for the study population sample size until the time of the development and full validation of automated analysis software. Real-time "eyeballing" the microcirculation by bedside assessment of MFI is a major advantage in the development of a bedside tool and showed good agreement with the gold standard offline analysis [27]. Post hoc analysis of our data confirmed 2.6 as the optimal cut-off for the discrimination between survivors and non-survivors. Finally, this was a pure observational study: patients were treated following the international guidelines and principles of good clinical practice, and clinicians had no information about the microcirculation during the study. Therefore, our study design is insufficient to draw conclusions on the applicability of microcirculatory monitoring as a tool to guide resuscitation. Even in the setting where there is an absence of additional prognostic information, derived from microcirculatory monitoring, the observation itself may contain valuable information about the underlying pathophysiologic mechanisms. For example, an increased lactate may adequately predict outcome, but does not reveal its underlying mechanism. Under these conditions, additional assessment of microvascular blood flow may not be useful to predict outcome, but may be helpful for the clinician to select the appropriate resuscitation strategy. Further research is needed to address this topic. Careful selection of subgroups and adequate timing remain of the essence in this process.

Conclusions

This MicroDAIMON study provides data about incidence of microcirculatory alterations in a heterogeneous group of critically ill patients. Microcirculatory flow abnormalities at the baseline were independently associated with an increased risk of unfavourable outcome. Simultaneous presence of tachycardia enhanced this predictive value. However, neither the evolution of MFI over time nor the development or new abnormalities after day 1 was associated with organ function or mortality in our population with a sample size limitation. Further studies are needed to incorporate microcirculatory monitoring into a set of currently available hemodynamic variables and to establish its value as a tool to guide specific resuscitation strategies.

Additional files

Additional file 1. Flow chart for patients' recruitment. A schema to clarify the procedures for the patients' recruitment for the study.

Additional file 2. Comparison between in-hospital survivors and non-survivors. The table illustrates the results of the univariable analysis for baseline clinical and microcirculatory variables between in-hospital survivors and non-survivors.

Additional file 3. Comparison between 90-day survivors and non-survivors. The table illustrates the results of the univariable analysis for baseline clinical and microcirculatory variables between 90-day survivors and non-survivors.

Abbreviations

SDF: Sidestream Dark Field; ICU: Intensive Care Unit; SOFA: sequential organ failure assessment; MFI: Microvascular Flow Index; PPV: proportion of perfused vessels; TVD: total vessel density; PVD: perfused vessel density; SD: standard deviation; IQR: interquartile range; OR: odds ratio; CI: confidence interval; APACHE II: acute physiology and chronic evaluation score; HR: heart rate; MAP: mean arterial pressure.

Authors' contributions

CS, AD, ED, RR, EA designed the study, contributed to the interpretation of the results and critically revised the manuscript. CS and ED performed the statistical analysis, drafted the manuscript and interpreted the data. ED, CS, RD, AC, SP, ST, VM, SC, MR, BM made a substantial contributions to the acquisition of the data and the analysis of SDF videos and revised the manuscript for important intellectual content. CB made a substantial contribution in drafting the manuscript and interpreting the results. CI made a substantial contribution in the study design and critically revised the manuscript for important intellectual content. All authors had full access to the data, take responsibility for the integrity of the data and the accuracy of the analysis. All authors read and approved the final manuscript.

Author details

[1] Anaesthesia and Intensive Care, Department of Biomedical Sciences and Public Health, Università Politecnica delle Marche, via Tronto 10/a, 60126 Ancona, Italy. [2] Department of Translational Physiology, Academic Medical Centre, University of Amsterdam, Meibergdreef 9, 1105 AZ Amsterdam, The Netherlands. [3] Department of Intensive Care, Medical Centre Leeuwarden, Henri Dunantweg 2, 8934 AD Leeuwarden, The Netherlands.

Acknowledgements

We would like to thank Luca Giovannelli, MD, and Marco Zacchilli, MD, Università Politecnica delle Marche, Department of Biomedical Science and Public Health, for the precious help in the SDF video analysis all the medical doctors, residents and nurses of the Clinic of General, Respiratory and Trauma Intensive Care of Ospedali Riuniti of Ancona for the kind support.

Competing interests

CI is the inventor of Sidestream Dark Field imaging technology. He has been a consultant for MicroVision Medical in the past but he has actually no contact with this company for more than 5 years, except that he still holds shares. He has no other competing interests in this field other than his commitment to promoting the importance of the microcirculation during patient care; and there are no other relationships or activities that could appear to have influenced the submitted work. The other authors have no competing interests to declare.

Funding

Local departmental funding.

References

1. Ince C. The microcirculation is the motor of sepsis. Crit Care. 2005;9(Suppl 4):S13–9.
2. Kanoore Edul VS, Ince C, Dubin A. What is microcirculatory shock? Curr Opin Crit Care. 2015;21(3):245–52.
3. Spanos A, Jhanji S, Vivian-Smith A, et al. Early microvascular changes in sepsis and severe sepsis. Shock. 2010;33(4):387–91.
4. Bateman RM, Sharpe MD, Ellis CG. Bench-to-bedside review: microvascular dysfunction in sepsis–hemodynamics, oxygen transport, and nitric oxide. Crit Care. 2003;7(5):359–73.
5. Tachon G, Harrois A, Tanaka S, et al. Microcirculatory alterations in traumatic hemorrhagic shock. Crit Care Med. 2014;42(6):1433–41.
6. van Genderen ME, Lima A, Akkerhuis M, et al. Persistent peripheral and microcirculatory perfusion alterations after out-of-hospital cardiac arrest are associated with poor survival. Crit Care Med. 2012;40(8):2287–94.
7. De Backer D, Donadello K, Sakr Y, et al. Microcirculatory alterations in patients with severe sepsis: impact of time of assessment and relationship with outcome. Crit Care Med. 2013;41(3):791–9.
8. Trzeciak S, Dellinger RP, Parrillo JE, et al. Early microcirculatory perfusion derangements in patients with severe sepsis and septic shock: relationship to hemodynamics, oxygen transport, and survival. Ann Emerg Med. 2007;49(1):88–98.
9. Jhanji S, Lee C, Watson D, et al. Microvascular flow and tissue oxygenation after major abdominal surgery: association with post-operative complications. Intensive Care Med. 2009;35(4):671–7.
10. den Uil CA, Lagrand WK, van der Ent M, et al. Impaired microcirculation predicts poor outcome of patients with acute myocardial infarction complicated by cardiogenic shock. Eur Heart J. 2010;31(24):3032–9.
11. Sakr Y, Dubois MJ, De Backer D, et al. Persistent microcirculatory alterations are associated with organ failure and death in patients with septic shock. Crit Care Med. 2004;32(9):1825–31.

12. Top APC, Ince C, de Meij N, et al. Persistent low microcirculatory vessel density in nonsurvivors of sepsis in pediatric intensive care. Crit Care Med. 2011;39(1):8–13.
13. Goedhart PT, Khalilzada M, Bezemer R, et al. Sidestream Dark Field (SDF) imaging: a novel stroboscopic LED ring-based imaging modality for clinical assessment of the microcirculation. Opt Express. 2007;15(23):15101–14.
14. De Backer D, Creteur J, Dubois MJ, et al. Microvascular alterations in patients with acute severe heart failure and cardiogenic shock. Am Heart J. 2004;147(1):91–9.
15. Vellinga NAR, Boerma EC, Koopmans M, et al. International study on microcirculatory shock occurrence in acutely ill patients. Crit Care Med. 2015;43(1):48–56.
16. Damiani E, Ince C, Scorcella C, et al. Impact of microcirculatory video quality on the evaluation of sublingual microcirculation in critically ill patients. J Clin Monit Comput. 2017;31(5):981–8.
17. Massey MJ, Shapiro NI. A guide to human in vivo microcirculatory flow image analysis. Crit Care. 2016;20:35.
18. De Backer D, Hollenberg S, Boerma C, et al. How to evaluate the microcirculation: report of a round table conference. Crit Care. 2007;11(5):R101.
19. Boerma EC, Mathura KR, van der Voort PHJ, et al. Quantifying bedside-derived imaging of microcirculatory abnormalities in septic patients: a prospective validation study. Crit Care. 2005;9(6):R601–6.
20. Pranskunas A, Koopmans M, Koetsier PM, et al. Microcirculatory blood flow as a tool to select ICU patients eligible for fluid therapy. Intensive Care Med. 2013;39(4):612–9.
21. Trzeciak S, McCoy JV, Phillip Dellinger R, et al. Early increases in microcirculatory perfusion during protocol-directed resuscitation are associated with reduced multi-organ failure at 24 h in patients with sepsis. Intensive Care Med. 2008;34(12):2210–7.
22. Hoke RS, Müller-Werdan U, Lautenschläger C, et al. Heart rate as an independent risk factor in patients with multiple organ dysfunction: a prospective, observational study. Clin Res Cardiol. 2012;101(2):139–47.
23. Schmittinger CA, Torgersen C, Luckner G, et al. Adverse cardiac events during catecholamine vasopressor therapy: a prospective observational study. Intensive Care Med. 2012;38(6):950–8.
24. Disegni E, Goldbourt U, Reicher-Reiss H, et al. The predictive value of admission heart rate on mortality in patients with acute myocardial infarction. SPRINT Study Group. Secondary Prevention Reinfarction Israeli Nifedipine Trial. J Clin Epidemiol. 1995;48(10):1197–205.
25. Bone RC, Balk RA, Cerra FB, et al. Definitions for sepsis and organ failure and guidelines for the use of innovative therapies in sepsis. The ACCP/SCCM Consensus Conference Committee. American College of Chest Physicians/Society of Critical Care Medicine. Chest. 1992;101(6):1644–55.
26. Edul VSK, Enrico C, Laviolle B, et al. Quantitative assessment of the microcirculation in healthy volunteers and in patients with septic shock. Crit Care Med. 2012;40(5):1443–8.
27. Arnold RC, Parrillo JE, Phillip Dellinger R, et al. Point-of-care assessment of microvascular blood flow in critically ill patients. Intensive Care Med. 2009;35(10):1761–6.

De-escalation of antifungal treatment in critically ill patients with suspected invasive *Candida* infection: incidence, associated factors, and safety

Karim Jaffal[1], Julien Poissy[1,2,3], Anahita Rouze[1,2,3], Sébastien Preau[1,2,3], Boualem Sendid[2,3,4], Marjorie Cornu[2,3,4] and Saad Nseir[1,2,3*]

Abstract

Background: Antifungal treatment is common in critically ill patients, but only a small proportion of patients receiving antifungals have a proven fungal infection. However, antifungal treatment has side effects such as toxicity, emergence of resistance, and high cost. Moreover, empirical antifungal treatment is still a matter for debate in these patients. Our study aimed to determine the incidence, associated factors, and safety of de-escalation of antifungals in critically ill patients.

Methods: This retrospective study was conducted in a 30-bed mixed ICU, from January 2012 through January 2013. Patients hospitalized for > 5 days and treated with antifungals for first suspected or proven invasive *Candida* infection were included. Exclusion criteria were prophylactic antifungals, suspected invasive aspergillosis, and neutropenia. De-escalation was defined as switch from initial systemic antifungals (except fluconazole) to triazoles, or stopping initial drugs within the 5 days following their initiation.

Results: One hundred and ninety patients were included. Antifungal treatment was empirical, preemptive, and targeted in 55, 27, and 24% of study patients, respectively. Caspofungin (53%), fluconazole (43%), voriconazole (4%), and liposomal amphotericin B (0.5%) were the more frequently used antifungals. De-escalation was performed in 38 (20%) patients. Invasive mechanical ventilation was independently associated with lower rates of de-escalation (OR 0.25 [95% CI 0.08–0.85], $p=0.013$). Total duration of antifungal treatment was significantly shorter in patients with de-escalation, compared with those with no de-escalation (med [IQR] 6 (5, 18) vs. 13 days (7, 25), $p=0.023$). No significant difference was found in duration of mechanical ventilation (22 [5–31] vs. 20 days [10–35], $p=0.43$), length of ICU stay (25 [14–40) vs. 25 days [11–40], $p=0.99$), ICU mortality (45 vs. 59%, $p=0.13$), or 1-year mortality (55 vs. 64%, $p=0.33$) between patients with de-escalation and those with no de-escalation, respectively.

Conclusions: De-escalation was performed in 20% of patients receiving systemic antifungals for suspected or proven invasive *Candida* infection. Mechanical ventilation was independently associated with lower rates of de-escalation. De-escalation of antifungal treatment seems to be safe in critically ill patients.

Background

Invasive fungal infections are common in critically ill patients [1–3]. Candidiasis is the most frequent fungal infection in hospitalized patients worldwide [4]. Despite a frequency twice less important than the frequency of bacteremia, mortality linked to candidemia is twice higher than that linked to bacteremia [5]. In case of septic shock, this mortality can reach 60% [6]. Despite the introduction of several extended-spectrum triazoles and echinocandin antifungal agents with superior safety,

*Correspondence: s-nseir@chru-lille.fr
[1] Critical Care Center, CHU Lille, 59000 Lille, France
Full list of author information is available at the end of the article

spectrum, and potency, the incidence of invasive *Candida* infection and the associated mortality have not decreased over the past two decades [2]. The high mortality rate is related to comorbidities and also to the difficulty in diagnosis coupled with challenges in prompt adequate antifungal therapy [7].

Clinical signs of invasive *Candida* infection are nonspecific, risk factors are common, the predictive positive value of all scores set to help clinicians remains insufficient [8, 9], and blood cultures have insufficient diagnostic accuracy [10, 11]. Because prompt antifungal treatment has a major impact on mortality [6, 12], guidelines recommend initiating systemic antifungal therapy, for critically ill patients with risk factors for invasive *Candida* infection and no other known cause for fever [13]. Criteria for initiating such therapy in clinical practice remain poorly defined. Consequently, the lack of rapid, sensitive, and specific diagnostic tests can lead to possible overuse of antifungal agents without further confirmation of invasive *Candida* infection [14]. Moreover, the overuse of antifungal agents is associated with increased prevalence of *Candida* non-albicans species and antifungal resistance [15–18]. Other potential consequences of inappropriate use of antifungals are increased cost, drug toxicity, and adverse drug interactions [19, 20].

A cross-sectional multicenter study showed that antifungal treatment was administered to 7.5% of ICU patients, although two-thirds of them had no documented invasive candidiasis [14]. In addition, recent studies suggested no benefit of empirical antifungal treatment in these patients [21, 22]. Reducing antifungal use in the ICU with an antifungal stewardship is feasible and would allow avoiding drawbacks. The European Society for Clinical Microbiology and Infectious Diseases (ESCMID) and the Infectious Diseases Society of America (IDSA) guidelines recommend a de-escalation strategy (5 days in stabilized patients for the IDSA and 10 days overall for the ESCMID) [13, 23], but the level of recommendations is low. The safety of de-escalation in the case of proven invasive *Candida* infection has been suggested by prospective recent studies [24–26]. However, some limitations, such as non-comparative or post hoc design, preclude definite conclusions. Therefore, we hypothesized that de-escalation of antifungal treatment might be safe in patients with suspected invasive *Candida* infection and conducted this retrospective study to identify the incidence and associated factors, and to assess safety of antifungal treatment de-escalation in ICU patients.

Methods

Study design

This retrospective observational study was performed in a 30-bed mixed ICU, located in the University Hospital of Lille, France. All data were retrospectively collected during a one-year period (from January 2012 through January 2013). The study was approved by the local Institutional Review Board (Comité de Protection des Personnes Nord-ouest IV). Because of the retrospective observational design of the study, and in accordance with the French law, written informed consent was not required by the local IRB.

Definitions and studied population

De-escalation of antifungal treatment was defined as either a switch from initial antifungals, except fluconazole, to triazoles, or discontinuation of initial antifungal treatment within the 5 days following their initiation [26]. Proven and suspected fungal infections were defined according to the revised criteria of the European Organization for Research and Treatment of invasive fungal infections Cooperative Group (EORTC) [27]. All patients hospitalized for more than 5 days and requiring systemic antifungal treatment for the first documented or suspected invasive *Candida* infection during their ICU stay were eligible. Patients receiving prophylactic antifungal treatment were excluded, as well as those with suspected mold infection, or neutropenia.

Study objectives

The primary objective was to evaluate the factors independently associated with antifungal de-escalation. Secondary objectives were to evaluate the incidence of de-escalation of antifungal treatment, and its impact on ICU length of stay, duration of mechanical ventilation, and mortality.

Data collection

All data were retrospectively recorded from archived medical records of University Hospital of Lille and its mycology laboratory. Patients were identified using the electronic pharmacy database setup to guide and monitor antifungal prescriptions. Only first episodes of proven or suspected invasive *Candida* infection were considered. Initial antifungal treatment was based on local guidelines, driven from international guidelines [28].

The following characteristics were recorded at ICU admission: age, gender, severity of acute illness based on simplified acute physiology score (SAPS) II, comorbidities (diabetes, chronic obstructive pulmonary disease (COPD), chronic heart failure, cirrhosis, chronic renal failure requiring dialysis, or immunosuppression), location before ICU admission, admission category (medical or surgical), reason for ICU admission (acute exacerbation of COPD, acute respiratory distress syndrome, pneumonia, congestive heart failure, neurologic failure, poisoning, shock, and infection), and prior antibiotic or antifungal treatment used in the last 3 months. During ICU stay, data were collected on type of antifungal treatment (empirical, preemptive, or curative), suspected (probable and possible categories of the EORTC definitions) or proven invasive *Candida* infection, successive antifungal treatments prescribed, duration of each antifungal treatment, total duration of antifungal therapy, and appropriateness of the initial antifungal treatment. The following data were collected regarding de-escalation: date of onset and reasons for de-escalation. We also collected the results of mycological cultures from sterile sites (blood, cerebrospinal, pleural, peritoneal and pericardial fluid, surgical site) and the sites usually checked for the multifocal colonization status (skin, urine, trachea, catheter, anus), and data on antibiotic treatment, severe sepsis, total parenteral nutrition, surgery, renal replacement therapy, length of mechanical ventilation, duration of treatment with vasoactive drugs, length of ICU stay, occurrence of apyrexia, ICU, and 30-day and 1-year mortality.

Statistical analysis

SPSS software (SPSS, Chicago, IL, USA) was used for data analysis. Categorical variables were described as frequency (%). Kolmogorov–Smirnov test was used to evaluate the distribution of continuous variables. Normally distributed and skewed continuous variables were described as mean ± standard deviation (SD), or as median and interquartile range (IQR), respectively.

To determine factors associated with de-escalation, patients with de-escalation were compared with those with no de-escalation using univariate and multivariate analyses. Student's *t* test or the Mann–Whitney *U* test was used to compare normally distributed and skewed continuous variables, respectively. The Chi-square (χ^2) test or Fischer's exact test was used to compare qualitative variables, as appropriate. The odds ratio (OR) and 95% confidence interval (CI) were calculated for all qualitative variables significant in univariate analysis and for all variables significant in multivariate analysis. Differences were considered significant if p values were < 0.05, with two-tailed tests. Exposure to potential factors associated with antifungal de-escalation was considered until the occurrence of de-escalation, or until ICU discharge in patients with no de-escalation. All variables with p values < 0.2 by univariate analysis were included in a backward multivariate logistic regression model. Potential interactions were tested, and the Hosmer–Lemeshow goodness of fit and *c*-statistics were calculated. Cox proportional hazards models were performed to determine factors associated with ICU mortality.

Results

Among the 582 patients hospitalized for > 5 days during the study period, 244 (42%) patients received antifungal treatment. Fifty-four (22%) patients were excluded, because they received prophylactic antifungal treatment ($n = 18$, 8%), had suspected filamentous fungal infection ($n = 20$, 8%), or were neutropenic ($n = 16$, 7%). The remaining 190 patients were all included in the study (Fig. 1). One hundred and five (55%), 52 (27%), and 46 (24%) patients received empirical, preemptive, and targeted treatment, respectively. Caspofungin ($n = 101$, 53%), fluconazole ($n = 81$, 43%), voriconazole ($n = 7$, 4%), and liposomal amphotericin B ($n = 1$, 0.5%) were the most frequently used antifungals.

Patient characteristics and incidence of de-escalation

De-escalation was performed in 38 (20%) of the 190 included patients. Initial antifungal treatment was stopped in 19 (50%) patients within 5 days and switched to an azole in 19 (50%) patients. Reasons for de-escalation were susceptible strain based on antifungal

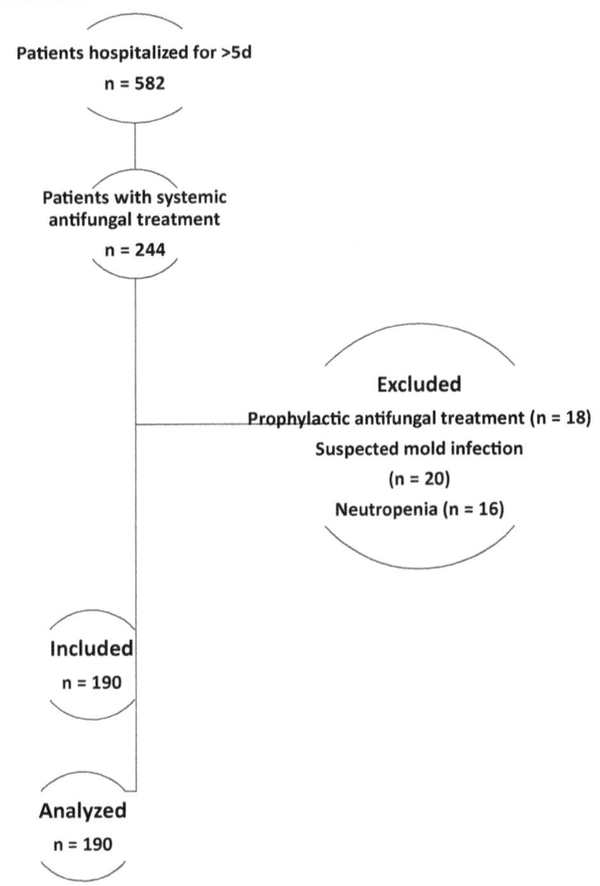

Fig. 1 Patient flowchart

susceptibility testing in 16 (42%) patients, proven bacterial infection with no evidence for fungal infection in 10 (26%) patients, and negative mycological investigations in 12 (32%) patients.

Patient characteristics are presented in Table 1.

Mycological results

Thirty-four (18%) of the 187 samples taken from sterile sites were positive, of which 26 (76%) were positive to *Candida albicans*, 2 (6%) to *Candida glabrata*, and 6 (18%) to other *Candida* species. Of 192 samples taken from non-sterile sites, 170 (89%) samples were positive, including 99 (58%) to *C. albicans*, 27 (16%) to *C. parapsilosis*, 20 (12%) to *C. glabrata*, 17 (10%) to *C. tropicalis*, and 7 (4%) to other *Candida* species.

Table 1 Characteristics of study patients at ICU admission

Characteristics	De-escalation		*p*
	Yes ($n=38$)	No ($n=152$)	
Age, years	63 [56–68]	63 [55–72]	0.57
Female gender *n* (%)	8 (21)	55 (36)	0.067
SAPS II	49 [30–68]	54 [36–71]	0.38
Comorbidities *n* (%)			
Diabetes	8 (21)	30 (20)	0.87
COPD	9 (24)	33 (22)	0.79
Chronic heart failure	8 (21)	30 (20)	0.87
Cirrhosis	4 (11)	10 (6)	0.49
Chronic dialysis	9 (24)	14 (9)	0.014*
Immunosuppression *n* (%)			
Chemotherapy	7 (18)	13 (9)	0.076
Corticosteroid therapy	9 (24)	29 (19)	0.53
Transfer from			0.66
Home	4 (11)	21 (14)	
Other wards	25 (66)	104 (68)	
Other ICUs	9 (24)	27 (18)	
Admission category			0.75
Medical	22 (58)	98 (64)	
Surgical	15 (39)	51 (34)	
Other (trauma, burn)	1 (3)	3 (2)	
Cause for ICU admission			
Acute exacerbation of COPD	3 (8)	26 (17)	0.16
Acute respiratory distress syndrome	12 (32)	41 (27)	0.57
Community-acquired pneumonia	11 (29)	32 (21)	0.30
Hospital-acquired pneumonia	6 (16)	38 (25)	0.23
Congestive heart failure	0 (0)	7 (5)	0.18
Neurologic failure	0 (0)	7 (5)	0.18
Poisoning	1 (3)	15 (10)	0.15
Septic shock	22 (58)	89 (59)	0.94
Infection at ICU admission	37 (97)	135 (89)	0.17
Prior antibiotic treatment	16 (42)	69 (45)	0.72
Prior antifungal treatment	5 (13)	15 (10)	0.56

Data are N (%), or median (interquartile range)

COPD chronic obstructive pulmonary disease, *ICU* intensive care unit, *SAPS* simplified acute physiology score

* Odds ratio (95% confidence interval) 3.1 (1.21–7.74)

Factors associated with antifungal de-escalation

By univariate analysis, factors associated with higher rate of de-escalation were chronic dialysis, negative mycological samples, proven bacterial infection, apyrexia for >72 h, and vasoactive drug discontinuation at 72 h after initiation of antifungal treatment. Multifocal *Candida* colonization, preemptive treatment, and mechanical ventilation were associated with significantly lower rate of de-escalation (Tables 1 and 2). By multivariate analysis, only mechanical ventilation was independently associated with de-escalation (OR 0.25 (95% CI 0.08–0.74), $p=0.023$; Hosmer–Lemeshow goodness-of-fit test, $p=0.95$, *c*-statistics 0.85).

Impact of de-escalation on outcomes

There was no significant impact of de-escalation on ICU length of stay, duration of mechanical ventilation, ICU mortality, 30-day mortality, or 1-year mortality rate (Table 3). In multivariable Cox proportional hazards model, only SAPS II and catecholamines withdrawal at day 3 were independently associated with ICU mortality, even when de-escalation was forced in the model (Table 4).

Discussion

Our results suggest that de-escalation is performed in 20% of critically ill patients receiving empirical, preemptive, or targeted antifungal treatment for suspected or proven invasive *Candida* infection. Mechanical ventilation was the only factor independently associated with lower rates of de-escalation of antifungal treatment. No negative impact of de-escalation was found on duration of mechanical ventilation, ICU length of stay, ICU mortality, 28-day mortality, or 1-year mortality rates.

The incidence of de-escalation of antifungal treatment in our study is in line with that reported recently by Bailly et al. (22%) [26]. In another recent retrospective study performed in 262 critically ill patients receiving empirical or targeted antifungal treatment, the incidence of de-escalation was lower at 10% [29]. Azoulay et al. performed a large multicenter cross-sectional one-day study to determine the incidence of ICU patients without documented antifungal infection who receive antifungals. Antifungal treatment was used in 154 (7.5%) of study patients, including 100 (65%) patients without documented fungal infection. These results suggest that de-escalation of antifungal treatment could probably be performed in a larger proportion of critically ill patients.

Table 2 Patient characteristics during ICU stay

Characteristics	De-escalation		p	OR [95% CI]
	Yes ($n=38$)	No ($n=152$)		
Multifocal colonization	19 (50)	115 (76)	0.002	0.32 [0.15–0.67]
Negative yeast samples	16 (42)	30 (20)	0.004	2.95 [1.4–6.3]
Empirical antifungal treatment	12 (32)	68 (45)	0.14	
Preemptive antifungal treatment	4 (11)	48 (32)	0.008	0.26 [0.09–0.78]
Targeted antifungal treatment	10 (26)	36 (24)	0.73	
Proven bacterial infection	10 (26)	0 (0)	<0.001	NA
Apyrexia >72 h	37 (97)	123 (81)	0.013	8.7 [1.2–66]
Catecholamine withdrawal at 72 h	29 (76)	89 (59)	0.026	2.57 [1.1–5.98]
Mechanical ventilation	30 (79)	142 (93)	0.006	0.26 [0.09–0.73]
Antibiotic treatment	38 (100)	150 (99)	0.96	
Total parenteral nutrition	18 (47)	81 (53)	0.51	
Surgery	21 (55)	76 (50)	0.56	
Renal replacement therapy	21 (55)	76 (50)	0.56	
Shock	31 (82)	121 (80)	0.79	

Data are N (%)

CI confidence interval, *OR* odds ratio

Table 3 Impact of de-escalation on outcome

Characteristics	De-escalation		p
	Yes ($n=38$)	No ($n=152$)	
Length of ICU stay	25 [14–40]	25 [14–40]	0.99
Duration of mechanical ventilation	22 [5–31]	20 [10–35]	0.43
Total duration of antifungal treatment	6 [5–18]	13 [7–25]	0.023
ICU mortality	17 (45)	89 (59)	0.13
30-day mortality	9 (24)	56 (37)	0.13
1-year mortality	21 (55)	97 (64)	0.33

Data are *N* (%), or median (interquartile range)

Invasive mechanical ventilation was the only factor independently associated with lower rates of de-escalation of antifungal treatment. This result could be related to the higher severity of patients receiving invasive mechanical ventilation, which might have prevented attending physicians from de-escalating antifungal treatment. The superiority of echinocandins over fluconazole has been demonstrated in a single head-to-head clinical trial of anidulafungin that showed significantly better overall response rates (76 vs. 60%; $p=0.01$) [30]. A further post hoc analysis showed better global responses (70.8 vs. 54.1%) and reduced 14-day all-cause mortality (10.1 vs. 20.3%, $p=0.08$) in critically ill patients [31]. However, a recent large multicenter observational study,

Table 4 Factors associated with ICU mortality by Cox proportional hazards models

Factors	Univariate analysis		Multivariate analysis	
	HR (95% CI)	p	HR (95% CI)	p
At ICU admission				
SAPS II	1.01* (1.004–1.02)	0.005	1.01* (1–1.02)	0.040
Surgical patients	0.46 (0.3–0.69)	<0.001	–	–
ARDS	1.81 (1.22–2.68)	0.003	–	–
During ICU stay				
Renal replacement therapy	1.64 (1.1–2.47)	0.018	–	–
Preemptive antifungal treatment	0.50 (0.32–0.80)	0.004	–	–
Apyrexia >72 h	0.36 (0.23–0.57)	<0.001	–	–
Catecholamine withdrawal at 72 h	0.35 (0.27–0.52)	<0.001	0.47 (0.29–0.76)	0.002
De-escalation of antifungal treatment**	0.75 (0.44–1.26)	0.28	–	–

ICU intensive care medicine, *SAPS* simplified acute physiology score, *ARDS* acute respiratory distress syndrome

* Per point of SAPS II; *HR* hazard ratio, *CI* confidence interval

** De-escalation of antifungal treatment was forced in the final Cox model using a propensity-score derived analysis, did not report increased mortality using fluconazole as empirical or targeted treatment, as compared with echinocandins, in adult patients with candidemia [32]. Similar results were also reported in the subgroup of patients with sepsis or septic shock.

Recent observational and randomized controlled studies have questioned the beneficial effects of empirical antifungal treatment on mortality, even in patients in septic shock with high colonization index [33, 34]. However, the randomized controlled EMPIRICUS trial found significantly reduced rate of invasive candidiasis in patients who received micafungin, as compared with those who received placebo [34]. Our results suggest that de-escalation of antifungal treatment is safe. Overall, our results confirm previous studies, suggesting that early de-escalation to azole is possible and safe. For proven invasive *Candida* infection, three studies reported that de-escalation is safe in *Candida spp.* fluconazole-sensitive infections [24, 25, 35]. Bailly et al. [26] also reported that de-escalation could be safely performed in critically ill patients, as no negative impact was found on ICU mortality, duration of mechanical ventilation, or length of ICU stay. In addition, antifungal de-escalation was associated with significant decrease in the antifungal consumption, which might be helpful in reducing toxicity, drug interaction, fungal resistance, and cost [36]. A recent randomized controlled trial aimed to determine the usefulness of fungal biomarkers in early discontinuation of empirical antifungal treatment [37]. Patients were randomized to receive routine care (control group) or biomarker-based strategy (intervention group), in which a recommendation was given based on (1,3)-β-D-glucan, mannan, and anti-mannan serum assays performed on day 0 and day 4. The percentage of patients with early discontinuation of empirical antifungal treatment was significantly higher in intervention, compared with control group (54 vs. 2%, $p < 0.0001$), with no negative impact on mortality or morbidity. However, this open-label study was performed in a single center, and patients with immunosuppression were excluded. Therefore, further randomized controlled trials are needed to confirm these results.

Our study has some limitations. First, it was a retrospective study performed in a single center. Therefore, our results could not be generalized and further prospective multicenter studies are needed to confirm these findings. Second, the number of patients with de-escalation was relatively low. Therefore, analysis of subgroups with early stop, or reduction in antifungal spectrum was not possible. Third, potential benefit of de-escalation of antifungal treatment on cost was not evaluated. However, given the significant reduction in duration of antifungal treatment of 6 days in patients with de-escalation, compared with those with no de-escalation, a lower cost could be expected in these patients. Finally, no data were collected on dose or duration of corticosteroids. Corticosteroids use is a risk factor for invasive Candida infection and could impact on prognosis of patients with these infections. However, it is unlikely that corticosteroids have influenced de-escalation of antifungal treatment.

Conclusions

De-escalation was performed in 20% of patients receiving systemic antifungals for suspected invasive *Candida* infection. Invasive mechanical ventilation was independently associated with reduced de-escalation of antifungal treatment. De-escalation was associated with decreased antifungal treatment duration. De-escalation of antifungal treatment seems to be feasible and safe in critically ill patients. However, further large prospective studies are required to confirm these findings.

Authors' contributions

KJ and SN designed the study. KJ and MC collected the data. SN performed the statistical analysis. KF and SN wrote the manuscript. All authors participated in the final revision of the manuscript. All authors read and approved the final manuscript.

Author details

[1] Critical Care Center, CHU Lille, 59000 Lille, France. [2] U995-LIRIC-Lille Inflammation Research International Center, Univ. Lille, 59000 Lille, France. [3] Inserm, U995, 59000 Lille, France. [4] Laboratory of Mycology and Parasitology, CHU Lille, 59000 Lille, France.

Acknowledgments

None.

Competing interests

SN, Medtronic, and MSD (lecture); CielMedical and Bayer (advisory board); other authors: none.

Funding

None.

References

1. León C, Ostrosky-Zeichner L, Schuster M. What's new in the clinical and diagnostic management of invasive candidiasis in critically ill patients. Intensive Care Med. 2014;40:808–19.
2. Lortholary O, Renaudat C, Sitbon K, Madec Y, Denoeud-Ndam L, Wolff M, et al. Worrisome trends in incidence and mortality of candidemia in intensive care units (Paris area, 2002–2010). Intensive Care Med. 2014;40:1303–12.
3. Leroy O, Bailly S, Gangneux J-P, Mira J-P, Devos P, Dupont H, et al. Systemic antifungal therapy for proven or suspected invasive candidiasis: the AmarCAND 2 study. Ann Intensive Care. 2016;6:2.
4. Vincent J-L, Rello J, Marshall J, Silva E, Anzueto A, Martin CD, et al. International study of the prevalence and outcomes of infection in intensive care units. JAMA. 2009;302:2323–9.

5. Kett DH, Azoulay E, Echeverria PM, Vincent J-L. Candida bloodstream infections in intensive care units: analysis of the extended prevalence of infection in intensive care unit study. Crit Care Med. 2011;39:665–70.
6. Bassetti M, Righi E, Ansaldi F, Merelli M, Trucchi C, Cecilia T, et al. A multicenter study of septic shock due to candidemia: outcomes and predictors of mortality. Intensive Care Med. 2014;40:839–45.
7. Ostrosky-Zeichner L, Kullberg BJ, Bow EJ, Hadley S, León C, Nucci M, et al. Early treatment of candidemia in adults: a review. Med Mycol. 2011;49:113–20.
8. Ostrosky-Zeichner L. Invasive mycoses: diagnostic challenges. Am J Med. 2012;125:S14–24.
9. León C, Álvarez-Lerma F, Ruiz-Santana S, León MÁ, Nolla J, Jordá R, et al. Fungal colonization and/or infection in non-neutropenic critically ill patients: results of the EPCAN observational study. Eur J Clin Microbiol Infect Dis. 2009;28:233–42.
10. Arvanitis M, Anagnostou T, Fuchs BB, Caliendo AM, Mylonakis E. Molecular and nonmolecular diagnostic methods for invasive fungal infections. Clin Microbiol Rev. 2014;27:490–526.
11. Clancy CJ, Nguyen MH. Finding the "missing 50%" of invasive candidiasis: how nonculture diagnostics will improve understanding of disease spectrum and transform patient care. Clin Infect Dis. 2013;56:1284–92.
12. Kollef M, Micek S, Hampton N, Doherty JA, Kumar A. Septic shock attributed to Candida infection: importance of empiric therapy and source control. Clin Infect Dis. 2012;54:1739–46.
13. Pappas PG, Kauffman CA, Andes DR, Clancy CJ, Marr KA, Ostrosky-Zeichner L, et al. Clinical practice guideline for the management of candidiasis: 2016 update by the infectious diseases society of America. Clin Infect Dis. 2016;62:e1–50.
14. Azoulay E, Dupont H, Tabah A, Lortholary O, Stahl J-P, Francais A, et al. Systemic antifungal therapy in critically ill patients without invasive fungal infection. Crit Care Med. 2012;40:813–22.
15. Arendrup MC, Dzajic E, Jensen RH, Johansen HK, Kjaeldgaard P, Knudsen JD, et al. Epidemiological changes with potential implication for antifungal prescription recommendations for fungaemia: data from a nationwide fungaemia surveillance programme. Clin Microbiol Infect. 2013;19:E343–53.
16. Ostrosky-Zeichner L. Candida glabrata and FKS mutations: witnessing the emergence of the true multidrug-resistant Candida. Clin Infect Dis. 2013;56:1733–4.
17. Lortholary O, Desnos-Ollivier M, Sitbon K, Fontanet A, Bretagne S, Dromer F, et al. Recent exposure to caspofungin or fluconazole influences the epidemiology of candidemia: a prospective multicenter study involving 2,441 patients. Antimicrob Agents Chemother. 2011;55:532–8.
18. Dannaoui E, Desnos-Ollivier M, Garcia-Hermoso D, Grenouillet F, Cassaing S, Baixench M-T, et al. *Candida* spp. with acquired echinocandin resistance, France, 2004–2010. Emerg Infect Dis. 2012;18:86–90.
19. Drgona L, Khachatryan A, Stephens J, Charbonneau C, Kantecki M, Haider S, et al. Clinical and economic burden of invasive fungal diseases in Europe: focus on pre-emptive and empirical treatment of Aspergillus and Candida species. Eur J Clin Microbiol Infect Dis. 2014;33:7–21. https://doi.org/10.1007/s10096-013-1944-3.
20. Valerio M, Rodriguez-Gonzalez CG, Munoz P, Caliz B, Sanjurjo M, Bouza E, et al. Evaluation of antifungal use in a tertiary care institution: antifungal stewardship urgently needed. J Antimicrob Chemother. 2014;69:1993–9.
21. Playford EG, Webster AC, Sorrell TC, Craig JC. Antifungal agents for preventing fungal infections in non-neutropenic critically ill and surgical patients: systematic review and meta-analysis of randomized clinical trials. J Antimicrob Chemother. 2006;57:628–38.
22. Schuster MG, Edwards JE, Sobel JD, Darouiche RO, Karchmer AW, Hadley S, et al. Empirical fluconazole versus placebo for intensive care unit patients: a randomized trial. Ann Intern Med. 2008;149:83–90.
23. Cornely OA, Bassetti M, Calandra T, Garbino J, Kullberg BJ, Lortholary O, et al. ESCMID guideline for the diagnosis and management of Candida diseases 2012: non-neutropenic adult patients. Clin Microbiol Infect. 2012;18:19–37.
24. Takesue Y, Ueda T, Mikamo H, Oda S, Takakura S, Kitagawa Y, et al. Management bundles for candidaemia: the impact of compliance on clinical outcomes. J Antimicrob Chemother [Internet]. 2015;70:587–93.
25. Vazquez J, Reboli AC, Pappas PG, Patterson TF, Reinhardt J, Chin-Hong P, et al. Evaluation of an early step-down strategy from intravenous anidulafungin to oral azole therapy for the treatment of candidemia and other forms of invasive candidiasis: results from an open-label trial. BMC Infect Dis. 2014;14:97.
26. Bailly S, Leroy O, Montravers P, Constantin J-M, Dupont H, Guillemot D, et al. Antifungal de-escalation was not associated with adverse outcome in critically ill patients treated for invasive candidiasis: post hoc analyses of the AmarCAND2 study data. Intensive Care Med. 2015;41:1931–40. https://doi.org/10.1007/s00134-015-4053-1.
27. De Pauw B, Walsh TJ, Donnelly JP, Stevens DA, Edwards JE, Calandra T, et al. Revised definitions of invasive fungal disease from the European Organization for Research and Treatment of Cancer/Invasive Fungal Infections Cooperative Group and the National Institute of Allergy and Infectious Diseases Mycoses Study Group (EORTC/MSG) Consensus Group. Clin Infect Dis. 2008;46:1813–21. https://doi.org/10.1086/588660.
28. Pappas PG, Kauffman CA, Andes D, Benjamin DK Jr, Calandra TF, Edwards JE Jr, et al. Clinical practice guidelines for the management of candidiasis: 2009 update by the infectious diseases society of America. Clin Infect Dis. 2009;48:503–35.
29. Zein M, Parmentier-Decrucq E, Kalaoun A, Bouton O, Wallyn F, Baranzelli A, et al. Factors predicting prolonged empirical antifungal treatment in critically ill patients. Ann Clin Microbiol Antimicrob. 2014;13:11.
30. Reboli AC, Rotstein C, Pappas PG, Chapman SW, Kett DH, Kumar D, et al. Anidulafungin versus fluconazole for invasive candidiasis. N Engl J Med. 2007;356:2472–82. https://doi.org/10.1056/NEJMoa066906.
31. Kett DH, Shorr AF, Reboli AC, Reisman AL, Biswas P, Schlamm HT. Anidulafungin compared with fluconazole in severely ill patients with candidemia and other forms of invasive candidiasis: support for the 2009 IDSA treatment guidelines for candidiasis. Crit Care. 2011;15:R253. https://doi.org/10.1186/cc10514.
32. López-Cortés LE, Almirante B, Cuenca-Estrella M, Garnacho-Montero J, Padilla B, Puig-Asensio M, et al. Empirical and targeted therapy of candidemia with fluconazole versus echinocandins: a propensity score-derived analysis of a population-based, multicentre prospective cohort. Clin Microbiol Infect. 2016;22(733):e1–8.
33. Bailly S, Bouadma L, Azoulay E, Orgeas MG, Adrie C, Souweine B, et al. Failure of empirical systemic antifungal therapy in mechanically ventilated critically ill patients. Am J Respir Crit Care Med. 2015;191:1139–46. https://doi.org/10.1164/rccm.201409-1701OC.
34. Timsit J-F, Azoulay E, Schwebel C, Charles PE, Cornet M, Souweine B, et al. Empirical micafungin treatment and survival without invasive fungal infection in adults with ICU-acquired sepsis, *Candida* colonization, and multiple organ failure. JAMA. 2016;316:1555.
35. Bal AM, Shankland GS, Scott G, Imtiaz T, Macaulay R, McGill M. Antifungal step-down therapy based on hospital intravenous to oral switch policy and susceptibility testing in adult patients with candidaemia: a single centre experience. Int J Clin Pract. 2014;68:20–7.
36. Rouzé A, Jaffal K, Nseir S. How could we reduce antifungal treatment in the intensive care unit. World J Clin Infect Dis. 2015;5:55–8.
37. Rouzé A, Loridant S, Poissy J, Dervaux B, Sendid B, Cornu M, et al. Biomarker-based strategy for early discontinuation of empirical antifungal treatment in critically ill patients: a randomized controlled trial. Intensive Care Med. 2017;43(11):1668–77.

11

High level of venous thromboembolism in critically ill trauma patients despite early and well-driven thromboprophylaxis protocol

S. R. Hamada[1*], C. Espina[2], T. Guedj[3], R. Buaron[3], A. Harrois[1], S. Figueiredo[1] and J. Duranteau[1]

Abstract

Background: Venous thromboembolism (VTE) is one of the most common preventable causes of in-hospital death in trauma patients surviving their injuries. We assessed the prevalence, incidence and risk factors for deep venous thrombosis (DVT) and pulmonary embolism (PE) in critically ill trauma patients, in the setting of a mature and early mechanical and pharmacological thromboprophylaxis protocol.

Methods: This was a prospective observational study on a cohort of patients from a surgical intensive care unit of a university level 1 trauma centre. We enrolled consecutive primary trauma patients expected to be in intensive care for ≥48 h. Thromboprophylaxis was protocol driven. DVT screening was performed by duplex ultrasound of upper and lower extremities within the first 48 h, between 5 and 7 days and then weekly until discharge. We recorded VTE risk factors at baseline and on each examination day. Independent risk factors were analysed using a multivariate logistic regression.

Results: In 153 patients with a mean Injury Severity Score of 23 ± 12, the prevalence of VTE was 30.7%, 95 CI [23.7–38.8] (29.4% DVT and 4.6% PE). The incidence was 18%, 95 CI [14–24] patients-week. The median time of apparition of DVT was 6 days [1; 4]. The global protocol compliance was 77.8% with a median time of introduction of the pharmacological prophylaxis of 1 day [1; 2]. We identified four independent risk factors for VTE: central venous catheter (OR 4.39, 95 CI [1.1–29]), medullar injury (OR 5.59, 95 CI [1.7–12.9]), initial systolic arterial pressure <80 mmHg (OR 3.64, 95 CI [1.3–10.8]), and pelvic fracture (OR 3.04, 95 CI [1.2–7.9]).

Conclusion: Despite a rigorous, protocol-driven thromboprophylaxis, critically ill trauma patients showed a high incidence of VTE. Further research is needed to tailor pharmacological prophylaxis and balance the risks and benefits.

Keywords: Severe trauma, Venous thromboembolism, Risk factors, Thromboprophylaxis, Duplex ultrasound

Background

Venous thromboembolism (VTE), comprising deep venous thrombosis (DVT) and pulmonary embolism (PE), is a potentially life-threatening complication in severe and multiple trauma patients [1]. It is one of the most common preventable causes of in-hospital death in trauma patients surviving their injuries [2]. It remains a challenging issue for the clinician as the clinical clues are rough and found in less than 5% of patients [3, 4], and the treatment should be balanced between risks and benefits [5, 6].

A number of risk factors and injury patterns have been identified to predict the occurrence of VTE [7, 8]. From the endothelial damage [9], to the activation of the coagulation system enhanced by the inflammatory state in association with hypotension, immobilization, stasis [10–12], and procoagulant therapies [13, 14], the whole system is unbalanced towards a predominant prohaemostatic state that remains for several days. As a consequence, VTE prophylaxis has to be started early and should combine mechanical and chemical prophylaxis

*Correspondence: sophiehamada@hotmail.com
[1] Department of Anaesthesia and Critical Care, AP-HP, Hôpital Bicêtre, Hôpitaux Universitaires Paris Sud, University Paris-Sud, 78 rue du Général Leclerc, 94275 Le Kremlin Bicêtre, France
Full list of author information is available at the end of the article

[15]. Some guidelines are available to help the clinicians, but the level of evidence remains fairly low [5, 8]. Recent literature nevertheless tends to push forward early chemical thromboprophylaxis, tempering the fears of haemorrhagic complications, especially in the setting of solid organ and brain injuries [16].

The aim of this study was to assess the epidemiology of DVT and associated PE by repeated compression duplex ultrasound (DUS), in severe trauma patients in the setting of a rigorous and early mechanical and pharmacological thromboprophylaxis protocol.

Methods

This prospective, 1-year observational study took place between February 2015 and 2016 in Bicêtre hospital, an academic level 1 trauma centre on the southern edge of Paris, with a 28-bed surgical and trauma intensive care unit (ICU), which receives an average of 500 suspected severe trauma patients per year. The local institutional review board approved the study and waived the need for informed consent ("Comité de Protection des Personnes", No. SC 14-019). Patients and families were informed of the protocol. All consecutive trauma patients directly admitted in the ICU trauma room, were assessed and included if they were more than 18 years old and were expected to be in ICU for more than 48 h. Patients transferred from the emergency department or from another hospital were not included.

Protocol

The local thromboprophylaxis protocol is extensively described in Appendix 1. DVT screening and follow-up were performed by DUS within the first 48 h, between 5 and 7 days and then weekly until ICU discharge. Both upper and lower extremities were examined: the internal jugular, subclavian, axillary, common femoral, superficial femoral and popliteal veins. Common iliac, internal and external iliac veins were also evaluated when possible (if no gas screen impeding penetration of US). A high-frequency transducer (5–10 MHz) was mostly used for upper extremities, but a 2–5-MHz transducer could also be used for lower extremities and abdominal imaging if necessary (Vivid I, GEMS Ultrasound, Tirat Carmel, Israel). The criteria to consider the diagnosis of a DVT were: non-compressibility of the vein (partial or total), direct visualization of the thrombus in the vein lumen and the absence of coloured or continuous Doppler flow. Each identified thrombus was categorized as "non-occlusive/mural", "floating" or "occlusive". Pulmonary embolism was diagnosed on CT angiography according to clinical suspicion.

For the purpose of the study, two practitioners (SH and CE) already experienced in ultrasound (US) imaging, received a complementary training with a radiologist specialized in US vascular imaging (TG) (10 complete examinations combined with theory). Every DVT diagnosis by SH and CE was confirmed by the radiologist (TG) either by a direct control or through several sequential video recordings.

To overcome some limitations of DUS screening, we planned a blind proofreading focused on DVT and PE of all contrast CT scans (including the initial injury assessment whole body CT scan with a biphasic injection) undergone by all patients enrolled in the study. A single, independent radiologist (RB) blinded of any medical history performed all the CT scan reviews.

All data were collected prospectively (Appendix 2).

Endpoints

The primary clinical endpoints were the prevalence and incidence of VTE (DUS diagnosed DVT and PE) in our cohort of trauma patients admitted in the surgical ICU.

The secondary endpoints were the calculation of the total prevalence of VTE with CT scan re-readings, the analysis of risk factors (among clinical factors, resuscitative strategies, transfusion and prophylaxis), morbidity and mortality analysis of VTE and early thromboprophylactic strategies.

Statistical analysis

Quantitative data are expressed as mean ± standard deviation or median [quartile 1; 3] according to their distribution. Categorical data are expressed as numbers and percentages. Two groups were identified: patients with VTE (group VTE+) and patients without any VTE (group VTE−). Statistical tests used for the univariate analysis were Student's *t* test, Mann–Whitney test, Chi-square or Fisher's exact test according to their validity conditions. For incidence and timing calculation, we only considered the first episode of DVT or PE. The probability of developing a VTE was estimated using a Kaplan–Meier method. Patients who died of other cause than VTE and patient who were discharged from the ICU were censored in the analysis. A multiple logistic regression was performed according to the standards and respectfully of validity conditions, to identify independent risk factors for VTE. The calibration (Hosmer–Lemeshow statistic) and discrimination (area under the curve, AUC) were calculated, and the model internally validated using a bootstrap methodology [17]. All variables were tested for interactions and collinearity. The variables were chosen for their clinical relevance and their pragmatism for daily use, prohibiting any pre-existing clinical score to enter into the model. They were chosen a priori if they were associated with VTE on the univariate analysis with a $p < 0.1$ and then assessed by a forward stepwise analysis to preserve a number of event-to-variable ratio around 10. The missing data were <1%.

All statistical analysis was performed using R 3.2.1 software (http://www.R-project.org/) and using a $p < 0.05$ as significant.

Results

Over the 513 trauma patients admitted in 1 year, 153 were included in the analysis (flow chart displayed in Fig. 1). Demographic and clinical characteristics of the cohort are presented in Table 1.

Primary endpoint

A total of 59 DVTs were diagnosed with DUS and one with CT angiography in 46 patients (30.1%). Eleven patients developed more than one DVT (average 1.3, maximum 4). Seven patients presented a PE (4.6%), including one patient having no DVT found on control examinations. So the prevalence of at least one episode of VTE in our cohort over the studied period was 30.7%, CI 95 [24–39] (47 patients), with a calculated incidence of 18%, CI 95 [14–24] patients-week (18 patients over 100 are diagnosed with VTE over a 1-week ICU follow-up).

Deep venous thrombosis (DVT)

The majority of DVT was asymptomatic (56/60, 93%). The median time of apparition of DVT was 6 days [1; 4]. The Kaplan–Meier curve of probability of presenting a VTE is displayed in Fig. 2. Patients were followed during a median of 7 days [4; 17]. Eighteen DVT (40%) disappeared during their follow-up in a median time of 22 days [13; 25]. The diagnosed DVT was essentially located in the femoral and internal jugular vein as presented in Fig. 3. The types of thrombus found on DUS were categorized as "non-occlusive/mural" in 81.4% ($n = 48$), "floating" in 11.9% ($n = 7$) and "occlusive" in 6.7% ($n = 4$).

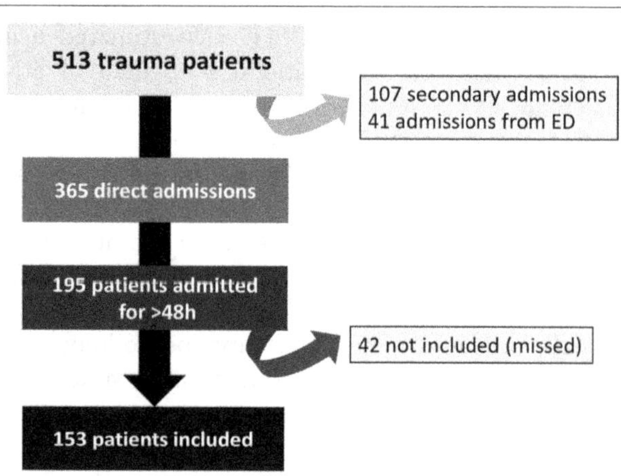

Fig. 1 Flow chart of the study. Patients missed because length of stay was underestimated, or because the investigators of the study were not present during the first 48 h of inclusion

Table 1 Demographic and clinical characteristics of included patients

Variable	All patients ($n = 153$)
Demographic characteristics	
Age (years)	44.6 ± 19.4
Sex (male)	72% (110)
BMI (kg/m²)	26.1 ± 6.5
Mechanism of injury	
MVA	26% (39)
Motorbike accident	21% (37)
Fall from high	25% (32)
Severity scores	
SOFA 24 h	6.4 ± 4.7
SAPS 2	34.9 ± 19.2
ISS	23.7 ± 12.7
Clinical presentation	
Initial GCS	12.4 ± 3.9
Vasopressor on day 1	22% (34)
RAP score	11.1 ± 5.6
ICU length of stay (days)	7 [4, 17]
Hospital length of stay (days)	26.5 ± 22. 9
Initiation of thromboprophylaxis (days)	2 ± 1
Mortality	11.8% (18)

Data expressed as mean ± SD or median [quartile 1; 3] according to distribution

Categorical variables expressed as percentage (*n*)

BMI body mass index, *MVA* motor vehicle accident, *ICU* intensive care unit, *GCS* Glasgow Coma Score, *SOFA* Sequential Organ Failure Assessment Score, *SAPS 2* Simplified Acute Physiology Score 2, *ISS* Injury Severity Score, *RAP score* Risk Assessment Profile

Deep venous thrombosis and catheters

Three-fourth of DVTs (44/59) were diagnosed on the location of a central venous catheter (CVC), either on site or within the week following its withdrawal. The details of the association between DVT and CVC are presented in Table 2. Among the DVT unrelated to CVC ($n = 16$, 25.4%), seven were found in the femoral vein, eight in the internal jugular and one in the subclavian vein. The median time of apparition of DVT was 8 days [4; 12] when developing on CVC and 5.5 days [1.5; 12] when developing out of CVC.

Deep venous thrombosis and anticoagulants

The compliance with the local thromboprophylaxis protocol was observed in 119 patients (77.8%). The median time of introduction of the anticoagulant prophylaxis was 1 day [1; 2], with 80.4% ($n = 123$) of the patients receiving their first injection within the initial 48 h. Only four

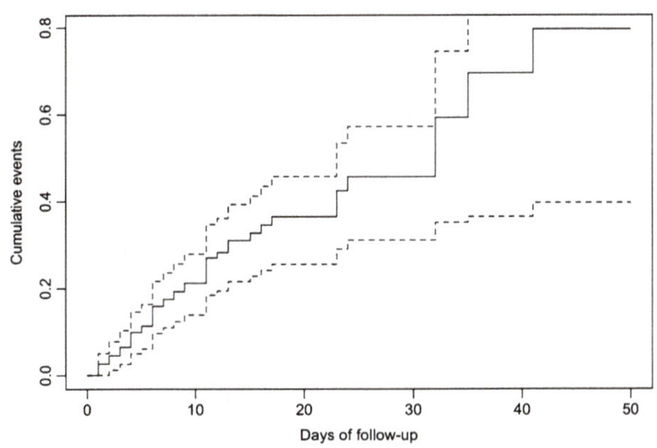

Fig. 2 Kaplan–Meier curve of cumulative thromboembolic events in the cohort. We decided to include all patients presenting even with early diagnosis of DVT (within 48 h) as none of them had known risk factors (past medical history of DVT, or family history, cancer, obesity), nor any symptoms identified before admission. They were severely injured patients and had either extended vehicle extrication time or prolonged surgery with potentially compression mechanism

patients (2.6%) received the first injection after the 96th hour. LMW heparin accounted for 86.9% of the initial prescription ($n = 133$), when unfractionated heparin represented 11.8% ($n = 18$). Two patients did not receive any heparin, one died before the introduction (day 3), and the other one was an haemophiliac (who developed a DVT on day 8). There was no significant difference in the application of the protocol between the two groups.

In patients diagnosed with asymptomatic VTE, the introduction of a therapeutic dose of heparin was discussed on a case-by-case basis and 21 patients (44.7%) were curatively treated (outcome presented in Additional file 1: Table S1). We identified no complication related to pharmacological thromboprophylaxis. We did not find any worsening neither in clinically available monitoring of haemorrhage (tubes, drainage devices or wounds) nor in radiological imaging (volume of contusion or haematoma, haemorrhage relapse). Three patients benefited from a vena cava filter as they presented a contraindication for continuous anticoagulant therapy. Two still

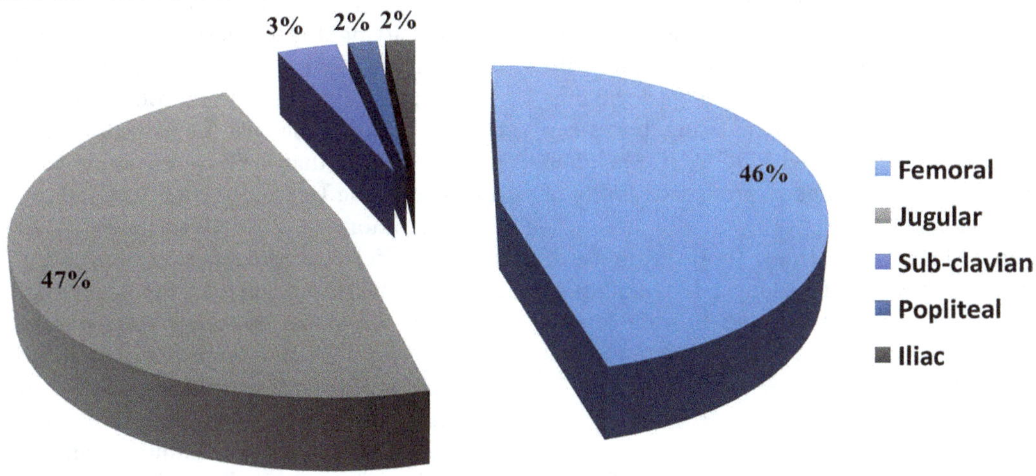

Fig. 3 Anatomical situation of DVT diagnosed with duplex US examination ($n = 59$ in 45 patients). Femoral ($n = 27$), internal jugular ($n = 29$), subclavian ($n = 2$), popliteal ($n = 1$), external iliac ($n = 1$)

Table 2 Relation between central venous catheter characteristics and DVT

Vein	Incidence of DVT (1000 catheter-days)	CVC (*n*) Patients (*n*)	DVT (*n*)	No. of days of catheterization	Length of catheterization (days)
Femoral	67.7	126/119	22	325	2 [1; 3]
I. jugular	47.5	53/47	21	442	8 [4.3; 12]
Subclavian	35.7	5/5	1	28	6 [4.8; 7.3]

No CVC ($n = 29$), 1 CVC ($n = 73$), 2 CVC (42), 3 CVC ($n = 9$)

Data expressed as median [quartile 1; 3]

I. Jugular internal jugular catheter, *DVT/1000 catheter-days* number of event/number of days of catheterization × 1000, *DVT* deep venous thrombosis, *CVC* central venous catheter necessitated potentially haemorrhagic surgery, and one had complex pelvic fracture associated with a large cerebral contusion.

CT scan review

A total of 205 CT scan angiograms were reviewed by the independent radiologist. Seven additional thromboembolic events were found in six patients: four segmental PE in patients who had no identified clinical symptom (outcome presented in Additional file 2: Table S2), and three DVT including one in internal jugular and two in common iliac veins. The overall prevalence was re-estimated at 34.6% ($n = 53$ patients).

VTE and risk factors and outcome

Table 3 presents the results of the univariate analysis between the groups VTE + and VTE-. The multivariate analysis found no significant interactions among risk factors or risk factors and time. Four independent risk factors were identified: pelvic fracture (OR 3.04, 95% confidence interval (CI) [1.2–7.9]), CVC (OR 4.39, 95% CI [1.1–29]), medullar injury (OR 4.59, 95% CI [1.7–12.9]) and hypotension below 80 mmHg during initial management (OR 3.64, 95% CI [1.3–10.8]). The Hosmer–Lemeshow test showed a convenient fitting of the model with the observations ($p = 0.94$). The predictive performance showed an AUC of 0.74 [0.66–0.82]. Using bootstrap validation, the optimism-corrected ROC AUC was 0.73 [0.65–0.82], which represents a good predictive ability of the model in future patients [18].

Regarding the clinical outcomes (bottom lines of Table 3), patients with VTE had a longer ICU length of stay (5.5 vs 18 days, $p < 0.001$) and longer hospital length of stay (17 vs 28 days, $p < 0.003$), but no difference was observed on mortality (14.9 vs 10.4%, ns).

Discussion

This study demonstrates that in a population of critically ill trauma patients receiving early and protocolized thromboprophylaxis, the prevalence of VTE with a weekly DUS screening was as high as 30%.

Epidemiology and prophylaxis in the literature

LMWH has been part of the standard of care for the prophylaxis of venous thromboembolism for more than 20 years. They have shown to be more effective than unfractionated heparin with an equal or even better level of safety. Several meta-analyses have confirmed a higher benefit/risk ratio. Major bleeding is less frequent. Heparin-induced thrombocytopenia is ten times less frequent with LMWH, and even in patients with renal insufficiency, they have demonstrated a higher ratio of efficacy/safety than unfractionated heparin [19]. In trauma patients, Geerts et al. [20] have shown that low molecular weight heparins were more effective than low-dose unfractionated heparin in preventing venous thromboembolism after major trauma.

The incidence in our study remains very high despite the protocol-driven early thromboprophylaxis (median time 1 day [1, 2]) and a satisfying global protocol compliance. Published incidences of VTE after trauma range from 4.6 to 28% [21–23] in patients receiving pharmacological and/or mechanical prophylaxis to 90% in patients receiving no pharmacological prophylaxis [24, 25]. In the largest reported venographic study, Geerts et al. [24] identified DVT in 58% of 349 trauma patients receiving no antithrombotic prophylaxis and undergoing contrast venography 1–3 weeks after admission. A recent Cochrane database review, including 16 studies ($n = 3005$ patients), concluded that any prophylaxis might reduce the risk of VTE: mechanical (RR 0.43, 95% CI [0.25–0.73]), pharmacological (RR 0.48, 95% CI [0.25–0.95]) or even better with both prophylaxis (RR 0.34, 95% CI [0.19–0.60]) [15]. The protocol we implemented in our unit combined all existing methods of prophylaxis, introduced as soon as possible for mechanical devices and specifying the earliest timing of introduction for the pharmacological prophylaxis. The median delay of introduction obtained in our cohort (1 day [1; 2]) is one of the shortest times we found in the literature. Hence, we can assume that VTE in our study was more due to a failure of the treatment than to a failure of treatment administration. In 2013, Gentile et al. [26] described a median delay of introduction of 13 days with 37% of trauma patients having no chemical prophylaxis. Nevertheless, the global trend is to start the antithrombotic prophylaxis more and more early, even in brain trauma patients [1, 16]. So far, providing LMWH within 36 h of trauma to all patients, including those with solid organ injuries or traumatic brain injuries, appears safe, effective and is recommended to reduce the incidence of DVT and VTE, without significant increase in bleeding [5, 27]. The optimal regimen dose is still debated: once or twice daily LMWH injections or twice daily unfractionated heparin. In a prospective cohort of 87 trauma patients, Ko et al. [28] showed that subprophylactic anti-Xa trough level was found in 73 of 87 patients (84%) with a twice daily 30-mg enoxaparin injection. This suggests that early monitoring and tailoring of anticoagulant prophylaxis in high-risk patients might be another research field to decrease the failure of VTE prevention.

Duplex US and diagnosis

Duplex US is the modality of choice for the diagnosis and follow-up of symptomatic DVT [8], but its use in screening asymptomatic patients is still controversial.

Table 3 Univariate analysis of patient characteristics according to the occurrence of thromboembolic events

Variables	TEE+ ($n = 47$)	TEE− ($n = 106$)	p
Demographic characteristics			
Age (years)	46.8 ± 18.4	43.6 ± 19.8	0.3505
Sex (male)	80.9% (38)	67.9% (72)	0.6140
BMI (kg/m^2)	26.6 ± 7.1	25.9 ± 6.2	0.5571
History of cancer	0% (0)	6 (5.7%)	0.2253
History of DVT	0% (0)	0% (0)	–
Injuries grading			
Initial GCS ≤ 8	29.8% (14)	17.9% (19)	0.1519
AIS thorax > 2	46.8% (22)	36.8% (39)	0.3230
AIS head > 2	40.4% (19)	43.4% (46)	0.8684
AIS abdomen > 2	27.6% (13)	17.9% (19)	0.2500
Pelvic fracture	29.8% (14)	12.3% (13)	0.0167
Lower limbs fracture	25.5% (12)	28.3% (30)	0.8746
Medullar injury	25.53% (12)	9.43% (10)	0.0179
Spine fracture	42.6% (20)	24.5% (26)	0.0402
Scores			
SAPS II	44.9 [38.7; 50.7]	30.4 [27.4; 34.1]	0.0001
ISS	28.9 [20; 34]	21.4 [13; 29]	0.0006
SOFA 24 h	8.3 [5; 11]	5.6 [1; 9.5]	0.0007
RAP score > 5	95.7% (45)	83% (88)	0.0582
RAP score > 10	70.2% (33)	39.6% (42)	0.0009
Clinical status			
SAP min (mmHg)	99 ± 28	111 ± 25	0.0083
Vasopressors	31.9% (15)	18.1% (19)	0.0594
Surgery > 2 h	46.8% (22)	30.2% (32)	0.0782
Central venous catheter	95.7% (45)	74.5% (79)	0.0041
Initial transfusion treatment (day 1)			
Transfusion > 4 RBC in 6 h	29.8% (14)	13.2% (14)	0.0264
Tranexamic acid	36.2% (17)	17.9% (19)	0.0246
Fibrinogen	31.9% (15)	13.2% (14)	0.0124
Thromboprophylactic procedure			
Compression stockings (absent)	8.5% (4)	9.5% (10)	0.9769
Pneumatic intermittent compression (no)	14.9% (7)	18.1% (19)	0.8877
Time before initiation of antithrombotic chemoprophylaxis	2 [1; 2]	1 [1; 2]	0.4533
Outcome			
ICU length of stay	18 [7; 32]	5.5 [3; 11]	<0.0001
Hospital length of stay	28 [15; 43]	17 [11; 28]	0.0027
Mortality	10.6% (5)	10.4% (11)	0.5976
Binarized characteristics			
ISS ≥ 16	87.2% (41)	69.6% (73)	0.0333
SAPS II ≥ 30	76.6% (36)	47.6% (49)	0.0016
SOFA 24 ≥ 5	80.9% (38)	50.9% (54)	0.0009
BMI ≥ 30 kg/m^2	23.9% (11)	24.7% (21)	1
Age ≥ 50 years	40.4% (19)	34.6% (36)	0.614
SAP min ≤ 80 mmHg	26.1 (12)	7.8% (8)	0.0061
GCS ≤ 8	25.5% (12)	18.9% (20)	0.4718

Continuous data are expressed as mean ± SD or median [quartile 1; 3] according to their distribution. Categorical data are expressed as percentage (n)

SAPS II Simplified Acute Physiology Score, *SOFA à 24 h* Sequential Organ Failure Assessment, *AIS* Abbreviated Injury Score, *ISS* Injury Severity Score, *RAP* Risk Assessment Profile, *DVT* deep venous thrombosis, *BMI* body mass index, *GCS* Glasgow Coma Score, *RBC* red blood cells, *systolic arterial pressure* minimal systolic arterial pressure recorded during transport, *ICU* intensive care unit

It remains an operator-dependant technique with varying reported performances between level I and level II studies (sensitivity 61–92%, respectively, and specificity 97–98%, respectively) [29]. Moreover, the use of US in screening asymptomatic patients is burdened by a low sensitivity when compared with venography [29, 30]. As a consequence, the incidence of DVT could just have been "underestimated" in our study. The double check allowed to minor the false positive, when false negative just relied on practitioners' US performance. Moreover, in patients with overlying orthopaedic devices (external fixators, splints, bandages), only available areas were imaged. These local constraints, the low sensitivity of calf US vascular imaging [31] and the unknown significance of calf DVT explain why we intentionally focused our investigations on femoral and popliteal veins for the lower limb. Another hypothesis to explain the differences in incidence and performance reports could come from the non-uniform definition of thrombosis. A small mural thrombus on a CVC scar is probably different from an occlusive thrombus developing by itself. In our study, we decided to describe all thrombi corresponding to the protocol definition ("Methods" section). Nevertheless, on a pragmatic point of view, we addressed differently the different types of thrombus. We treated all floating and occlusive DVT without debating. Mural thrombi led to discuss the benefits/risks balance and really depended on the beliefs of the practitioner in charge.

Risk factors

The risk factors identified in our study were in accordance with some of the risk factors identified in the trauma literature [7, 8, 23, 32]. The univariate analysis highlights the link between the severity of the patients and the exposition to transfusion and prothrombotic treatment and the risk of developing a VTE. Surprisingly, head AIS > 2 or GCS ≤ 8 was not associated with VTE. We might explain this observation by the fact that every patient, even those presenting severe traumatic brain injury, received a rather early chemical thromboprophylaxis, which is often not the case in other studies [1]. The individual risk factors (obesity, cancer, coagulation disorders or age) were not significantly associated with VTE because our cohort gathered mostly young patients, with little comorbidities. So if we had screened "high-risk patients" on the RAP score > 10, like Thorson et al. [23], we would have missed 14 patients (30%) what is, in an absolute point of view, quite consistent.

Our results also identified CVC as an independent risk factor for VTE (OR 4.1). This is a well-described risk factor in the trauma population, generally declined according to the insertion site. In our population, the femoral catheters were at highest risk of VTE (Table 3) as it was the emergency access (allowing simultaneous access of vein and artery for invasive arterial pressure monitoring), with delicate asepsis conditions and during the most prothrombotic period. The femoral site is known to be at higher risk of VTE in numerous studies (4, 37, 38), even in non-trauma patients [33].

Strength

Concerning the method of selection of variables for the multiple logistic regression, we wanted a pragmatic, easy-to-use tool to identify patients at high risk of VTE. We excluded all pre-existing processed calculations (ISS, SAPS II, RAP, SOFA), and we focused on transfusion strategy, easy-to-identify injury pattern and resuscitation management. The CVC represents probably here a surrogate of global severity of the patient. As an inherent limit of this statistical tool, we could not prove causation but just identify association and adjust confounding factors one to the other. We could not test our model on a prospective validation cohort in this study.

Limits

The limits of our study are inherent to its design. First, it is a prospective, single-centre, exploratory cohort study, which does not allow projecting the results over all trauma populations with different case mix and different prevention policies. Nevertheless, the baseline characteristics of our trauma population depict a cohort of classical, blunt, male, rather young trauma patients and our thromboprophylaxis protocol is detailed to allow sharing of information. Second, all the categories of DVT were pooled together, and occlusive thrombosis was the only symptomatic and was only 6.7. Third, this is a modest cohort of 153 patients that does not allow building up a robust predictive score, which was not the purpose of the study. Nevertheless, we tried to extract a signal for the clinicians to arise their awareness on the patients' main risk of VTE. Fourth, and the most striking, is that the observed incidence is suspected to be rather "underestimated" by all the study bias. These statements highlight the failure of VTE prophylaxis in trauma patients, which is incentive to explore how to tailor adequate thromboprophylaxis in these patients [34, 35].

Conclusion

We found that the prevalence of VTE among trauma patients remaining in the ICU for more than 48 h and receiving protocolized early thromboprophylaxis was 31% (incidence 18% patients-week). Main identified independent risk factors were CVC, pelvic fracture, medullar injury or hypotension <80 mmHg during initial management. Further research is needed to determine whether a more intensified thromboprophylaxis regime would be safe and effective in severe trauma patients.

Abbreviations
DVT: deep venous thrombosis; VTE: venous thromboembolism; PE: pulmonary embolism; 95 CI: 95% confidence interval; GCS: Glasgow Coma Scale; SAP: systolic arterial pressure; SOFA: Sequential Organ Failure Assessment; ISS: Injury Severity Score; RAP score: Risk Assessment Profile; CVC: central venous catheter; LMWH: low molecular weight heparin; CT: computed tomography; AIS: Abbreviated Injury Scale; SAPS II: Simplified Acute Physiology Score; US: ultrasound; DUS: venous duplex ultrasound.

Authors' contributions
Sophie Rym Hamada contributed to the study design, data collection, data analysis and interpretation, literature search and writing. *Caroline Espina* contributed to the study design, data collection, data analysis and interpretation, literature search and writing. *Thierry Guedj* contributed to the study design, data collection and interpretation. *Raphael Buaron* contributed to data collection, analysis and interpretation. *Samy Figueiredo* contributed to data collection and critical revision. *Anatole Harrois* contributed to data collection and critical revision. *Jacques Duranteau* contributed to study design, critical revision and writing. All authors read and approved the final manuscript.

Author details
[1] Department of Anaesthesia and Critical Care, AP-HP, Hôpital Bicêtre, Hôpitaux Universitaires Paris Sud, University Paris-Sud, 78 rue du Général Leclerc, 94275 Le Kremlin Bicêtre, France. [2] Department of Anaesthesia and Critical Care, AP-HP, Hôpital Cochin, Hôpitaux Universitaires Paris Centre, University Paris Descartes, 27 Rue du Faubourg Saint-Jacques, 75014 Paris, France. [3] Department of Radiology, Hôpital Bicêtre, Hôpitaux Universitaires Paris Sud, University Paris-Sud, 78 rue du Général Leclerc, 94275 Le Kremlin Bicêtre, France.

Acknowledgements
We thank Pr Charles Marc Samama for his expertise and careful advising.

Competing interests
The authors declare that they have no competing interests.

Funding
No funding source.

Appendix 1: Venous thromboembolism prophylaxis protocol

- All patients receive elastic stockings and tight-and-leg intermittent pneumatic compression device as soon as possible after the second survey (excluding anatomical constraints).
- If patients have an immediate surgery or interventional radiology procedure, the intermittent pneumatic compression devices are set up post-operatively.
- The chemical prophylaxis by low-dose heparin, either unfractionated (5000 UI subcutaneous injection (SC)/12 h) or low molecular weight heparin (enoxaparin 40 mg SC/24 h), according to renal function, is started after 6 h post-operatively or following any invasive procedure in the absence of brain injury or latent haemorrhagic risk.
- For patients weighting more than 100 kg, heparin doses are increased to 5000 UI/8 h and enoxaparin 60 mg/24 h.
- For patients in haemorrhagic shock, heparin is started after bleeding control and restoration of biological haemostasis (platelets > 80.000/mm^3, prothrombin time > 40%).
- For patients having a latent haemorrhagic risk (large solid organ contusion without embolization procedure, comminutive pelvic fracture, refractory epistaxis, etc.), the chemical prophylaxis is started after the first 24 h.
- For patients having spine or intracranial injuries, heparin is started 48 h after injury or neurosurgical intervention when a head CT scan shows stability of brain injuries and restoration of biological haemostasis (platelets > 100.000/mm^3, prothrombin time > 60%).
- In case of an existing medical history of coagulopathy, the chemical prophylaxis is discussed on a case-by-case basis with haematologists.

Appendix 2: List of data collected

- Demographic data including age, gender, weight and height for body mass index calculation (BMI kg/m^2).
- Clinical data concerning comorbidities and medical history of thrombosis.
- Complete injury assessment (Abbreviated Injury Score of all body regions).
- Trauma management: injury mechanism, clinical data on scene and during transport (arterial pressure, Glasgow Coma Score, fluid load, vasopressor use), initial hospital coagulation and transfusion strategy (plasma, platelets, red blood cells, tranexamic acid, fibrinogen, activated factors), length of initial surgery.
- Severity (as day 1 scores): Injury Severity Score (ISS), Simplified Acute Physiologic Score (SAPS II), Sequential Organ Failure Assessment (SOFA) and Risk Assessment Profile (RAP) scores.
- Protocol compliance: elastic stockings (presence and timing), tight-and-leg intermittent pneumatic compression device (presence and timing).
- Modality of initial thromboprophylaxis (date of introduction of heparin, type of heparin, dose and respect of the protocol timing).
- All central venous catheters were identified and followed for insertion sites and length of maintenance.
- Clinical examination and coagulation screening tests (prothrombin time, fibrinogen, activated partial thromboplastin time and platelet count) on each day of DVT ultrasound screening.

References
1. Nyquist P, Bautista C, Jichici D, Burns J, Chhangani S, DeFilippis M, et al. Prophylaxis of venous thrombosis in neurocritical care patients: an evidence-based guideline: A Statement for Healthcare Professionals from the Neurocritical Care Society. Neurocrit Care. 2016;24:47–60.

2. Acosta JA, Yang JC, Winchell RJ, Simons RK, Fortlage DA, Hollingsworth-Fridlund P, et al. Lethal injuries and time to death in a level I trauma center. J Am Coll Surg. 1998;186:528–33.
3. Norwood SH, McAuley CE, Berne JD, Vallina VL, Kerns DB, Grahm TW, et al. A potentially expanded role for enoxaparin in preventing venous thromboembolism in high risk blunt trauma patients. J Am Coll Surg. 2001;192:161–7.
4. Knudson MM, Collins JA, Goodman SB, McCrory DW. Thromboembolism following multiple trauma. J Trauma. 1992;32:2–11.
5. Foreman PM, Schmalz PGR, Griessenauer CJ. Chemoprophylaxis for venous thromboembolism in traumatic brain injury: a review and evidence-based protocol. Clin Neurol Neurosurg. 2014;123:109–16.
6. Kwiatt ME, Patel MS, Ross SE, Lachant MT, MacNew HG, Ochsner MG, et al. Is low-molecular-weight heparin safe for venous thromboembolism prophylaxis in patients with traumatic brain injury? A Western Trauma Association multicenter study. J. Trauma Acute Care Surg. 2012;73:625–8.
7. Gearhart MM, Luchette FA, Proctor MC, Lutomski DM, Witsken C, James L, et al. The risk assessment profile score identifies trauma patients at risk for deep vein thrombosis. Surgery. 2000;128:631–40.
8. Rogers FB, Cipolle MD, Velmahos G, Rozycki G, Luchette FA. Practice management guidelines for the prevention of venous thromboembolism in trauma patients: the EAST practice management guidelines work group. J Trauma Acute Care Surg. 2002;53:142–64.
9. Bagot CN, Arya R. Virchow and his triad: a question of attribution. Br J Haematol. 2008;143:180–90.
10. Brohi K, Cohen MJ, Ganter MT, Matthay MA, Mackersie RC, Pittet J-F. Acute traumatic coagulopathy: initiated by hypoperfusion: modulated through the protein C pathway? Ann Surg. 2007;245:812–8.
11. Engelman DT, Gabram SG, Allen L, Ens GE, Jacobs LM. Hypercoagulability following multiple trauma. World J Surg. 1996;20:5–10.
12. Selby R, Geerts W, Ofosu FA, Craven S, Dewar L, Phillips A, et al. Hypercoagulability after trauma: hemostatic changes and relationship to venous thromboembolism. Thromb Res. 2009;124:281–7.
13. Schöchl H, Voelckel W, Maegele M, Kirchmair L, Schlimp CJ. Endogenous thrombin potential following hemostatic therapy with 4-factor prothrombin complex concentrate: a 7-day observational study of trauma patients. Crit Care Lond Engl. 2014;18:R147.
14. Kornblith LZ, Kutcher ME, Redick BJ, Calfee CS, Vilardi RF, Cohen MJ. Fibrinogen and platelet contributions to clot formation: implications for trauma resuscitation and thromboprophylaxis. J Trauma Acute Care Surg. 2014;76:255–63.
15. Barrera LM, Perel P, Ker K, Cirocchi R, Farinella E, Morales Uribe CH. Thromboprophylaxis for trauma patients. Cochrane Database Syst Rev. 2013;(3):CD008303. doi:10.1002/14651858.CD008303.pub2.
16. Shahan CP, Magnotti LJ, McBeth PB, Weinberg JA, Croce MA, Fabian TC. Early antithrombotic therapy is safe and effective in patients with blunt cerebrovascular injury and solid organ injury or traumatic brain injury. J Trauma Acute Care Surg. 2016;81:173–7.
17. Steyerberg EW, Harrell FE, Borsboom GJ, Eijkemans MJC, Vergouwe Y, Habbema JDF. Internal validation of predictive models: efficiency of some procedures for logistic regression analysis. J Clin Epidemiol. 2001;54:774–81.
18. Faraklas I, Stoddard GJ, Neumayer LA, Cochran A. Development and validation of a necrotizing soft-tissue infection mortality risk calculator using NSQIP. J Am Coll Surg. 2013;217(153–160):e3.
19. Mismetti P, Laporte S, Darmon JY, Buchmüller A, Decousus H. Meta-analysis of low molecular weight heparin in the prevention of venous thromboembolism in general surgery. Br J Surg. 2001;88:913–30.
20. Geerts WH, Jay RM, Code KI, Chen E, Szalai JP, Saibil EA, et al. A comparison of low-dose heparin with low-molecular-weight heparin as prophylaxis against venous thromboembolism after major trauma. N Engl J Med. 1996;335:701–7.
21. Lu J-P, Knudson MM, Bir N, Kallet R, Atkinson K. Fondaparinux for prevention of venous thromboembolism in high-risk trauma patients: a pilot study. J Am Coll Surg. 2009;209:589–94.
22. Velmahos GC, Kern J, Chan LS, Oder D, Murray JA, Shekelle P. Prevention of venous thromboembolism after injury: an evidence-based report—part II: analysis of risk factors and evaluation of the role of vena caval filters. J Trauma. 2000;49:140–4.
23. Thorson CM, Ryan ML, Van Haren RM, Curia E, Barrera JM, Guarch GA, et al. Venous thromboembolism after trauma: a never event?*. Crit Care Med. 2012;40:2967–73.
24. Geerts WH, Code KI, Jay RM, Chen E, Szalai JP. A prospective study of venous thromboembolism after major trauma. N Engl J Med. 1994;331:1601–6.
25. Shackford SR, Davis JW, Hollingsworth-Fridlund P, Brewer NS, Hoyt DB, Mackersie RC. Venous thromboembolism in patients with major trauma. Am J Surg. 1990;159:365–9.
26. Gentile A, Petit L, Masson F, Cottenceau V, Bertrand-Barat J, Freyburger G, et al. Subclavian central venous catheter-related thrombosis in trauma patients: incidence, risk factors and influence of polyurethane type. Crit Care. 2013;17:1.
27. Cupitt JM. Prophylaxis against thromboembolism in patients with traumatic brain injury: a survey of UK practice. Anaesthesia. 2001;56:780–5.
28. Connelly CR, Van PY, Hart KD, Louis SG, Fair KA, Erickson AS, et al. Thrombelastography-based dosing of enoxaparin for thromboprophylaxis in trauma and surgical patients: a randomized clinical trial. JAMA Surg. 2016;151:e162069.
29. Agnelli G, Radicchia S, Nenci GG. Diagnosis of deep vein thrombosis in asymptomatic high-risk patients. Haemostasis. 1995;25:40–8.
30. Wells PS, Lensing AW, Davidson BL, Prins MH, Hirsh J. Accuracy of ultrasound for the diagnosis of deep venous thrombosis in asymptomatic patients after orthopedic surgery. A meta-analysis. Ann Intern Med. 1995;122:47–53.
31. Comerota AJ, Katz ML, White JV. Why does prophylaxis with external pneumatic compression for deep vein thrombosis fail? Am J Surg. 1992;164:265–8.
32. Haut ER, Chang DC, Pierce CA, Colantuoni E, Efron DT, Haider AH, et al. Predictors of posttraumatic deep vein thrombosis (DVT): hospital practice versus patient factors-an analysis of the National Trauma Data Bank (NTDB). J Trauma. 2009;66:994–1001.
33. Merrer J, De Jonghe B, Golliot F, Lefrant JY, Raffy B, Barre E, et al. Complications of femoral and subclavian venous catheterization in critically ill patients: a randomized controlled trial. JAMA. 2001;286:700–7.
34. Rostas JW, Brevard SB, Ahmed N, Allen J, Thacker D, Replogle WH, et al. Standard dosing of enoxaparin for venous thromboembolism prophylaxis is not sufficient for most patients within a trauma intensive care unit. Am Surg. 2015;81:889–92.
35. Ko A, Harada MY, Barmparas G, Chung K, Mason R, Yim DA, et al. Association between enoxaparin dosage adjusted by anti-factor Xa trough level and clinically evident venous thromboembolism after trauma. JAMA Surg. 2016;151(11):1006–13.

12

Association between elevated central venous pressure and outcomes in critically ill patients

Dong-kai Li†, Xiao-ting Wang† and Da-wei Liu*

Abstract

Background: Some prior studies have shown that elevated mean central venous pressure in certain patient populations and disease processes may lead to poor prognosis. However, these studies failed to generalize the concept of elevated central venous pressure (ECVP) load to all patients in critical care settings because of the limited cases and exclusive cohorts. The aim of the study was to investigate the association between elevated central venous pressure and outcomes in critical care.

Methods: We performed a retrospective analysis on a single-center public database (MIMIC) of more than 9000 patients and more than 500,000 records of central venous pressure measurement. We evaluated the association between mean central venous pressure level and 28-day mortality after intensive care unit admission. The secondary outcomes were duration of mechanical ventilation, vasoactive drug use, laboratory results related to organ dysfunction and length of intensive care unit hospitalization. Accordingly, we proposed the concept of $ECVP_{10}$ (the time sum of CVP above 10 mmHg) and investigated its association with outcome.

Results: There were 1645 deaths at 28 days after admission. Compared with the lowest quartile of mean central venous pressure [mean (SD) 7.4 (1.9) mmHg], the highest quartile [17.4 (4.1) mmHg] was associated with a 33.6% (95% CI 1.117–1.599) higher adjusted risk of death. Poor secondary outcomes were also associated with higher quartiles of elevated mean central venous pressure. After stratification by mean central venous pressure, elevated duration of central venous pressure above 10 mmHg was significantly higher in the non-survival group than in the survival group.

Conclusions: Elevated central venous pressure level correlated with poor outcomes and prolonged treatment in critical care settings. Level and duration of elevated central venous pressure should be both evaluated to establish its cause and apply appropriate treatment.

Keywords: Central venous pressure, Survival, Critical care

Background

Elevated right atrial pressure or central venous pressure (CVP) occurs frequently in critical care settings [1–4] and may be caused by several conditions, such as congestive heart failure syndrome, constrictive pericardial disease, tension pneumothorax, and resuscitation/evacuation phases of septic shock. Although CVP has been utilized as a surrogate of intravascular volume in critically ill patients, recent studies have challenged the validity of elevated CVP (ECVP) in critical care settings [5–9]. Based on rationale provided by the Starling curves and Guyton model on cardiac function, CVP is determined by the interaction of cardiac function and the return of blood to the heart. An ECVP might indicate an impediment to the venous return and microcirculatory blood flow as well as accompanying lung edema and splanchnic congestion [3, 10], which may further worsen the potential organ failure in critical patients.

*Correspondence: pumchicuky@163.com
†Dong-kai Li and Xiao-ting Wang contributed equally to this study and share first authorship
Department of Critical Care Medicine, Peking Union Medical College Hospital, Peking Union Medical College, Chinese Academy of Medical Science, 1 Shuaifuyuan, Dongcheng District, Beijing 100730, China

Some prior studies have shown that increased mean CVP in certain patient populations and disease processes may lead to poor prognosis. In septic patients, increased mean CVP was associated with worse outcome, including increased 28-day mortality as well as the development and progression of acute kidney injury [6, 7, 11]. For patients with cardiovascular diseases, ECVP might be associated with impaired hepatic and renal function and may be independently related to all-cause mortality [8, 9]. These studies, however, could not generalize the concept of elevated central venous pressure (ECVP) load to all patients in critical care settings because of the limited cases and exclusive cohorts. Besides, the importance of ECVP duration was underestimated in estimating the ECVP load and analyzing its relationship with outcome, which is only accessible with the advantage of "big data" technology [12].

By using the large, public, de-identified clinical database, Multi-parameter Intelligent Monitoring in Intensive Care (MIMIC-III) [13], we evaluated the effect of ECVP on all patients in critical care settings, for whom CVP data were carefully recorded. We aimed to further characterize the association between mean CVP level and outcome as well as treatment received in the intensive care unit (ICU). Specifically, we investigated the potential effect of ECVP duration on outcome when mean CVP were stratified at different levels.

Methods

Data source

We conducted a large-scale, single-center, retrospective cohort study using data collected from the MIMIC-III open source clinical database (version 1.3, released on December 10, 2015), which was developed and maintained by the Massachusetts Institute of Technology (MIT), Philips Healthcare, and Beth Israel Deaconess Medical Center (BIDMC) [13]. Information derived from the electronic medical records of 46,476 unique critical care patients admitted to the ICUs at BIDMC between 2001 and 2012 was included in this free accessible database. Use of the MIMIC-III database has been approved by the Institutional Review Boards of BIDMC and MIT, and waiver of informed consent was granted.

Patient population

All patients in the database were screened. The inclusion criteria in this study were as follows: (1) adults ($\geq$18 years of age) at ICU admission, with complete medical records including available CVP measurement records; (2) ICU stay $\geq$72 h; and (3) consecutive CVP monitoring $\geq$12 h. For patients with multiple ICU stays, only data related the first ICU admission were considered.

All available CVP measurements recorded during ICU stay were extracted. Other variables including ICU type, demographic data, age, sex, Elixhauser comorbid conditions [14] and admission illness severity scores [including the Simplified Acute Physiology Score (SAPS) [15] and Sequential Organ Failure Assessment (SOFA) [16]] were extracted from the database. Additionally, data on use of vasopressors, mechanical ventilation, laboratory results related to organ dysfunction and length of ICU stay and hospitalization were extracted from the database.

Exposure

The primary exposure was the mean CVP during the first 72 h after ICU admission. We also calculated the duration of $ECVP_{10}$ as the time of CVP above the level of 10 mmHg, which was considered as a relatively higher CVP level that might by unbeneficial for patients in critical care settings [17], and used it as an alternative indicator of the mean CVP level to estimate the association between ECVP load and outcome in the critical care settings.

Outcome

The primary outcome was 28-day mortality after ICU admission. The secondary outcomes included duration of mechanical ventilation and vasoactive drug use (epinephrine, norepinephrine, vasopressin, dopamine, dobutamine, milrinone and phenylephrine), laboratory results related to organ dysfunction and the length of ICU admission and hospitalization. For some patients, whose death occurred outside the hospital, the Social Security Death Index was linked to the database for investigations related to mortality.

Statistical analysis

Baseline characteristics were stratified by quartiles of mean CVP during the first 72 h after ICU admission. Cox regression analyses were undertaken to compare the 28-day mortality among different mean CVP quartiles. All other covariates, which comprised demographic characteristics, ICU type, SAPS II score at admission, comorbidities and mean duration of CVP measurement, were included into the multivariable regression model. We also compared the survivors and non-survivors for their $ECVP_{10}$ duration with the outcome independently through the stratification on mean CVP.

The results are expressed as mean $\pm$ SD (standard deviation) for normally distributed data or median [interquartile range (IQR)] for non-normally distributed data. Continuous variables were compared using one-way analysis of variance for normally distributed quantitative data, and Mann–Whitney *U* test for non-normally distributed quantitative data to determine differences between groups. All statistical analyses were performed by using the IBM® SPSS® Statistics version 22 (SPSS Inc., Chicago, IL, USA). Any *p* value <0.05 was considered statistically significant.

Subset and sensitivity analyses

Since the mean CVP level can only describe the overall level of CVP, in sensitivity analyses, we replaced the mean CVP level with the duration of $ECVP_{10}$ as an alternative indicator to estimate the association between ECVP load and outcome in the critical care settings.

We examined whether elevated mean CVP level in the highest quartile was associated with poor outcome compared to the other quartiles in patients with and without sepsis, which was defined as suspected or documented infection and an acute increase of ≥ 2 SOFA points infection [18], and AKI, as defined by either a greater than or equal to 0.3 mg/dL increase within 48 h or a greater than or equal to 50% increase within 7 days of ICU admission, or acute dialysis, in keeping with the Kidney Disease Outcome Quality Initiative guidelines [19]. We individually tested association between elevated mean CVP and these variables in adjusted analysis and provided graphical representation of the stratified risks.

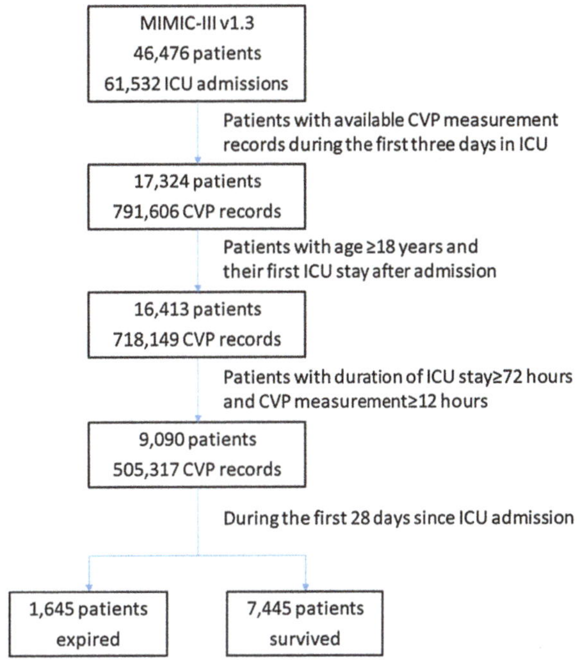

Fig. 1 Flowchart showing step-by-step selection on patients included in the study. *CVP* central venous pressure, *ICU* intensive care unit

Results

Baseline characteristics

Among the 46,476 ICU patients and 61,532 ICU admissions in the MMIC-III v1.3, 17,324 patients underwent CVP measurement during the first 3 days of the ICU hospitalization and 791,606 CVP records were available in the database. Sequentially, we excluded 911 patients whose age at admission was below 18 years, 7323 patients with ICU stay less than 3 days and CVP measurement duration of less than 12 h, as illustrated in Fig. 1. The final cohort comprised 9090 patients with their first ICU admission and the corresponding 505,317 records of CVP measurement. The mean ($\pm$SD) interval between two consecutive CVP measurements was 0.9 ± 1.2 h, and the mean ($\pm$SD) duration of CVP measurement during the first 72 h in ICU hospitalization was 49.5 ± 18.8 h.

In the 9090 critically ill patients included in the study, the mean ($\pm$ SD) CVP level was 11.8 ± 4.0 mmHg and median (IQR) $ECVP_{10}$ duration of 23.0 (9.0, 43.8) h. As shown in Table 1, patients in the highest quartile of mean CVP level presented greater SOFA score and more comorbidities. The mean duration of CVP measurement and $ECVP_{10}$ duration were also increased in higher quartiles of mean CVP level.

Mean CVP level and outcome

During the first 28 days after ICU admission, 1645 patients died. Higher quartiles of mean CVP level during the first 3 days after ICU admission were associated with higher unadjusted mortality. After adjusting for sex, age, gender, ethnicity, congestive heart failure, cardiac arrhythmias, hypertension, valvular disease, pulmonary circulation disease, renal failure and other 24 Elixhauser comorbidities, ICU type, SAPS II score at admission and duration of CVP measurement, the mean CVP level remained a significant predictor of 28-day mortality, as shown in Table 2. The other potential determinants are shown in Additional file 1: Supplement Table 1. The survival curve of 28-day mortality by the quartiles of mean CVP level is shown in Fig. 2, and the detailed comparison of 28-day mortality between the deciles of mean CVP level is shown in Additional file 1: Supplement Table 2 .

In addition to the 28-day mortality, we investigated the association between quartiles of mean CVP level and secondary ICU outcomes, which included length of hospitalization, treatment received in ICU and laboratory results related to organ dysfunction, as shown in Table 1. The result showed that prolonged ICU stay and hospitalization were required for patients with higher mean CVP level during the first 3 days from ICU admission, and the duration of vasopressor or mechanical ventilation treatment also was prolonged. Furthermore, leukocytosis, higher serum bilirubin, creatinine, and lactate were all more commonly seen in the higher mean CVP quartiles.

Subset and sensitivity analyses

Duration of $ECVP_{10}$ was investigated between 28-day survival and non-survival patients. After stratification by different levels of mean CVP, as in Additional file 1: Supplement Figure 2, the results showed that the $ECVP_{10}$

Table 1 General patient characteristics stratified by quartiles of mean CVP level during the first 72 h from ICU admission

	Quartiles of mean CVP level			
	1 ($n = 2281$)	2 ($n = 2269$)	3 ($n = 2277$)	4 ($n = 2263$)
Mean CVP/mmHg	7.4 (1.9)	10.6 (1.9)	13.1 (2.2)	17.4 (4.1)
Median CVP/mmHg	7	10	13	16
Age (years)	67.1 (15.8)	66.9 (15.9)	65.8 (15.5)	64.4 (15.4)
Sex, male	1070 (57.9%)	1088 (58.9%)	1046 (56.7%)	1007 (54.6%)
Ethnicity, *n* (%)				
Asian	33 (1.8%)	40 (2.2%)	21 (1.1%)	37 (2.0%)
Black	101 (5.5%)	114 (6.2%)	99 (5.4%)	119 (6.4%)
White	1326 (71.8%)	1301 (70.5%)	1297 (70.3%)	1293 (70.1%)
Latino	47 (2.5%)	41 (2.2%)	58 (3.1%)	57 (3.1%)
Other	341 (18.5%)	350 (19.0%)	370 (20.1%)	339 (18.4%)
ICU type				
Medical	437 (23.6%)	440 (23.8%)	481 (26.1%)	601 (32.6%)
Surgical	335 (18.1%)	238 (12.9%)	272 (14.7%)	293 (15.9%)
Trauma surgical	227 (12.3%)	198 (10.7%)	203 (11.0%)	167 (9.1%)
Cardiac surgery recovery	647 (35.0%)	739 (40.0%)	654 (35.4%)	558 (30.2%)
Coronary	202 (10.9%)	231 (12.5%)	235 (12.7%)	226 (12.2%)
Comorbidities				
Congestive heart failure	265 (14.3%)	277 (15.0%)	359 (19.5%)	363 (19.7%)
Cardiac arrhythmias	288 (15.6%)	291 (15.8%)	328 (17.8%)	408 (22.1%)
Hypertension	134 (7.3%)	170 (9.2%)	162 (8.8%)	659 (34.2%)
Valvular disease	88 (4.8%)	78 (4.2%)	117 (6.3%)	119 (6.4%)
Pulmonary circulation disease	63 (3.4%)	54 (2.9%)	78 (4.2%)	100 (5.4%)
Renal failure	167 (9.0%)	199 (10.8%)	202 (10.9%)	310 (16.8%)
Admission status				
Admission SAPS, points	20.6 (4.7)	21.2 (4.8)	21.9 (4.9)	23.0 (4.9)
Mean duration of CVP measurement (h)	40.55 (19.78)	22.88 (10.27)	51.25 (16.97)	60.24 (12.56)
Mean duration of $ECVP_{10}$ (h)	5.65 (6.10)	20.60 (11.54)	35.70 (16.06)	47.90 (17.55)
ICU outcome				
28-day mortality (%)	15.4	16.8	17.3	22.8
Length of hospitalization (day)	15.4 (14.1)	15.4 (13.4)	16.1 (13.3)	17.8 (15.8)
Length of ICU stay (day)	6.9 (7.1)	7.8 (8.0)	9.3 (9.7)	11.0 (10.9)
Selected laboratory test				
WBC max, k/μL	19.1 (9.7)	19.9 (11.1)	20.4 (16.2)	21.4 (12.7)
Lactate max (mmol/L)	2.9 (2.6)	3.2 (3.1)	3.6 (3.2)	4.9 (4.5)
Creatinine max (mg/dL)	1.9 (1.9)	2.1 (2.0)	2.3 (3.5)	2.8 (2.7)
Total bilirubin max (μmol/L)	1.7 (4.8)	1.8 (4.3)	2.4 (5.9)	4.0 (8.2)
Treatment received				
Duration of vasopressor (day)	1.8 (4.4)	2.6 (5.4)	3.6 (7.1)	4.9 (8.4)
Duration of ventilator (day)	3.8 (6.9)	4.8 (8.0)	6.5 (9.7)	7.9 (11.0)
Fluid balance [L, Median (IQR)]	3.9 (0.7, 8.0)	4.6 (1.3, 9.0)	5.3 (2.0, 10.1)	6.8 (3.0, 12.8)

Values are presented as mean (SD), unless otherwise stated

CVP central venous pressure, *IQR* interquartile range, *ICU* intensive care unit, *WBC* white blood cell, *SAPS* Simplified Acute Physiology Score

duration in non-survival group was significantly higher than in the survival group. Replacement of mean CVP with $ECVP_{10}$ duration as indicator of ECVP load did not meaningfully change the association between ECVP load and 28-day mortality (odds ratio in the highest quartile, 1.354, 95% CI 1.151–1.594, $p < 0.001$).

To examine whether the higher mean CVP level remained associated with increased 28-day mortality

Table 2 Association between $ECVP_{10}$ load during the first 3 days from ICU admission and mortality in 28 days

	Hazard ratio 28-Day mortality by quartiles of mean CVP level			
	Quartiles of mean CVP level			
	1	2	3	4
Mean CVP (SD)/mmHg	7.4 (1.9)	10.6 (1.9)	13.1 (2.2)	17.4 (4.1)
Deaths, *n* (%)	245 (13.3%)	273 (14.8%)	337 (17.5%)	433 (23.5%)
Unadjusted	1.00 (Ref.)	1.127 (0.949–1.340) $p = 0.173$	1.264 (1.068–1.496) $p = 0.006$	1.887 (1.613–2.207) $p < 0.005$
Adjusted*	1.00 (Ref.)	1.017 (0.848–1.219) $p = 0.426$	1.216 (1.018–1.451) $p = 0.046$	1.336 (1.117–1.599) $p < 0.005$

Hazard ratios (95% CI) provided. *Adjusted for sex, age, gender, ethnicity, congestive heart failure, cardiac arrhythmias, hypertension, valvular disease, pulmonary circulation disease, renal failure and other 24 Elixhauser comorbidities, ICU type, SAPS II score at admission and duration of CVP measurement

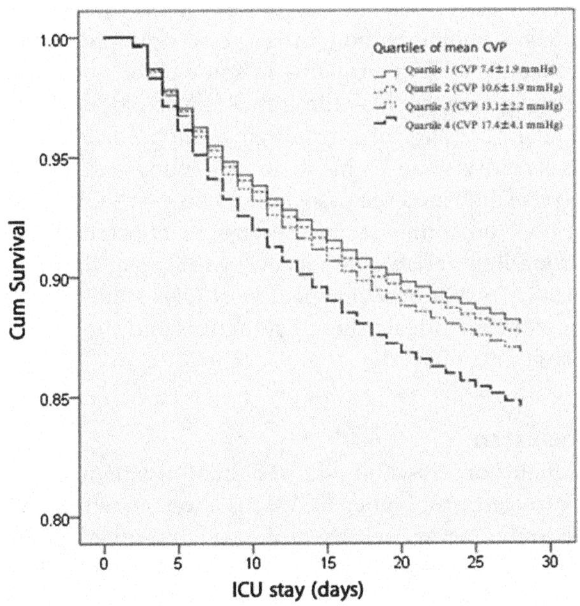

Fig. 2 Survival curve of 28-day mortality by the quartiles of mean CVP level in the patients in the critical care settings. *CVP* central venous pressure

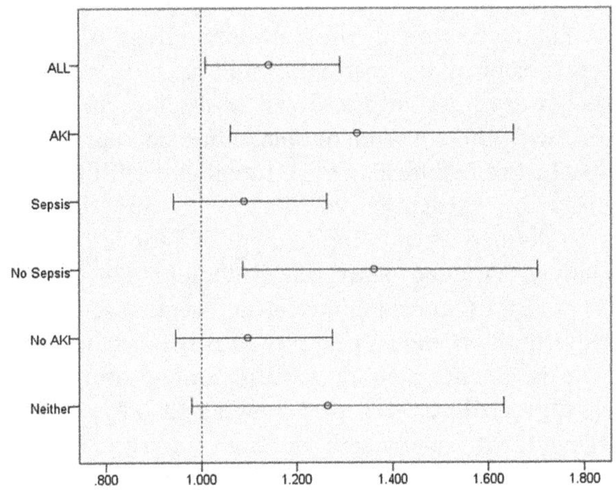

Fig. 3 Forest plot for adjusted odds ratio value of higher mean CVP level (≥10 mmHg) and 28-day mortality per subgroup. Adjusted for age, gender, ethnicity, ICU type, congestive heart failure, cardiac arrhythmias, hypertension, valvular disease, pulmonary circulation disease, renal failure and other 24 Elixhauser comorbidities, ICU type, SAPS II score at admission and duration of CVP measurement. *AKI* acute kidney injury

across subset of patients, we explored multiplicative interaction terms with and without sepsis and AKI. No significant effect of ECVP on mortality was observed in patients with sepsis [$n = 5121$, odds ratio (OR) 1.090, 95% CI 0.941–1.263, $p = 0.252$] and without AKI [$n = 6131$, odds ratio (OR) 1.097, 95% CI 0.945–1.274, $p = 0.224$], while there was a significant trend toward increased mortality from higher ECVP load in patients without sepsis [$n = 3969$, odds ratio (OR) 1.36, 95% CI 1.087–1.702, $p = 0.007$], as illustrated in Fig. 3.

Discussion

This study investigated the association between ECVP load and outcomes of patients in critical care setting. Based on comparison among patients with different levels of mean CVP, which is a measurement of ECVP load, we found that the higher mean CVP level was associated with increased 28-day mortality. Further investigation on length of hospitalization, duration of vasopressor treatment and mechanical ventilation, and laboratory results related to organ dysfunction also demonstrated that higher mean CVP level was associated with poor ICU outcome for patients in critical care settings.

In contrast to the common misleading statement of increasing CVP to a higher level to increase cardiac output, Starling curves, with the contribution of Guyton's work, did not suggest any causal relationship between CVP and cardiac output, but emphasized the comprehensive role in the interaction between cardiac function and venous return of CVP. Recent studies have showed that not only the CVP failed as a useful measure for the assessment of preload and fluid responsiveness [20], but that the ECVP is independently associated with a higher mortality and increased risk of AKI in patients with sepsis and heart failure [7, 9, 11]. These results indicated that the CVP should be considered part of the evaluation in patients with hemodynamic instability. Furthermore, an ECVP may signify an impediment to venous return [3].

Based on the study for the consensus of congestive heart failure treatment, the pathophysiology of chronic systemic venous congestion should include decreased cardiac output from increased resistance to venous return, with the subsequent splanchnic damage and tissue perfusion insufficiency [1]. Integrated with the Starling–Guyton cardiac curve, the direct cause of ECVP may be defined as "the impediment to venous return by a relatively fatigued heart" [3]. Therefore, the potential causes of ECVP may include elevated venous return, cardiac dysfunction, increased vascular resistance, increased pericardial or intrapleural pressure, among other conditions. Our study showed that a higher $ECVP_{10}$ load was associated with prolonged duration of treatment and length of ICU hospitalization. In sensitivity analysis, the result showed that impact of ECVP on mortality was limited in some subgroup patients, especially in the sepsis group, which was inconsistent with previous result [11]. Considering the difference in enrolling criteria, our result indicated that for the sepsis patients who survived the resuscitation phase, the benefit from successful resuscitation, which was always presented as higher CVP level, may attenuate the impact of ECVP on outcome and did not lead to statistically significant result. The fluid balance, mean CVP level and duration of ECVP10 result in different subgroups, and outcome (survival and non-survival) is shown in Additional file 1: Supplement Table 3.

In contrast to the long-term influence of systemic venous hypertension caused by cardiac dysfunction such as right heart failure, pericardial effusion and other conditions, the pathophysiological changes that occur with ECVP, as manifestation of systemic venous congestion, generally have acute consequences in patients being treated in critical care settings. Based upon the significance of association between ECVP load and ICU outcome, we also showed that the ECVP load should be considered and corrected in two independent aspects, level and duration, because both played important pathophysiological roles. According to the present results, we suggest that ECVP, with its association with worse outcome in critical care settings, should be considered seriously and further actions should be undertaken to discover potential causes and treatment. Our study was based on data extracted from electronic medical records in the MIMIC-III v1.3 [13], a large, open clinical database, which allowed precise research on ECVP load. To our knowledge, this study is the first to evaluate ECVP on a large population of patients managed in critical settings. More than 500,000 CVP records and 9000 patients were involved in our study. Furthermore, the use of database technologies and statistics played a critical role in reaching a meaningful conclusion in the present study. Given the extreme complexity and diversity of critically ill patients and their treatment, the traditional approach of knowledge discovery may not satisfy the need to address clinical concerns, and further efforts should be made to organize, share and analyze the "big data" in critical care [21].

This study has several limitations. First, our study is limited by its retrospective nature and the source of data used. For this reason, no causal relationships could be established. Additionally, CVP records could only be assessed in critical care patients with central venous catheter and we only extracted data from the first 3 days of ICU admission. Thus, our conclusions cannot be generalized to patients treated in a setting other than a critical care setting or without opportunities of continuous treatment during the first 3 days in ICU, for the latter of which extremely low or high CVP values may occur during the rescue/emergency phase of certain disease or pathophysiology process. Second, unlike the other studies on elevated mean CVP in certain patient populations and disease processes [5–9], we focused on a relatively long phase (72 h from ICU admission) during the general management of patients in critical care settings. Besides, it should be noted that we do not oppose to the significance of CVP targeting in some emergency events of critical care, such as the initial resuscitation phase of septic shock [2]. Third, although some predictors of illness severity were included in our study and adjusted analysis confirmed the association between $ECVP_{10}$ load and poor outcome, our results may be affected by other confounding variables associated with organ damage or mortality. Additional prospective studies should be performed to investigate these parameters and the potential causes of ECVP load.

Conclusion

In conclusion, this study showed that for patients in critical care settings, higher ECVP load was associated with poor outcome as well as prolonged treatment in ICU. Level and duration of ECVP should be evaluated, and more effort should be made to establish the cause and appropriate treatment of ECVP.

Abbreviations

CVP: central venous pressure; ECVP: elevated CVP; ICU: intensive care unit; MIT: Massachusetts Institute of Technology; BIDMC: Beth Israel Deaconess Medical Center; MIMIC: Multi-parameter Intelligent Monitoring in Intensive Care; SAPS: Simplified Acute Physiology Score; SOFA: Sequential Organ Failure Assessment; IQR: interquartile range; SD: standard deviation.

Authors' contributions

LDK and WXT contributed equally to the study, and they designed the study and performed data analysis and manuscript preparation. LDW conceived the study and helped in the result interpretation. All authors read and approved the final manuscript.

Acknowledgements
The authors acknowledge all of those involved in the design, construction and maintenance of the open access MIMIC-III database at the MIT Laboratory of Computational Physiology as well as the online community at Open Data Stack Exchange (http://opendata.stackexchange.com) and GitHub (https://github.com/MIT-LCP/mimic-code/issues).

Competing interests
The authors declare that they have no competing interests.

Funding
The authors declare that they have no relative funding support.

References

1. Marik PE. Iatrogenic salt water drowning and the hazards of a high central venous pressure. Ann Intensive Care. 2014;4(1):1–9.
2. Dellinger RP, Levy MM, Rhodes A, Annane D, Gerlach H, Opal SM, et al. Surviving Sepsis Campaign: international guidelines for management of severe sepsis and septic shock, 2012. Intensive Care Med. 2013;39(2):165–228.
3. Berlin DA, Bakker J. Starling curves and central venous pressure. Crit Care. 2015;19(1):1–8.
4. Malbrain ML, Marik PE, Witters I, Cordemans C, Kirkpatrick AW, Roberts DJ, et al. Fluid overload, de-resuscitation, and outcomes in critically ill or injured patients: a systematic review with suggestions for clinical practice. Anaesthesiol Intensive Ther. 2014;46(5):361–80.
5. Semler MW, Wheeler AP, Thompson BT, Bernard GR, Wiedemann HP, Rice TW. Impact of initial central venous pressure on outcomes of conservative versus liberal fluid management in acute respiratory distress syndrome. Crit Care Med. 2016;44(4):782–9.
6. Wang XT, Yao B, Liu DW, Zhang HM. Central venous pressure dropped early is associated with organ function and prognosis in septic shock patients: a retrospective observational study. Shock. 2015;44:426–30.
7. Legrand M, Dupuis C, Simon C, Gayat E, Mateo J, Lukaszewicz AC, et al. Association between systemic hemodynamics and septic acute kidney injury in critically ill patients: a retrospective observational study. Crit Care. 2013;17(6):1–8.
8. Damman K, van Deursen VM, Navis G, Voors AA, van Veldhuisen DJ, Hillege HL. Increased central venous pressure is associated with impaired renal function and mortality in a broad spectrum of patients with cardiovascular disease. J Am Coll Cardiol. 2009;53:582–8.
9. Mullens W, Abrahams Z, Francis GS, Sokos G, Taylor DO, Starling RC. Importance of venous congestion for worsening of renal function in advanced decompensated heart failure. J Am Coll Cardiol. 2009;53:589–96.
10. Vellinga NAR, Ince C, Boerma EC. Elevated central venous pressure is associated with impairment of microcirculatory blood flow in sepsis: a hypothesis generating post hoc analysis. BMC Anesthesiol. 2013;13(1):1–7.
11. Boyd JH, Forbes J, Nakada TA, Walley KR, Russell JA. Fluid resuscitation in septic shock: a positive fluid balance and elevated central venous pressure are associated with increased mortality. Crit Care Med. 2011;39(2):259–65.
12. Pinsky MR, Dubrawski A. Gleaning knowledge from data in the intensive care unit. Am J Respir Crit Care Med. 2014;190:606–10.
13. Johnson AE, Pollard TJ, Shen L, Lehman LWH, Feng M, Ghassemi M, et al. MIMIC-III, a freely accessible critical care database. Sci Data. 2016;3:160035.
14. Elixhauser A, Steiner C, Harris DR, Coffey RM. Comorbidity measures for use with administrative data. Med Care. 1998;36:8–27.
15. Le Gall JR, Loirat P, Alperovitch A, Glaser P, Granthil C, Mathieu D, et al. A simplified acute physiology score for ICU patients. Crit Care Med. 1984;12:975–7.
16. Vincent JL, Moreno R, Takala J, Willatts S, De Mendonça A, Bruining H, et al. The SOFA (Sepsis-related Organ Failure Assessment) score to describe organ dysfunction/failure. Intensive Care Med. 1996;22:707–10.
17. Magder S, Bafaqeeh F. The clinical role of central venous pressure measurements. J Intensive Care Med. 2007;22:44–51.
18. Singer M, Deutschman CS, Seymour CW, Shankar-Hari M, Annane D, Bauer M, et al. The third international consensus definitions for sepsis and septic shock (sepsis-3). JAMA. 2016;315(8):801–10.
19. Palevsky PM, Liu KD, Brophy PD, Chawla LS, Parikh CR, Thakar CV, et al. KDOQI US commentary on the 2012 KDIGO clinical practice guideline for acute kidney injury. Am J Kidney Dis. 2013;61:649–72.
20. Marik PE, Cavallazzi R. Does the central venous pressure predict fluid responsiveness? An updated meta-analysis and a plea for some common sense. Crit Care Med. 2013;41:1774–81.
21. Ghassemi M, Celi LA, Stone DJ. State of the art review: the data revolution in critical care. Crit Care. 2015;19:118.

Feasibility and safety of virtual-reality-based early neurocognitive stimulation in critically ill patients

Marc Turon[1,2,3*], Sol Fernandez-Gonzalo[2,4], Mercè Jodar[3,4,5], Gemma Gomà[2,6], Jaume Montanya[1], David Hernando[7], Raquel Bailón[7], Candelaria de Haro[6], Victor Gomez-Simon[6], Josefina Lopez-Aguilar[1,2], Rudys Magrans[1,2], Melcior Martinez-Perez[1,6], Joan Carles Oliva[2] and Lluís Blanch[1,2,6]

Abstract

Background: Growing evidence suggests that critical illness often results in significant long-term neurocognitive impairments in one-third of survivors. Although these neurocognitive impairments are long-lasting and devastating for survivors, rehabilitation rarely occurs during or after critical illness. Our aim is to describe an early neurocognitive stimulation intervention based on virtual reality for patients who are critically ill and to present the results of a proof-of-concept study testing the feasibility, safety, and suitability of this intervention.

Methods: Twenty critically ill adult patients undergoing or having undergone mechanical ventilation for ≥24 h received daily 20-min neurocognitive stimulation sessions when awake and alert during their ICU stay. The difficulty of the exercises included in the sessions progressively increased over successive sessions. Physiological data were recorded before, during, and after each session. Safety was assessed through heart rate, peripheral oxygen saturation, and respiratory rate. Heart rate variability analysis, an indirect measure of autonomic activity sensitive to cognitive demands, was used to assess the efficacy of the exercises in stimulating attention and working memory.

Results: Patients successfully completed the sessions on most days. No sessions were stopped early for safety concerns, and no adverse events occurred. Heart rate variability analysis showed that the exercises stimulated attention and working memory. Critically ill patients considered the sessions enjoyable and relaxing without being overly fatiguing.

Conclusions: The results in this proof-of-concept study suggest that a virtual-reality-based neurocognitive intervention is feasible, safe, and tolerable, stimulating cognitive functions and satisfying critically ill patients. Future studies will evaluate the impact of interventions on neurocognitive outcomes.

Trial registration Clinical trials.gov identifier: NCT02078206

Keywords: Neurocognitive impairments, Critically ill patients, Neurocognitive stimulation, Virtual reality, Early intervention, ICU

Background

Growing evidence suggests that critical illness often results in significant long-term morbidities. One-third of patients in intensive care units (ICU) develop neurocognitive impairments in a magnitude similar to mild–moderate dementia [1] persisting for years after hospital discharge [2, 3]. ICU-related neurocognitive impairments are particularly pronounced in regard to memory, executive functions, attentional functions, and processing speed [1, 3–10]. These impairments have far-reaching consequences and adversely impact patients' lives, contributing to impaired ability to perform

*Correspondence: mturon@tauli.cat
[2] Institut d'Investigació i Innovació Parc Taulí (I3PT), Fundació Parc Taulí, Sabadell, Spain
Full list of author information is available at the end of the article

activities of daily living, to decreased quality of life for patients and relatives, to increased medical costs, and to inability to return to work [11, 12]; however, patients rarely undergo rehabilitation during or after critical illness.

Rehabilitation strategies during the ICU stay have mainly involved physical interventions such as early mobilizations [13–16] to enhance functional recovery. Other strategies include early detection and treatment of delirium [17], and occupational therapy [18]. Recently, early rehabilitation strategies in the ICU have been extended beyond physical therapy to include cognitive interventions [19].

Physical and cognitive rehabilitation tools based on new technologies are being used successfully in patients with dementia, traumatic brain injury, stroke [20], and schizophrenia [21]. However, critically ill patients are usually bedridden and often unable to communicate verbally, posing special challenges for the development and use of technologies for cognitive intervention. Thus, we sought to design a virtual-reality-based intervention that could be used to provide critically ill patients with neurocognitive stimulation early in the ICU stay.

Another challenge in this context is determining whether an intervention actually results in brain stimulation. Heart rate variability (HRV), a surrogate marker of sympathetic and vagal activity, is a particularly sensitive index of the changes in the neural network in response to cognitive requirements. The magnitude of the changes in HRV is inversely related to the individual level of cognitive effort during cognitive tasks. HRV decreases during tasks involving specifically selective and maintained attention [22, 23] and executive functions [24, 25]. Thus, HRV analysis seems useful to confirm that neurocognitive intervention results in brain stimulation in critically ill patients.

This paper describes a virtual-reality-based early neurocognitive stimulation intervention in critically ill patients and presents preliminary results of a proof-of-concept study to assess the feasibility and safety of the intervention, its tolerability in terms of difficulty and cognitive load, and the effectiveness of the cognitive exercises in stimulating the brain. Some of these results have been presented in abstract form [26–28].

Methods

Inpatient early neurocognitive intervention

An interdisciplinary team of neuropsychologists, nurses, critical care physicians, and biomedical engineers designed the *Early Neurocognitive Rehabilitation in Intensive Care* (ENRIC) platform for neurocognitive stimulation in critically ill patients. This platform uses stimulation software with low cognitive load exercises specifically designed or adapted for critically ill patients. The stimulation software is based on virtual reality techniques immersing patients in a relaxing environment; a virtual avatar accompanies patients, orienting them in time, delivering instructions, motivating them to complete exercises, and encouraging them to relax. Different exercises based on exercises proven effective in cognitive rehabilitation programs for acquired brain injury focus on attention and executive functions [20]. Details about the stimulation software and videos are reported in the Additional files 1 and 2. The ENRIC platform consists of a central processing unit, a flat-screen TV, and a motion sensor (Kinect® Microsoft, Redmond, Washington, USA) placed on a medical cart to allow it to be moved easily to each ICU bed. The system captures and interprets patient movements through smart middleware connecting the cognitive stimulation software with input from the motion sensor. This approach to patient–system interaction avoids the risk of cross-infections inherent in sharing physical devices such as joysticks and touch tablets. The platform also incorporates a system to collect and store physiological data (BetterCare®, Barcelona, Spain) from bedside monitors and ventilators [29] that could be used to adapt the level of cognitive stimulation to patients' clinical condition (Fig. 1). The ENRIC platform turns on when it is plugged in. Before each session, it is necessary to calibrate the Kinect® motion sensor and to adjust the distance between the patient and sensor; patients are asked to raise their hands in front of the sensor to check detection and motion recognition. Sometimes, the ICU bed needs to be raised or lowered. Bed adjustments and sensor calibration take less than 2 min. Although patients have no physical contact with any components of the device at any time, for reasons of infection control, the device is cleaned and disinfected after each session when it is used in isolated patients.

Patients

Patients were recruited from a mixed medical/surgical ICU with 16 beds in single rooms at a university teaching hospital. Patients aged 18–85 years old who were undergoing or had undergone invasive mechanical ventilation for $\geq$24 h were eligible. Patients with a history of neurologic disease, dementia, focal brain injury at ICU admission, serious psychiatric disorders, or mental retardation were excluded. Deaf and/or blind patients were also excluded. Eligible patients were screened daily and invited to participate when they achieved minimum levels of consciousness to interact with the ENRIC platform [Glasgow Coma Scale (GCS) $\geq$13] and sedation (Richmond Agitation–Sedation Scale (RASS) -1 to $+1$).

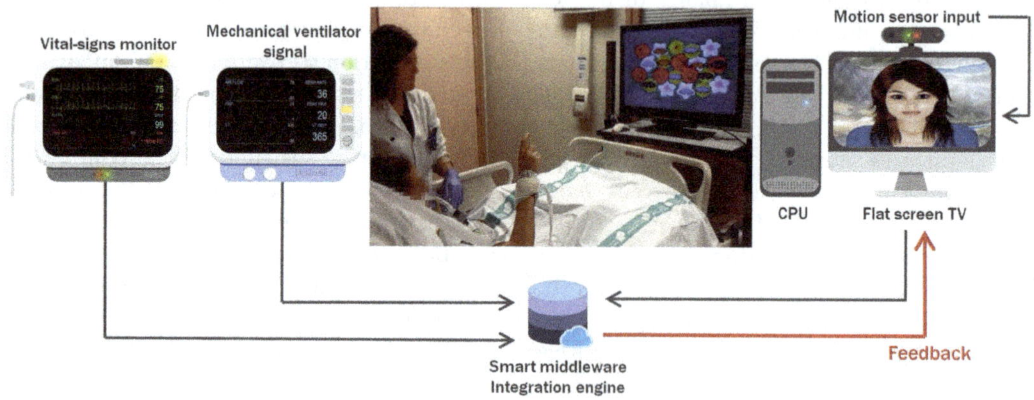

Fig. 1 Schematic diagram of the smart middleware connecting ENRIC platform, bedside monitor and ventilator (screenshots of bedside monitor and ventilator courtesy of BetterCare®, Barcelona, Spain). The platform uses smart middleware to connect the cognitive stimulation software with input from a motion sensor (Kinect®, Microsoft, Redmond, Washington, USA) that captures and interprets patient movements. The platform also incorporates a system to collect and store physiological data (BetterCare®, Barcelona, Spain) from bedside monitors and ventilators that could be used to adapt the level of cognitive stimulation to patients' clinical condition

Procedure

Demographic data and severity (Acute Physiologic and Chronic Health Evaluation II (APACHE-II) and Sequential Organ Failure Assessment (SOFA) scores) were recorded at inclusion. Level of consciousness was assessed daily from ICU admission to initiation of the intervention. Upon reaching GCS ≥13, patients were screened daily for delirium using the Spanish version of the Confusional Assessment Method for the Intensive Care Unit (CAM-ICU) and for level of alertness using the RASS.

Patients received the neurocognitive stimulation sessions each day in their own beds when they were alert and calm (RASS −1 to +1) until discharge from the ICU. Sessions were guided by a neuropsychologist and supervised by an ICU nurse. Sessions aimed to provide cognitive stimulation and engagement through exercises, not necessarily obtaining correct answers. The exercises included in each session were determined by patients' alertness level and ability to raise each arm separately with elbow straight against gravity (see Additional file 3: Figure S1 for a detailed description of the protocol). The clinical team predefined the length of the session as a minimum of 15 and maximum of 20 min. However, whenever clinical conditions allowed it, patients were encouraged to continue as long as they could without fatigue. Physiological data were recorded 20 min before sessions, during sessions, and after sessions.

Before this proof-of-concept study, six healthy volunteers tested the ENRIC platform in a session simulating ICU patients' situation and then rated their experience on a five-point Likert scale. The first six patients included in the study also completed the same ad hoc survey about their experience with the ENRIC platform. Finally, ICU personnel, including nurses, physicians, and physiotherapists, were asked to complete an acceptance survey, giving their opinions about the compatibility of the ENRIC platform with ICU workload (see Additional file 4).

Measures

Feasibility was assessed in terms of the practicability of delivering neurocognitive stimulation early during critical illness: rates of patients eligible to receive the intervention and of patients who underwent the intervention, number of sessions performed, timing of initiation, and duration of each session.

Safety was assessed by considering the sessions that had to be stopped early for clinical reasons, through analyses of heart rate (HR), peripheral oxygen saturation (SpO_2), and respiratory rate (RR). The safety analysis was based on expert consensus criteria for unsafe active mobilization of mechanically ventilated critically ill patients [30]: $SpO_2 < 90\%$, RR > 35 breaths per minute, and HR > 150 beats per minute, all during ≥5 min. When out-of-range values were present at the beginning of the session, changes >20% from baseline in any physiological parameter were also considered unsafe events requiring the session to be stopped.

Tolerability was assessed in terms of the extent to which sessions were completed and to which patients tolerated the difficulty and cognitive load of the exercises included. Thus, we recorded number of interrupted sessions and cause of interruption, as well as the type of exercises in each session.

The effectiveness in stimulating the brain was assessed in terms of autonomic reactivity during sessions using

HRV frequency-domain analyses [31]. Spectral analysis was performed over consecutive 2-min R–R intervals series with an overlap of 1 min to ensure an analysis interval as stationary as possible. HRV was derived from the detected normal beat occurrence time series using the integral pulse frequency modulation (IPFM) model, which takes ectopic beats into accounts [32]. Since the mean heart rate is not constant (it evolves continuously in challenging situations, such as physical and mental effort, especially in critically ill patients), the HRV signal was corrected by the time-varying mean heart rate [33], yielding the modulating signal which, according to the IPFM model, represents autonomic nervous system modulation over the sinoatrial node. The modulating signal was sampled at 4 Hz, and its power spectral density was estimated. Low-frequency (LF) power and high-frequency (HF) power were computed by integrating the area under the power spectral density in the LF and HF bands, respectively. The LF band was 0.04–0.15 Hz. The HF band was centered on the respiratory frequency, and bandwidth ranged from 0.15 to 0.3 Hz in function of respiratory stability. We also included total power, an index of overall autonomic modulation summing the power in the LF and HF bands. LF values were normalized (LFn) by total power to exclusively reflect sympathetic modulation [31] and were expressed in normalized units, while HF values were expressed in adimensional units to reflect parasympathetic activity.

Statistical analysis

Mean scores on the satisfaction survey were computed from the individual raw scores for all items included in each category after converting scores of negatively worded items to positives. Mean scores were analyzed using the Mann–Whitney *U* test.

No formal power calculations were undertaken; rather sufficient participants were recruited during ~9 months to determine factors such as recruitment rates in relation to feasibility outcomes.

Feasibility, safety, and tolerability outcomes were analyzed using descriptive statistics. To analyze whether the intervention actually stimulated the brain, LFn, HF, and total power indices during the sessions were compared with baseline values using the Wilcoxon signed-rank test, because values for these variables were not normally distributed. Because patients received the total range of neurocognitive exercises during the first three sessions, to avoid potential effects on autonomic reactivity due to the lack of novelty in subsequent sessions, HRV analysis was limited to the first three sessions.

All analyses were performed with SPSS version 19.0 (IBM, Armonk, NY); significance was set at 0.05. Results are presented as means and ranges or n/N (%), unless otherwise noted.

Results

Patients' clinical and sociodemographic characteristics

Between April 2014 and December 2014, 193 patients were admitted to the ICU; 148 met at least one exclusion criterion. Of the 45 eligible patients, 25 were excluded for the following reasons: 12 were discharged within 48 h, 7 remained unconscious, 4 were transferred to other centers, and 2 did not consent (Fig. 2). Thus, 20 patients received the early neurocognitive intervention; Table 1 summarizes their clinical and sociodemographic characteristics.

Feasibility of early neurocognitive stimulation

All 20 patients (100%) received the early neurocognitive intervention on at least one study day. The first session was delivered 10.0 (2.0–23.0) days after ICU admission. Once patients started the intervention, sessions were delivered on 74.3% (25.0–100.0%) of the eligible study days until ICU discharge.

During the study, 76 sessions were delivered [mean number of sessions per patient, 3.8 (1.0–8.0); mean duration of each session, 17.5 (12.0–31.0) minutes].

Safety of early neurocognitive stimulation

Table 2a, b summarizes HR, RR, and SpO_2 at baseline, during the session, and after the session and indicates the percentage of patients who were mechanically ventilated during each session. No unsafe HR values were observed in recordings at baseline or during the session; after the first session, unsafe HR values lasting less than 5 min were observed in one patient (1/20, 5%) after the first session and in another patient (1/11, 9.1%) after the fourth. During sessions, some patients reached unsafe minimum SpO_2 values lasting less than 5 min (session #1: 2/20, 10%; session #2: 1/17, 5.9%; session #3: 1/13, 7.7%; and session #4: 1/11, 9.1%), and some patients reached unsafe RR (session #1: 6/20, 30%; session #2: 11.8%; session #3: 2/13, 15.4%; session #4: 3/11, 27.3%; session #5: 4/8, 50%; session #6: 1/4, 25%; and session #7: 1/2, 50%). Nevertheless, no sessions were stopped early for safety concerns, and no adverse events (e.g., inadvertent removal of catheters or endotracheal tubes) occurred. No changes in physiological parameters ≥20% from baseline were observed during the sessions. No patients received vasoactive agents during sessions.

Tolerability of early neurocognitive stimulation

Patients completed 66/76 (86.8%) of possible neurocognitive stimulation sessions. Most (70%) incomplete sessions

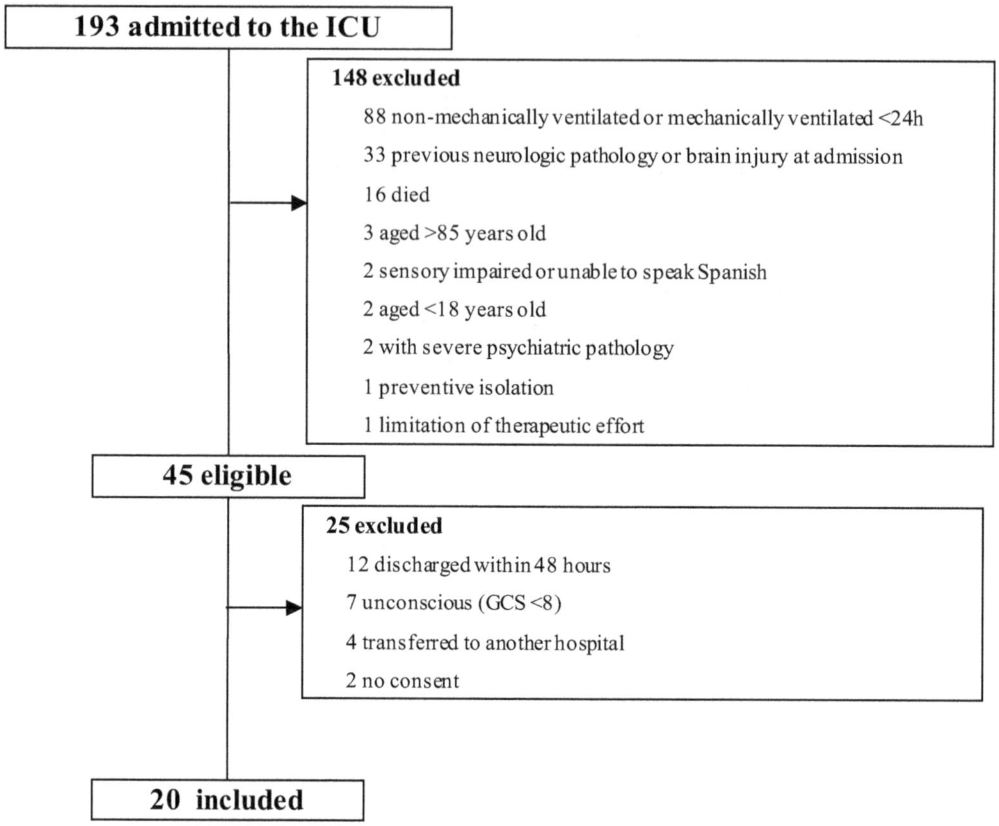

Fig. 2 Flow diagram of sample. During a period comprising ~9 months, 193 patients were admitted to the ICU; 148 met at least one exclusion criterion. Of the 45 eligible patients, 25 were finally excluded. Thus, 20 patients received the early neurocognitive intervention

occurred on the first day. Reasons for discontinuing a session were fatigue (50%), extreme sleepiness (20%), competing medical procedures (20%), and confusion (10%). Discontinuation did not preclude participation in subsequent sessions.

Figure 3 illustrates the composition of the first five sessions, with progressively more challenging exercises. In the first session, *passive exercises* requiring simple attention and gross motor functions accounted for 55.6% of the total time. In subsequent sessions, the time spent on *passive exercises* gradually decreased, while the time spent on exercises requiring more complex cognitive effort (*selective attention* and *working memory exercises*) increased. Patients correctly followed the neuropsychologist's orders in the *guided-observation exercises*, which represented 34.2% of the total session time. *Selective attention exercises* accounted for 10.2% of the total time. The most complex exercises, focusing on *working memory*, were only performed from the third session, and the time assigned for these exercises was increased progressively with each session. In the fifth session, equal time was assigned to each type of exercises.

Effectiveness of neurocognitive exercises in stimulating the brain

Table 3 displays the results of HRV analysis for the three main frequency-domain indices. In session #1, LFn was lower ($p = 0.02$) than baseline values. In session #2, all indices were lower than baseline (LFn, $p = 0.01$; HF, $p = 0.03$; and total power, $p = 0.01$). In session #3, total power was lower than baseline ($p = 0.02$).

Satisfaction and acceptance survey results

Table S1 compares satisfaction survey scores between healthy volunteers and critically ill patients (see Additional file 4). Patients scored higher than volunteers for *relaxation* ($p = 0.002$) and *system interaction* ($p = 0.004$) and lower for *boredom* ($p = 0.041$). Additional file 4: Table S2 reports the scores on the acceptance survey for ICU personnel, including the overall mean as well as mean scores for physicians, nurses, and physiotherapists. The lowest rated item was *Compatibility with physical infrastructure and ICU facilities*, and the highest rated items were *Compatibility with pharmacologic treatment* and *Compatibility with physiotherapy*.

Table 1 Clinical and sociodemographic characteristics of critically ill patients undergoing early neurocognitive intervention (n = 20)

Age, years (M, SD)	65	10
Sex (N, %)		
Male	14	63.66
Female	6	27.33
Diagnosis (N, %)		
Medical		
Pneumonia	3	15
Septic shock	3	15
Acute respiratory failure	1	5
ARDS	1	5
Pancreatitis	1	5
Toxic intake	1	5
Unplanned surgery		
Peritonitis	3	15
Multiple trauma	2	10
Intestinal perforation	2	10
Pneumoperitoneum	1	5
Planned surgery		
Hemorrhagic shock	1	5
Esophageal perforation	1	5
Receiving MV at inclusion (N, %)	7	35
APACHE-II (M, SD)	24.84	9.04
SOFA (M, SD)	9.58	4.23
GCS (M, SD)	10.33	5.91
ICU LoS, days (Md, IQR)	16.00	2.00
Total MV time, days (Md, IQR)	9.50	1.00
Sedation, days (Md, IQR)	5.00	0.00
Delirium, days (Md, IQR)	1.39	0.80
Septic shock (N, %)	12	60
Cardiac arrest (N, %)	1	5

APACHE-II Acute Physiology and Chronic Health Evaluation II, *ARDS* acute respiratory distress syndrome, *GCS* Glasgow Coma Scale, *ICU* intensive care unit, *IQR* interquartile range, *LoS* length of stay, *M* mean, *Md* median, *MV* mechanical ventilation, *SD* standard deviation

Discussion

Our results indicate that this virtual-reality-based neurocognitive intervention is feasible, safe, and tolerable for critically ill patients (including mechanically ventilated patients) and that the exercises used provide cognitive stimulation. The satisfaction and acceptance surveys found that critically ill patients considered the sessions enjoyable and relaxing without being overly fatiguing. Furthermore, ICU personnel considered the neurocognitive intervention compatible with the routine workload and the usual treatments prescribed in the ICU.

Neurocognitive impairments in ICU survivors may be understood as a manifestation of occult brain damage resulting from pathophysiological mechanisms related to critical illness and crosstalk between organs [34, 35]. Therefore, it might be interesting to consider ICU patients as a subset of brain-injured patients and treat them with tools such as cognitive stimulation that have proven effective in treating neurocognitive impairments in outpatient populations [36]. However, neurocognitive stimulation techniques commonly used in post-acute patients are often unfeasible in critically ill patients, who may be bedridden, have low awareness levels that fluctuate during the day, have reduced mobility due to myopathy and ICU-acquired weakness, and are unable to communicate verbally because they are receiving mechanical ventilation. To overcome these barriers to implementing neurocognitive interventions in the ICU, clinicians need safe, feasible, and easy-to-use tools for neurocognitive stimulation. To our knowledge, this study is the first to establish a proof of concept for virtual-reality-based neurocognitive stimulation in critically ill patients.

The motion sensor in the ENRIC platform provides a feasible solution to mobility and communication problems in early neurocognitive stimulation for critically ill patients. Brummel et al. [19] started an intervention combining physical therapy and cognitive therapy within 72 h after ICU admission when patients achieved RASS −3 to −2, but their cognitive protocol started only when they achieved RASS −1 to +1. In our study, neurocognitive stimulation started when patients reached RASS −1 to +1 (median, 10 days after ICU admission; range 2–23 days), suggesting that deep-sedation strategies, in addition to leading to increased prevalence of brain dysfunction in ICU [37], are the most important barrier to this kind of interventions in the ICU. In a pilot study of feasibility of physical interventions in critically ill patients, profound levels of sedation made 27% of physical sessions impossible [38]; protocols reducing sedation could help enable both physical and neurocognitive interventions in the ICU. Nonetheless, patients in our study successfully received neurocognitive stimulation during 74.3% of their time in the ICU, reflecting a wide therapeutic window for treatment.

No sessions were stopped early for safety concerns, and no adverse events (e.g., inadvertent removal of catheters or endotracheal tubes) occurred. Patients' tolerance to increasingly difficult exercises in neurocognitive stimulation sessions increased as patients' physical and cognitive status improved, showing that the intervention is safely adaptable to each patient's physical and cognitive condition from the first day to ICU discharge.

Importantly, the intervention seems effective in stimulating the brain. Our HRV analysis found an overall decrease in the spectral components of HRV during the neurocognitive stimulation intervention. Since HRV decreases when attentional [22, 23] and executive

Table 2 Values of physiological parameters at baseline, during session, and post-session

	Session 1			Session 2			Session 3			Session 4		
	(n = 20; MV in 35%)			(n = 17; MV in 35%)			(n = 13; MV in 38%)			(n = 11; MV in 36%)		
	Baseline	Session	Post	Baseline	Session	Post	Baseline	Session	Post	Baseline	Session	Post
(a)												
HR, Md (IQR)	92 (14)	92.5 (15.75)	91 (10.5)	82 (23)	84 (21.25)	81.5 (25.5)	96 (19)	90 (15)	90 (15)	86 (31.75)	67 (34.5)	90.5 (35.5)
Range	67–120	70–119	70–153[a]	56–127	68–126	65–125	69–134	72–137	72–137	62–128	59–129	67–168[a]
SPO_2, Md (IQR)	96 (5)	95.5 (4.25)	95 (5)	94.5 (3.75)	94.5 (4.5)	94 (3.75)	96 (4)	96 (2)	96 (2)	97 (2.75)	97 (2.75)	97 (2.5)
Range	88[b]–100	89[b]–100	90–100	89[b]–100	89[b]–100	89[b]–100	90–100	89[b]–100	90–100	91–100	89[b]–100	90–100
RR, Md (IQR)	22 (13)	24 (12)	22 (13.5)	22.5 (12.25)	23.5 (11)	24 (10.75)	25 (14)	25 (9)	22 (8)	20.5 (16.25)	21.5 (11.5)	24.5 (15)
Range	11–54[c]	10–41[c]	10–54[c]	9–46[c]	9–40[c]	9–44[c]	12–47[c]	12–37[c]	12–41[c]	12–42[c]	12–41[c]	9–43[c]
	Session 5			Session 6			Session 7			Session 8		
	(n = 8; MV in 50%)			(n = 4; MV in 50%)			(n = 2; MV in 100%)			(n = 1; MV in 100%)		
	Baseline	Session	Post	Baseline	Session	Post	Baseline	Session	Post	Baseline	Session	Post
(b)												
HR, Md (IQR)	102 (25.5)	103 (27.5)	101 (24)	108 (12)	110 (16)	111 (8.5)	112.5 (4.75)	115 (1.25)	111 (1)	126 (4)	123 (2)	127 (3)
Range	61–139	63–138	64–128	79–118	78–121	88–120	104–123	93–123	107–114	121–134	119–125	117–134
SPO_2, Md (IQR)	98 (2)	97 (1.5)	97 (2.5)	97 (4)	97 (2.5)	98 (2)	99.5 (1.25)	98.5 (1.25)	98 (1)	98 (1)	98 (0)	99 (1)
Range	89[b]–100	91–100	92–100	90–100	91–100	90–100	97–100	95–100	95–100	94–99	98–99	96–100
RR, Md (IQR)	21 (15)	23 (13)	23 (15.5)	25 (6)	25 (6.5)	26 (6)	26.5 (7)	27.5 (6.5)	29 (2)	27 (3)	26 (3)	25 (6)
Range	11–40[c]	10–39[c]	10–50[c]	13–38[c]	13–36[c]	13–37[c]	19–40[c]	18–37[c]	18–39[c]	14–33	20–33	12–40[c]

MV mechanical ventilation, *Md* median, *IQR* interquartile range, *HR* heart rate, *SpO_2* peripheral oxygen saturation, *RR* respiratory rate

[a] HR $\geq$ 150 bpm

[b] $SpO_2 \leq 90\%$

[c] RR $\geq$ 35 breaths/min

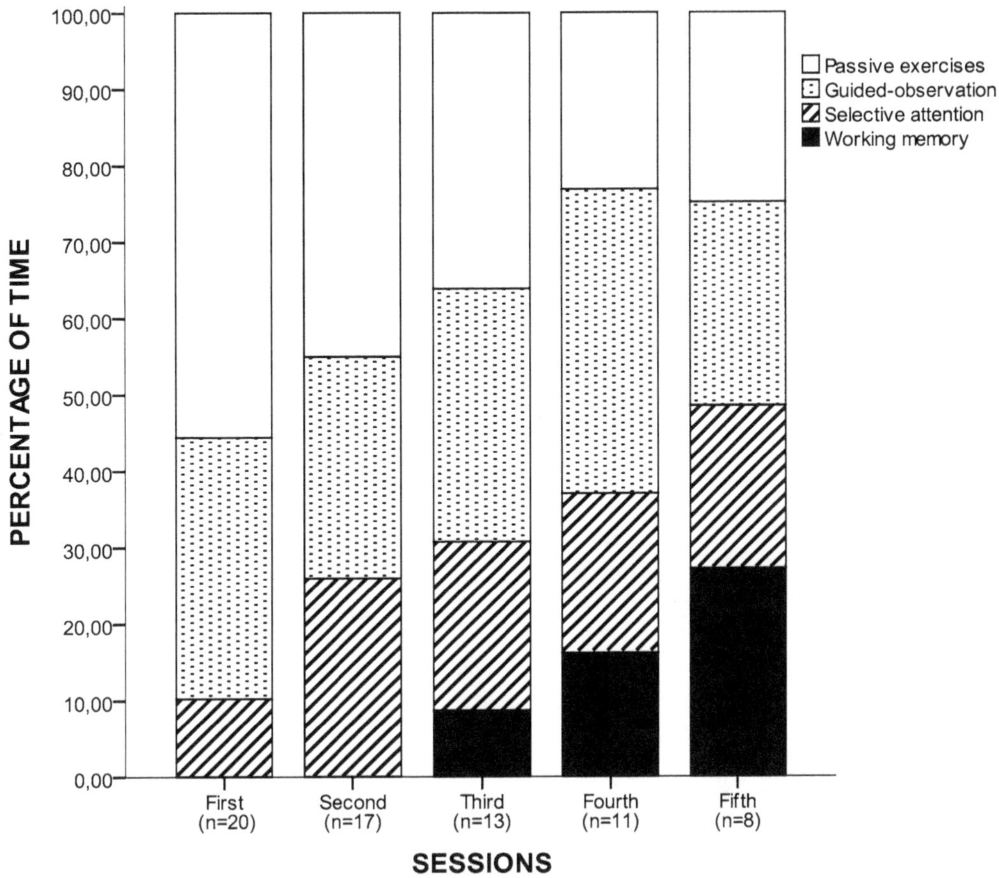

Fig. 3 Time distribution (%) of neurocognitive exercises for each session during the first five sessions. In the first session, *passive exercises* requiring simple attention and gross motor functions were the most performed exercises. In subsequent sessions, the time spent on *passive exercises* gradually decreased, while the time spent on exercises focusing on *selective attention* and *working memory* increased. *Guided-observation exercises* were well tolerated for patients from the first session. The most complex exercises, focusing on *working memory*, were only performed from the third session, and the time assigned for these exercises was increased progressively with each session. *Note* that in the fifth session, equal time was assigned to each type of exercises

functions [24, 25] are stimulated, these results indicate that the intervention stimulated these cognitive functions in our critically ill patients, including those with low alertness levels.

There is some evidence that neurocognitive interventions can help mitigate long-term ICU-related neurocognitive deficits. Jackson et al. [39] found that combined cognitive and physical therapy improved executive function and instrumental activities of daily living in a sample of ICU survivors. However, delaying interventions until after ICU discharge may be less effective, and introducing interventions only when cognitive and physical decline has already appeared seems insufficient to completely reverse deficits [40]. Early neurocognitive stimulation promises to improve outcomes in critically ill patients, potentially decreasing the incidence and duration of delirium, shortening ICU and hospital stays, and ultimately reducing costs while improving cognitive function and quality of life after discharge. Nevertheless, neurocognitive interventions are rarely routinely delivered during hospitalization. Our small sample from a single center limits the generalizability of our specific findings. However, this proof-of-concept study aimed only to assess feasibility of neurocognitive stimulation in the ICU. Therefore, many key questions were not addressed (e.g., the best type of intervention or exercises for cognitive stimulation, the optimal time to start neurocognitive interventions, the optimal duration and intensity of interventions, and impact of interventions on long-term outcomes). These questions should be assessed in larger samples. Ultimately, HRV can be influenced by certain drugs typically prescribed in ICU, among which include anticholinergic drugs, agents with effect on adrenergic receptors, angiotensin-converting enzyme inhibitors, or even calcium channel blockers, so the effect should be considered cautiously while interpreting HRV results.

Table 3 Heart rate variability indices at baseline and during session

	Session 1		p	Session 2		p	Session 3		p
	Baseline	Session		Baseline	Session		Baseline	Session	
LFn, Md (IQR)	3.87×10^{-5} (2.03×10^{-4})	3.02×10^{-5} (8.64×10^{-5})	0.02	7.44×10^{-5} (4.68×10^{-4})	6.91×10^{-5} (3.79×10^{-4})	0.01	9.17×10^{-5} (5.31×10^{-4})	6.74×10^{-5} (3.85×10^{-4})	0.23
HF, Md (IQR)	1.63×10^{-3} (1.64×10^{-1})	6.48×10^{-5} (2.31×10^{-1})	0.65	2.84×10^{-5} (5.17×10^{-5})	2.64×10^{-5} (2.05×10^{-4})	0.03	6.94×10^{-5} (1.21×10^{-3})	6.19×10^{-5} (8.71×10^{-4})	0.11
Total, Md (IQR)	2.88×10^{-3} (1.64×10^{-1})	2.25×10^{-4} (2.32×10^{-1})	0.38	9.85×10^{-5} (4.31×10^{-4})	9.81×10^{-5} (6.43×10^{-4})	0.01	2.44×10^{-4} (1.46×10^{-3})	1.08×10^{-4} (2.26×10^{-3})	0.02

LFn power in low-frequency band expressed in normalized units, *HF* power in high-frequency band expressed in adimensional units, *Total* total power expressed in adimensional units, *Md* median, *IQR* interquartile range

p values for nonparametric Wilcoxon signed-rank test

Conclusions

This proof-of-concept study shows that virtual-reality-based neurocognitive interventions are feasible, safe, and tolerable for critically ill patients. It also shows that the ENRIC platform stimulates cognitive functions and was well received by patients. These preliminary results lay the groundwork for implementing such interventions on a larger scale to evaluate their efficacy.

Additional files

Additional file 1: Video 1. Neurocognitive stimulation session with mechanically ventilated patient.

Additional file 2: Video 2. Details of neurocognitive stimulation software and system interaction.

Additional file 3: Figure S1. Diagram of sessions planning based on alertness and mobility parameters. RASS score and the ability to raise autonomously each arm separately with their elbow straight against gravity determined the intensity of stimulation and which exercises to include in each session.

Additional file 4: Table S1. Satisfaction survey scores in healthy volunteers versus critically ill patients. **Table S2.** Acceptance survey scores in physicians, nurses, and physiotherapists.

Abbreviations

APACHE-II: Acute Physiologic and Chronic Health Evaluation II; CAM-ICU: Confusional Assessment Method for ICU; ENRIC: Early Neurocognitive Rehabilitation in Intensive Care; GCS: Glasgow Coma Scale; HF: high frequency; HR: heart rate; HRV: heart rate variability; ICU: intensive care unit; IPFM: integral pulse frequency modulation; LF: low frequency; LFn: normalized low frequency; RASS: Richmond Agitation–Sedation Scale; RR: respiratory rate; SOFA: Sequential Organ Failure Assessment; SpO_2: oxygen peripheral saturation.

Authors' contributions

MT, SFG, MJ, VGS, MMP, and LB were involved in conception and design; MT, SFG, GG, and CdH were involved in realization; MT, DH, RB, JM, RD, and JCO analyzed and interpreted the data; MT, SFG, JLA, MJ, CdH, RM, and LB drafted the manuscript for important intellectual content. All authors read and approved the final manuscript.

Author details

[1] Centro de Investigación Biomédica En Red en Enfermedades Respiratorias (CIBERES), Instituto de Salud Carlos III, Madrid, Spain. [2] Institut d'Investigació i Innovació Parc Taulí (I3PT), Fundació Parc Taulí, Sabadell, Spain. [3] Department of Clinical and Health Psychology, Universitat Autònoma de Barcelona, International Excellence Campus, Bellaterra, Spain. [4] Centro de Investigación Biomédica En Red en Salud Mental (CIBERSAM), Instituto de Salud Carlos III, Madrid, Spain. [5] Neurology Department, Parc Taulí Hospital Universitari, Institut d'Investigació i Innovació Parc Taulí (I3PT), Universitat Autònoma de Barcelona, Sabadell, Spain. [6] Critical Care Department, Parc Taulí Hospital Universitari, Institut d'Investigació i Innovació Parc Taulí (I3PT), Universitat Autònoma de Barcelona, Sabadell, Spain. [7] BSICOS Group, 13A, Universidad de Zaragoza&CIBER-BBN, Saragossa, Spain.

Acknowledgements

The authors thank Mr. John Giba for his invaluable support in editing the manuscript.

Competing interests

LB is inventor of one Corporació Sanitaria Parc Taulí owned US patent: "Method and system for managed related patient parameters provided by a monitoring device," US Patent No. 12/538,940. LB is founder of BetterCare S.L., which is a research and development spin-off of Corporació Sanitària Parc Taulí (Spain). The authors declare that they have no competing interests.

Funding

This work has been financially supported by Fundació La Marató TV3 (181/U/2011), Instituto de Salud Carlos III de Madrid (PI13/02204), CIBER Enfermedades Respiratorias (ES15PINT007) and Fundació Parc Taulí (CIR2014/028). No funding organization or sponsor was involved in the preparation, review, or approval of the manuscript.

References

1. Jackson JC, Hart RP, Gordon SM, Shintani A, Truman B, May L, Ely EW. Six-month neuropsychological outcome of medical intensive care unit patients. Crit Care Med. 2003;31:1226–34.
2. Rothenhaüsler HB, Ehrentraut S, Stoll C, Schelling G, Kapfhammer HP. The relationship between cognitive performance and employment and health status in long-term survivors of the acute respiratory distress syndrome: results of an exploratory study. Gen Hosp Psychiatry. 2001;23:90–6.
3. Hopkins RO, Weaver LK, Collingridge D, Parkinson RB, Chan KJ, Orme JF Jr. Two-year cognitive, emotional, and quality-of-life outcomes in acute respiratory distress syndrome. Am J Respir Crit Care Med. 2005;171:340–7.
4. Hopkins RO, Weaver LK, Chan KJ, Orme JF. Quality of life, emotional and cognitive functions following acute respiratory distress syndrome. J Int Neuropsychol Soc. 2004;10:1005–17.
5. Sukantarat KT, Burguess PW, Williamson RC, Brett SJ. Prolonged cognitive dysfunction in survivors of critical illness. Anaesthesia. 2005;60:847–53.
6. Jones C, Griffits RD, Slater T, Benjamin KS, Wilson S. Significant cognitive dysfunction in non-delirious patients identified during and persisting following critical illness. Intensive Care Med. 2006;32:923–6.
7. Mikkelsen ME, Shull WH, Biester RC, Taichman DB, Lynch S, Demissie E, Hansen-Flaschen J, Christie JD. Cognitive, mood and quality of life impairments in a select population of ARDS survivors. Respirology. 2009;14:76–82.
8. Mikkelsen ME, Christie JD, Lanken PN, Biester RC, Thompson BT, Bellamy SL, Localio AR, Demissie E, Hopkins RO, Angus DC. The adult respiratory distress syndrome cognitive outcomes study: long-term neuropsychological function in survivors of acute lung injury. Am J Respir Crit Care Med. 2012;185:1307–15.
9. Woon FL, Dunn CB, Hopkins RO. Predicting cognitive sequelae in survivors of critical illness with cognitive screening tests. Am J Respir Crit Care Med. 2012;186:333–40.
10. Pandharipande PP, Girard TD, Jackson JC, Morandi A, Thompson JL, Pun BT, Brummel NE, Hughes CG, Vasilevskis EE, Shintani AK, Moons KG, Geevarghese SK, Canonico A, Hopkins RO, Bernard GR, Dittus RS, Ely EW. Long-term cognitive impairment after critical illness. N Engl J Med. 2013;369:1306–16.
11. Herridge MS, Tansey CM, Matté A, Tomlinson G, Diaz-Granados N, Cooper A, Guest CB, Mazer CD, Mehta S, Stewart TE, Kudlow P, Cook D, Slutsky AS, Cheung AM, Canadian Critical Care Trials Group. Functional disability 5 years after acute respiratory distress syndrome. N Engl J Med. 2011;364:1293–304.
12. Norman BC, Jackson JC, Graves JA, Girard TD, Pandharipande PP, Brummel NE, Wang L, Thompson JL, Chandrasekhar R, Ely EW. Employment outcomes after critical illness: an analysis of the bringing to light the risk factors and incidence of neuropsychological dysfunction in ICU survivors cohort. Crit Care Med. 2016;44:2003–9.
13. Gosselink R, Bott J, Johnson M, Dean E, Nava S, Norrenberg M, Schönhofer B, Stiller K, van de Leur H, Vincent JL. Physiotherapy for adult patients with critical illness: recommendations of the European Respiratory Society and European Society of Intensive Care Medicine Task Force on physiotherapy for critically ill patients. Intensive Care Med. 2008;34:1188–99.

14. Burtin C, Clerckx B, Robbeets C, Ferdinande P, Langer D, Troosters T, Hermans G, Decramer M, Gosselink R. Early exercise in critically ill patients enhances short-term functional recovery. Crit Care Med. 2009;37:2499–505.
15. Morris PE, Goad A, Thompson C, Taylor K, Harry B, Passmore L, Ross A, Anderson L, Baker S, Sanchez M, Penley L, Howard A, Dixon L, Leach S, Small R, Hite RD, Haponik E. Early intensive care unit mobility therapy in the treatment of acute respiratory failure. Crit Care Med. 2008;36:2238–43.
16. Bailey P, Thomsen GE, Spuhler VJ, Blair R, Jewkes J, Bezdjian L, Veale K, Rodriquez L, Hopkins RO. Early activity is feasible and safe in respiratory failure patients. Crit Care Med. 2007;35:139–45.
17. Brummel NE, Girard TD. Preventing delirium in the intensive care unit. Crit Care Clin. 2013;29:51–65.
18. Schweickert WD, Pohlman MC, Pohlman AS, Nigos C, Pawlik AJ, Esbrook CL, Spears L, Miller M, Franczyk M, Deprizio D, Schmidt GA, Bowman A, Barr R, McCallister KE, Hall JB, Kress JP. Early physical and occupational therapy in mechanically ventilated, critically ill patients: a randomized controlled trial. Lancet. 2009;373:1874–82.
19. Brummel NE, Girard TD, Ely EW, Pandharipande PP, Morandi A, Hughes CG, Graves AJ, Shintani A, Murphy E, Work B, Pun BT, Boehm L, Gill TM, Dittus RS, Jackson JC. Feasibility and safety of early combined cognitive and physical therapy for critically ill medical and surgical patients: the Activity and Cognitive Therapy in ICU (ACT-ICU) trial. Intensive Care Med. 2014;40:370–9.
20. Bogdanova Y, Yee MK, Ho VT, Cicerone KD. Computerized cognitive rehabilitation of attention and executive function in acquired brain injury: a systematic review. J Head Trauma Rehabil. 2016;31:419–33.
21. Fernandez-Gonzalo S, Turon M, Jodar M, Pousa E, Hernandez-Rambla C, García R, Palao D. A new computerized cognitive and social cognition training specifically designed for patients with schizophrenia/schizoaffective disorder in early stages of illness: a pilot study. Psychiatry Res. 2015;228:501–9.
22. Park G, Vasey MW, Van Bavel JJ, Thayer JF. Cardiac vagal tone is correlated with selective attention to neutral distractors under load. Psychophysiology. 2013;50:398–406.
23. Duschek S, Muckenthaler M, Werner N, del Paso GA. Relationships between features of autonomic cardiovascular control and cognitive performance. Biol Psychol. 2009;81:110–7.
24. Mathewson KJ, Jetha MK, Drmic IE, Bryson SE, Goldberg JO, Hall GB, Santesso DL, Segalowitz SJ, Schmidt LA. Autonomic predictors of Stroop performance in young and middle-aged adults. Int J Psychophysiol. 2010;76:123–9.
25. Thayer JF, Hansen AL, Saus-Rose E, Johnsen BH. Heart rate variability, prefrontal neural function, and cognitive performance: the neurovisceral integration perspective on self-regulation, adaptation, and health. Ann Behav Med. 2009;37:141–53.
26. Fernandez-Gonzalo S, Turon M, Gomà G, Martínez-Pérez M, De Haro C, Montanyà J, Jodar M, López-Aguilar J, Blanch L. Early neurocognitive rehabilitation in critically ill patients during ICU stay: a safety study. Intensive Care Med Exp. 2015;3:A994.
27. Turon M, Hernando D, Fernandez-Gonzalo VS, Bailón R, Gomà G, Lázaro J, Montanyà J, Gil E, Martinez-Perez M, de Haro C, López-Aguilar J, Martinez-Rubio A, Jodar M, Laguna P, Blanch L. Effect of an early neurocognitive rehabilitation on autonomic nervous system in critically ill patients. Intensive Care Med Exp. 2015;3:A989.
28. Hernando D, Turon M, Bailón R, Fernandez-Gonzalo S, Lázaro J, Gomà G, Gil E, Montanyà J, López-Aguilar J, de Haro C, Laguna P, Blanch L. Autonomic nervous system assessment in critically ill patients undergoing a cognitive rehabilitation therapy. Proc Comput Cardiol. 2015;42:785–8.
29. Blanch L, Sales B, Montanya J, Lucangelo U, Garcia-Esquirol O, Villagra A, Chacon E, Estruga A, Borelli M, Burgueño MJ, Oliva JC, Fernandez R, Villar J, Kacmarek R, Murias G. Validation of the Better Care® system to detect ineffective efforts during expiration in mechanically ventilated patients: a pilot study. Intensive Care Med. 2012;38:772–80.
30. Hodgson CL, Stiller K, Needham DM, Tipping CJ, Harrold M, Baldwin CE, Bradley S, Berney S, Caruana LR, Elliott D, Green M, Haines K, Higgins AM, Kaukonen KM, Leditschke IA, Nickels MR, Paratz J, Patman S, Skinner EH, Young PJ, Zanni JM, Denehy L, Webb SA. Expert consensus and recommendations on safety criteria for active mobilization of mechanically ventilated critically ill adults. Crit Care. 2014;18:658.
31. Task Force of the European Society of Cardiology, and the North American Society of Pacing and Electrophysiology. Heart rate variability. Standards of measurement, physiological interpretation, and clinical use. Eur Heart J. 1996;17:354–81.
32. Mateo J, Laguna P. Analysis of heart rate variability in the presence of ectopic beats using the heart timing signal. IEEE Trans Biomed Eng. 2003;50:334–43.
33. Bailon R, Laouini G, Grao C, Orini M, Laguna P, Meste O. The integral pulse frequency modulation model with time-varying threshold: application to heart rate variability analysis during exercise stress testing. IEEE Trans Biomed Eng. 2011;58:642–52.
34. Quílez ME, López-Aguilar J, Blanch L. Organ crosstalk during acute lung injury, acute respiratory distress syndrome, and mechanical ventilation. Curr Opin Crit Care. 2012;18:23–8.
35. Blanch L, Quintel M. Lung-brain cross talk in the critically ill. Intensive Care Med. 2017;43:557–9.
36. Turon M, Fernandez-Gonzalo S, Gomez-Simon V, Blanch L, Jodar M. Cognitive stimulation in ICU patients: should we pay more attention? Crit Care. 2013;17:158.
37. Fernandez-Gonzalo S, Turon M, de Haro C, Lopez-Aguilar J, Jodar M, Blanch L. Do sedation and analgesia contribute to long-term cognitive dysfunction in critical care survivors? Med Intensiva. 2017. doi:10.1016/j.medin.2017.06.010.
38. Zanni JM, Korupolu R, Fan E, Pradhan P, Janjua K, Palmer JB, Brower RG, Needham DM. Rehabilitation therapy and outcomes in acute respiratory failure: an observational pilot project. J Crit Care. 2010;25:254–62.
39. Jackson JC, Ely EW, Morey MC, Anderson VM, Denne LB, Clune J, Siebert CS, Archer KR, Torres R, Janz D, Schiro E, Jones J, Shintani AK, Levine B, Pun BT, Thompson J, Brummel NE, Hoenig H. Cognitive and physical rehabilitation of intensive care unit survivors: results of the RETURN randomized controlled pilot investigation. Crit Care Med. 2012;40:1088–97.
40. Mehlhorn J, Freytag A, Schmidt K, Brunkhorst FM, Graf J, Troitzsch U, Schlattmann P, Wensing M, Gensichen J. Rehabilitation interventions for postintensive care syndrome: a systematic review. Crit Care Med. 2014;42:1263–7.

14

Patient-important outcomes in randomized controlled trials in critically ill patients

Stéphane Gaudry[1,2,3*], Jonathan Messika[1,4,5], Jean-Damien Ricard[1,4,5], Sylvie Guillo[2,3,6,7], Blandine Pasquet[6,7], Emeline Dubief[1], Tanissia Boukertouta[1], Didier Dreyfuss[1,4,5] and Florence Tubach[2,3,6,7,8]

Abstract

Background: Intensivists' clinical decision making pursues two main goals for patients: to decrease mortality and to improve quality of life and functional status in survivors. Patient-important outcomes are gaining wide acceptance in most fields of clinical research. We sought to systematically review how well patient-important outcomes are reported in published randomized controlled trials (RCTs) in critically ill patients.

Methods: Literature search was conducted to identify eligible trials indexed from January to December 2013. Articles were eligible if they reported an RCT involving critically ill adult patients. We excluded phase II, pilot and physiological crossover studies. We assessed study characteristics. All primary and secondary outcomes were collected, described and classified using six categories of outcomes including patient-important outcomes (involving mortality at any time on the one hand and quality of life, functional/cognitive/neurological outcomes assessed after ICU discharge on the other).

Results: Of the 716 articles retrieved in 2013, 112 RCTs met the inclusion criteria. Most common topics were mechanical ventilation (27%), sepsis (19%) and nutrition (17%). Among the 112 primary outcomes, 27 (24%) were patient-important outcomes (mainly mortality, 21/27) but only six (5%) were patient-important outcomes besides mortality assessed after ICU discharge (functional disability = 4; quality of life = 2). Among the 598 secondary outcomes, 133 (22%) were patient-important outcomes (mainly mortality, 92/133) but only 41 (7%) were patient-important outcomes besides mortality assessed after ICU discharge (quality of life = 20, functional disability = 14; neurological/cognitive performance = 5; handicap = 1; post-traumatic stress = 1). Seventy-three RCTs (65%) reported at least one patient-important outcome but only 11 (10%) reported at least one patient-important outcome besides mortality assessed after ICU discharge.

Conclusion: Patient-important outcomes are rarely primary outcomes in RCTs in critically ill patients published in 2013. Among them, mortality accounted for the majority. We promote the use of patient-important outcomes in critical care trials.

Keywords: Patient-important outcome, Critical care, Quality of life

Background

The paternalistic model of patient care has also encompassed the field of research in critical care for many years. To change this paradigm, some clinicians and researchers recently advocated for "the patient at the center" of medical decision making. They suggested recommending interventions, not when the magnitude of the effect was "clinically relevant" but when it was "patient important" [1]. The notion of "Patient-important" sheds light on the individual clinical encounter and the preeminence of patient's value and preferences within that encounter. In

*Correspondence: stephanegaudry@gmail.com
[1] Service de Réanimation Médico-Chirurgicale, Hôpital Louis Mourier, AP-HP, 178 rue des Renouillers, 92700 Colombes, France
Full list of author information is available at the end of the article

clinical research, a patient-important outcome has been previously defined as: "a characteristic or variable that reflect how a patient feels, functions or survives" [2, 3].

The principal goal of implementing intensive care units (ICU) was to save the life of critically ill patients (i.e., decrease mortality). This goal has been reached in many clinical situations such as septic shock or acute respiratory failure, owing to progress in symptomatic and etiologic treatments of shock and in mechanical ventilation [4, 5]. Although this goal remains a major objective for intensivists, other priorities have emerged. In particular, the importance of assessing mean and long-term outcome in survivors has been underlined [6]. Critical illness is indeed associated with a wide array of long-term sequelae (physical and psychical) that impact functional status and quality of life [7–11]. To account for the patient perspective, clinical decision making by ICU physicians now pursues the goal of improving mean and long-term outcomes in survivors in addition to increasing their chance of survival. In case these goals cannot be reached, an alternative goal is improving the quality of death and dying in ICU.

In addition to mortality, assessing mean to long-term outcomes (after ICU and hospital discharge) could help define the usefulness of an intervention, taking into account what might be relevant and advantageous for the patients [12].

Numerous questions around outcomes used in randomized controlled trials (RCTs) in critically ill patients led us to conduct this systematic review. The core question of this review was guided, however, by patients' priorities. We chose to define patient-important outcomes according to these patients' priorities (survival, quality of life, functional, cognitive and neurological performance assessed after ICU discharge) as it has been done in other fields such as diabetes [13].

The main objective of this systematic review was to investigate whether RCTs in critically ill patients published in 2013 assess the patient-important outcomes.

Methods

To perform the systematic review on the 1-year period of 2013, we followed the PRISMA (Preferred Reporting Items for Systematic Reviews and Meta-Analysis) statement guidelines [14].

Outcome classification

Our outcome classification was developed according to previous work on patient-important outcome in various medical domains [3, 13, 15].

A scientific committee [including three intensivists (SG, J-DR and DD) and 1 methodologist (FT) particularly involved in designing and conducting RCTs in critically ill patients] established a classification of outcome categories relevant to ICU trials.

The experts identified six outcome categories:

Patient-important outcomes that included two entities: on the one hand, mortality at any time and on the other, quality of life, functional/cognitive/neurological outcomes assessed after ICU discharge.

Clinical outcomes in ICU and hospital organ failure, complication/adverse outcomes (for instance: drug induced skin reaction or hypotension during renal replacement therapy), healthcare-associated outcomes (nosocomial pneumonia, catheter-related infections), delirium, clinical events (such as venous thromboembolism, myocardial infarction), pain (in ICU), anxiety (in ICU), conscience level, return to spontaneous circulation, muscle strength/circumference, sleep duration, National Institute of Health Stroke Score (NIHSS) (for acute phase of stroke), clinical response to antibiotics, dyspnea (in ICU), noninvasive ventilation tolerance.

Biological/physiological/radiological outcomes such as brain natriuretic peptide (BNP), neutrophil gelatinase-associated lipocalin (NGAL), total lung capacity, chest X-ray severity score.

Care provider decision-related outcomes e.g., mechanical ventilation duration, length of stay, antibiotic exposure, volume of fluid resuscitation, intubation or reintubation, number of gastric tubes for aspiration, sedation exposure (dose/time), renal replacement therapy, ICU readmission, noninvasive ventilation, tracheostomy, transfusion, use of a prokinetic agent, need for surgery, dose of local anesthesia, hospital discharge disposition.

Care performance outcomes care procedure quality and noise/light exposure.

Other outcomes family satisfaction, physician/nurse or other provider satisfaction, cost/charges, withholding/withdrawal of care, patient judgment about his readiness to discharge, workload for staff team, compliance to a care protocol, medicolegal conflict.

Besides, for primary outcomes, we defined a "surrogate outcome" as an outcome measuring a substitute for some other variable (e.g., a biomarker intended to substitute for a clinical endpoint) [2].

Article eligibility criteria

Articles were eligible if they met the following criteria: article published between January 2013 and December 2013; reporting an RCT involving critically ill adult patients (i.e., adults hospitalized in ICU); written in English.

We considered only the first report of the trial results and trial extension follow-up, i.e., we excluded articles reporting post hoc analyses and sub-analyses of RCTs.

Indeed, our aim was to focus on the RCTs' initial objective. We also excluded phase II studies, pilot studies and physiological crossover studies because studies at this stage of clinical research are expected to explore mainly physiological and feasibility outcomes.

Search strategy and article selection

Main literature search (for the January 2013 to December 2013 period) was conducted on the July 16, 2014, in MEDLINE (via Pubmed®) to identify eligible articles indexed between January 2013 and December 2013. The search strategy relied on two algorithms, one dedicated to articles indexed with Mesh terms and the other dedicated to articles not indexed (at the time of the search), using exclusively free text. Terms related to intensive care were combined with terms related to RCTs. Details regarding the literature search strategy and the terms used are provided in Additional file 1.

Two senior intensivists (SG and JM) independently screened the titles and abstracts for the eligibility criteria, to identify articles to be read in full text. Definite article selection was only achieved after examination of the full text confirmed that inclusion criteria were met.

Data collection

A standardized extraction form (available from the corresponding author) was established from a literature review and a priori discussion. This extraction form was pretested by two authors (SG and JM) independently, in a set of ten articles. This test enabled to identify items needing rewording to avoid any confusion. Disagreements were discussed with an epidemiologist (last author, FT), to ensure similar understanding. Once all litigious points were settled, two reviewers (SG and JM) independently extracted the following data from the selected articles (using the full text and the Additional file 1): general data (funding source, geographical origin, topic, number of centers), methods (intervention assessed, study design, randomization design), quality assessment (by use of the risk of bias tool [16]), trial characteristics (inclusion period, length of follow-up, number of randomized patients) and outcomes (time from randomization to assessment for primary outcome, type and characteristic of all outcomes, see paragraph above).

For all articles included in the systematic review, disagreements between the two reviewers (SG and JM) were resolved by consensus. In case of persistent disagreement, arbitration by a third reviewer (FT) settled the discrepancy.

Statistical analyses

A 1-year time frame was chosen because it yielded a convenient study sample. Because of the significant lag in study indexation, the closest complete year available at the time of the literature search was 2013.

Continuous variables are described with median and interquartile range (IQR). Categorical variables are described with frequencies and percentages. Distribution of outcomes into the six categories (patient-important outcomes, clinical outcomes, bio/physio/radio outcomes, care provider decision-related outcomes, care performance outcomes and others outcomes) is presented as radar plot. For primary and secondary outcomes, distribution is presented for all outcomes and according to three major topics.

Trial characteristics associated with the presence of at least one patient-important outcome (primary or secondary outcome) were identified in univariate analysis, using Chi-square test or Fisher's test for categorical variables and Student's test or Wilcoxon's test for continuous variables.

Inter-reviewer agreement was measured by the kappa statistic for the following categorical variables: funding source, geographical origin, intervention assessed, unit of randomization and primary outcome category.

Statistical analysis was performed with GraphPad Prism 5 (GraphPad Software, San Diego, USA) and SAS version 9.3 (SAS Institute Inc, Cary, NC).

Results

Selection of articles and inter-reviewer agreement

The electronic search identified 716 articles. Four hundred and eighty were excluded on the basis of the title and abstract, and 124 after reading the full text. A total of 112 articles reporting RCTs in critically ill patients were finally included and analyzed (see Fig. 1 for PRISMA flow diagram).

Inter-reviewer agreement before consensus for categorical variables was very good [17]: The median kappa value was 0.89 [0.83–0.95] for funding source, 0.99 [0.96–1.00] for geographical origin, 0.83 [0.68–0.99] for unit of randomization and 0.95 [0.91–0.99] for primary outcome category; and good for intervention assessed (median kappa 0.74 [0.65–0.82]).

Characteristics of the 112 RCTs

Table 1 summarizes RCTs characteristics. Mechanical ventilation (27%), sepsis (18%) and nutrition (17%) were the most common topics of these trials. Therapeutic strategy (41%), drug (33%) and device (11%) evaluation were the most frequent types of intervention.

Follow-up period was defined until a fixed time point for 44 (39%) RCTs (median [IQR] 3 [1–6] months of follow-up), until ICU discharge for 14 (12%) RCTs and until hospital discharge for 15 (13%) RCTs. Follow-up period was unclear for 39 (35%) RCTs.

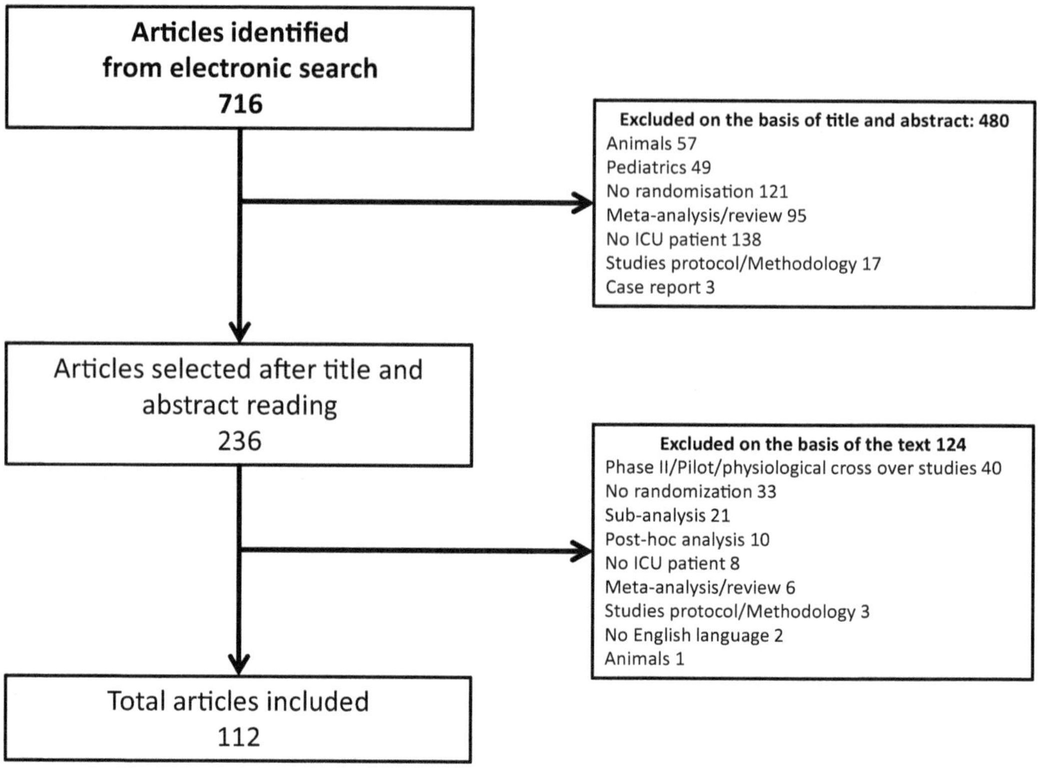

Fig. 1 PRISMA flow diagram

Quality assessment

Quality of the trials using the risk of bias tool is shown in Fig. 2. The absence of blinding of allocated intervention was the most frequent methodological component introducing a high risk of bias.

Primary outcomes

Seventy-three (65%) RCTs assessed the primary outcome after a median [IQR] fixed time point of 7 [2–28] days (from randomization) and only 13 (12%) assessed the primary outcome beyond 30 days (Fig. 3). The other RCTs assessed the primary outcome at ICU discharge ($n = 25$, 22%) or hospital discharge ($n = 9$, 8%). Five (4%) did not specify the time from randomization to primary outcome assessment.

Among the 112 primary outcomes, 27 (24%) were patient-important outcomes. Most of them were mortality (21/27, 78%) and only 6/27 (22%) were quality of life, functional/cognitive/neurological outcomes assessed after ICU discharge (functional disability = 4; quality of life = 2).

Among the 21 mortality outcomes, 18 were assessed after a fixed time point of 28 [28–60] days. The other three were assessed at ICU discharge. Among the six quality of life, functional/cognitive/neurological outcomes, two were assessed at hospital discharge and four after a fixed time point (6, 12, 12, 14 months). Figure 4 shows the distribution of the 112 primary outcomes and according to the three major topics (mechanical ventilation, sepsis, nutrition). Besides, 45 (40%) primary outcomes were surrogate endpoints.

Secondary outcomes

Among 598 secondary outcomes identified, 133 (22%) were patient-important outcomes. Most of them were mortality (92/133, 69%) and only 41 (31%) were quality of life, functional/cognitive/neurological outcomes assessed after ICU discharge (quality of life = 20, functional disability = 14; neurological/cognitive performance = 5; handicap = 1; post-traumatic stress = 1).

Among the 92 mortality outcomes, 43 were assessed after a fixed time point of 28 [28–90] days. The others were assessed at ICU discharge ($n = 26$) or at hospital discharge ($n = 23$). Among the 41 quality of life, functional/cognitive/neurological outcomes, 37 were assessed at a fixed time point of 365 [319–380] days and four at hospital discharge.

Figure 5 shows the distribution of the 598 secondary outcomes and according to the three major topics (mechanical ventilation, sepsis, nutrition).

Table 1 Characteristics of RCTs in critically ill adult patients

Characteristic	RCTs without any patient-important outcomes no. (%)	RCTs reporting at least one patient-important outcome no. (%)	*P* value
Total–*n*	39	73	
Funding			0.04
Public	14 (36)	42 (57)	
Industry	6 (15)	8 (11)	
Both public and private	18 (46)	10 (14)	
Not reported or unclear	1 (3)	13 (18)	
Geographical area			
Europe	12 (31)	34 (47)	
Asia	18 (46)	19 (26)	
North America	4 (10)	16 (22)	
Oceania	3 (8)	9 (12)	
South America	2 (5)	8 (11)	
Africa	0 (0)	5 (7)	
International (>1 country)	0 (0)	18 (25)	
Number of center(s)			0.005
Monocenter	29 (74)	33 (45)	
Multicenter	8 (21)	38 (52)	
Unclear	2 (5)	2 (3)	
Sample size			0.01
<50	16 (41)	16 (22)	
50–100	7 (18)	14 (19)	
100–150	6 (15)	5 (7)	
150–500	7 (18)	20 (27)	
>500	3 (8)	18 (25)	
Topic of the study[a]			
Mechanical ventilation	14 (36)	16 (22)	0.011
Sepsis	2 (5)	19 (26)	0.007
Nutrition	5 (13)	14 (19)	0.39
Infection	8 (21)	10 (14)	
Hemodynamics	2 (5)	4 (5)	
ARDS	2 (5)	7 (10)	
Cardiac arrest	2 (5)	4 (5)	
Trauma	3 (8)	3 (4)	
Sedation	2 (5)	1 (1)	
Acute kidney injury	1 (3)	3 (4)	
Pain	2 (5)	2 (3)	
Neurocritical care	1 (3)		
Hematological issue	1 (3)	2 (3)	
Rehabilitation/physical and/or cognitive therapy	2 (5)		
Metabolic disorder	1 (3)		
Burns	0 (0)	1 (1)	
ECMO	0 (0)	1 (1)	
Electric muscle stimulation	1 (3)		
Music	1 (3)		
Type of intervention			0.37
Therapeutic strategy	14 (36)	32 (44)	
Drug	13 (33)	24 (33)	
Device	6 (15)	7 (10)	

Table 1 continued

Characteristic	RCTs without any patient-important outcomes no. (%)	RCTs reporting at least one patient-important outcome no. (%)	*P* value
Monitoring	2 (5)	1 (1)	
Diagnostic strategy	0 (0)	4 (5)	
Other	4 (10)	5 (7)	
Unit of randomization			0.74
Patient	35 (90)	67 (92)	
Service	2 (5)	3 (4)	
Time	1 (3)	1 (1)	
Other	1 (3)	2 (3)	
Type of trial			1.00
Superiority	38 (97)	70 (96)	
Equivalence or non-inferiority	1 (3)	3 (4)	
Follow-up			
Fixed time point	22 (56)	41 (56)	
Median months [IQR]	0.5 [0.5–1]	3 [1–9]	0.0002
ICU	7 (18)	7 (10)	
Hospital	3 (8)	12 (16)	
Unreported	7 (18)	13 (18)	

The numbers in parentheses mean the percentage; ECMO: extracorporeal membrane oxygenation

A study can appear in more than one row for geographical area

[a] One study could have more than one topic

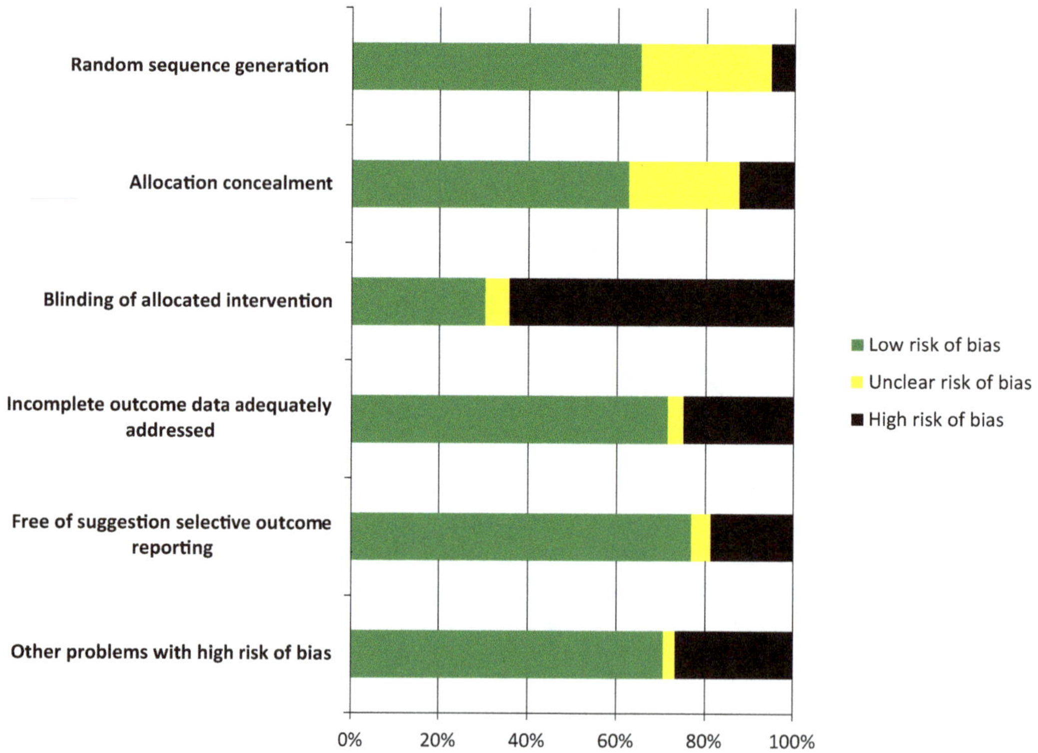

Fig. 2 RCTs quality assessment by risk of bias tool [16]. Methodological quality of the trials included in the systematic review assessed by six points: random sequence generation, allocation concealment, blinding of allocation intervention, incomplete data adequately addressed, free of suggestion selective outcome reporting and other problems. Horizontal axis represents the ratio (%) distribution among "low risk of bias" (*green*), "high risk of bias" (*red*) and "unclear risk of bias" (*yellow*)

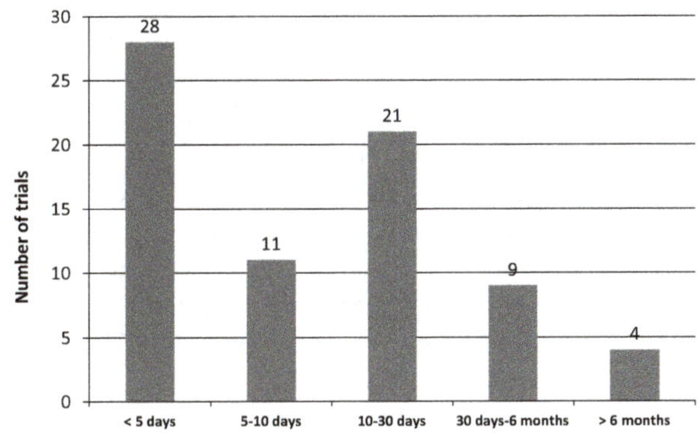

Fig. 3 Time from randomization to assessment of primary outcome. This figure represents the distribution of the time from randomization to assessment of primary outcome for the 73 RCTs that assessed the primary outcome after a fixed time point

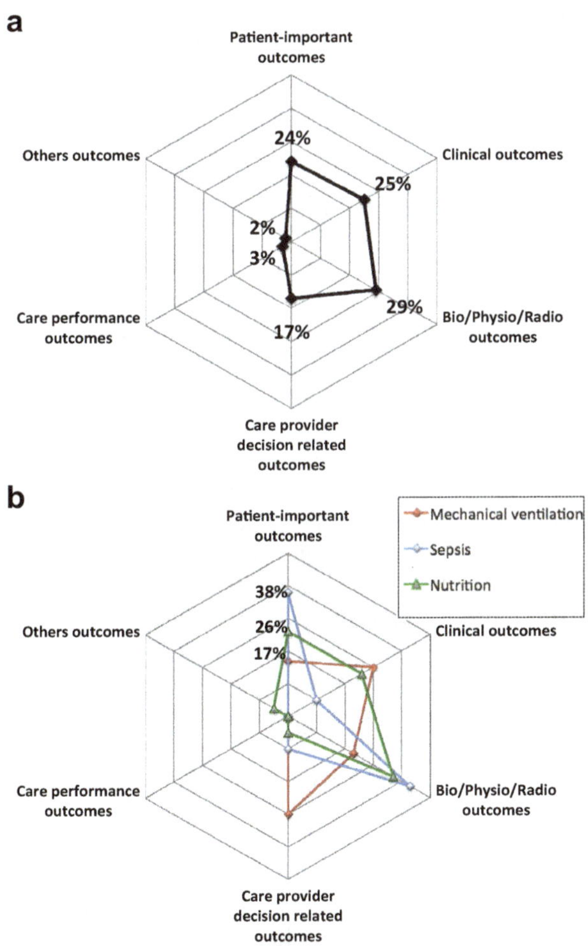

Fig. 4 Distribution of primary outcomes. **a** Distribution of 112 primary outcomes, percentage of primary outcomes by outcome category, **b** distribution of primary outcomes according to three major topics (mechanical ventilation, sepsis and nutrition), percentage of primary outcomes by outcome category

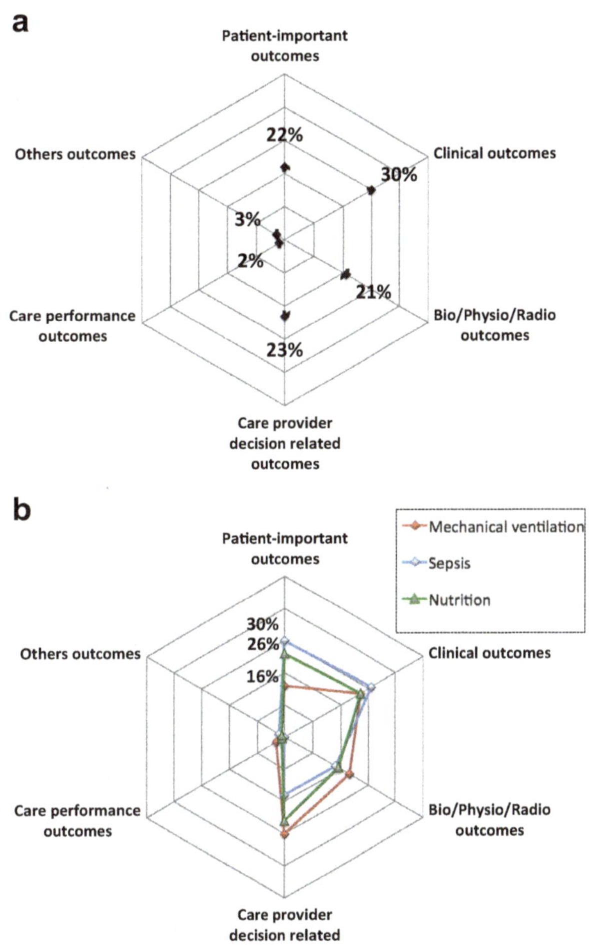

Fig. 5 Distribution of secondary outcomes. **a** Distribution of 598 secondary outcomes, percentage of secondary outcomes by outcome category, **b** distribution of secondary outcomes according to three major topics (mechanical ventilation, sepsis and nutrition), percentage of secondary outcomes by outcome category

Trial characteristics associated with the presence of at least one patient-important outcome (primary or secondary)

Among the 112 RCTs, 73 (65%) reported at least one patient-important outcome (primary or secondary outcomes) but only 11 (10%) reported at least one quality of life, functional/cognitive/neurological outcomes assessed after ICU discharge. Characteristics of these RCTs are provided in Table 1.

Discussion

We found that, during the 1-year survey period of RCTs performed in critically ill patients, a minority of outcomes used in these RCTs were patient-important outcomes. They accounted for 24 and 22% of primary and secondary outcomes, respectively. Mortality accounted for the vast majority of reported patient-important outcomes, whereas other patient-important outcomes (such as quality of life, functional/cognitive/neurological outcomes assessed after ICU discharge) were scarcely used (7% of all outcomes). Moreover, only 10% of surveyed RCTs reported at least one patient-important outcome besides mortality (quality of life, functional/cognitive/neurological outcomes assessed after ICU discharge). This is at striking contrast with clinical decision making of ICU physicians, which is felt to be in line with these crucial outcomes. In addition, we were cautious to retain only those RCTs for which patient-important outcomes were reasonably expected. Indeed, studies for which patient-important outcomes were less likely to be present (phase II studies, pilot studies and physiological crossover studies) were not included.

Our study is the first to explore the place of patient-important outcomes and how well they are reported in RCTs in critically ill patients. We derived the definition of patient-important outcome for critically ill patients from the definition used in other fields [3, 13, 15]. Mortality is obviously essential, and we considered that quality of life, functional/cognitive/neurological outcomes assessed after ICU discharge also qualified for patient-important outcome. Indeed, the potential adverse consequences of an ICU stay are best evaluated after ICU discharge and even more after hospital discharge since critical illness is associated with long-term sequelae. Survivors of critical care experience profound changes in their lives because of many forms of deficit in one or more domains [18] of physical [19, 20], psychological [11, 21, 22] or cognitive functioning [22–25]. These numerous symptoms led to define the new entity of "post-intensive care syndrome" [26].

This study is the first to use a definition of patient-important outcomes for critically ill patients. This definition is open to criticism on two points. Firstly, it includes exogenous measures of symptoms that may not perfectly capture how patients feel or how symptoms impact their overall quality of life. We could have restricted the definition to patient-reported outcomes [27]. Nevertheless, doing this, the message of this study would have been the same. Indeed, among the 27 primary outcomes, which were patient-important outcomes, four were classified as functional disability and two of those were not patient-reported outcomes. Secondly, besides mortality outcomes, we chose to restrict the patient-important outcomes to the post-ICU period (leaving out pain, anxiety and dyspnea which might have occurred during the ICU stay). However, in the present systematic review, "pain, anxiety and dyspnea in ICU" accounted for only two (1.8%) primary outcomes and four (0.7%) secondary outcomes. If we had considered these outcomes as patient-important outcomes, the results of this study would have been very similar.

To perform this systematic review, we developed an outcome classification relevant to the context of critical care, involving six categories (patient-important outcomes, clinical outcomes in ICU and hospital, biological/physiological/radiological outcomes, care provider decision-related outcomes, care performance outcomes and others). A systematic review is the first step to establish a core outcome set and our outcome classification could help researchers to clarify the place of patient-important outcomes in core outcome sets for future RCTs in critically ill patients. To date, there is no taxonomy of outcomes studied in critically ill patients, nor core outcome set. This may cause inconsistencies in outcome reports and difficulties in comparing these outcomes across studies and to combine them in systematic reviews and meta-analyses [28]. With the aim to facilitate the development and application of agreed standardized sets of outcomes, the Core Outcome Measures in Effectiveness Trials (COMET) initiative was initiated in [29]. In the field of critical care, the Core Outcomes in Ventilation Trials (COVenT) is in progress [30]. This systematic review can be the first step to develop other core outcome sets in other topics of critical care and to establish a core outcome set involving patients' opinion for future RCTs.

An inherent limitation of a systematic review of published trials is that it is performed at a given period (here 2013). The search led to identify 112 eligible RCTs, which provides a very large panel of ICU trials and thus robust information on the prevalence of patient-important outcomes in RCTs in critically ill patients. Many systematic reviews rely issues on a 1-year literature search [31, 32]. Our goal was to capture the most recent practices in trials as the literature on patient-important outcomes in other medical field and the growing interest for the patients' perspective may have had an impact.

Patient-important outcomes are gaining wide acceptance in some fields of clinical research [33–35]. Additionally, a recent survey from 2036 patients with diabetes showed that most of them (>75%) chose patient-important outcomes rather than HbA1c as their first choice for a trial primary outcome [36]. Patients understand the reality of their condition and disease's impact on their lives better than physicians can do [37]. James Lind Alliance in the UK [38, 39] and the Patient-Centered Outcome Research Institute in the USA [40–43] showed the mismatch between questions patients and clinicians needed an answer for on the one hand and those that were investigated by researchers on the other. This led some opinion leaders to call for a patient revolution [44]. Patients who survive after a critical illness may experience many sequelae after ICU or hospital discharge. In our study, only 10% of RCTs reported at least one non-mortality patient-centered outcome assessed after ICU discharge. It seems therefore desirable that more long-term outcomes be assessed in ICU studies.

Reasons explaining this small percentage of RCTs assessing patient-important outcomes and in particular the impressive scarcity of outcomes assessed after ICU discharge are diverse. One of them is the difficulty to ascertain mean and long-term follow-up of patients. The preference of researchers and funding agencies for rapidly obtained results favors short-term outcomes. This could be a shortcoming since paradoxical short- and long-term effects after certain interventions have been described [45, 46]. For instance, after acute myocardial infarction flecainide decreased arrhythmias but has been associated with increased mortality [45]. In critical illness, growth hormone improved nitrogen balance but has been also associated with increased mortality [47]. Moreover, many proposed short-term endpoints in critical care have not been formally evaluated for surrogacy [48] precluding any strong conclusion on the effect on patient-important outcomes. For example, acute organ dysfunction in ICU does not appear to have significant long-term implications for patient-important outcomes [49]. In our systematic review, we found that 40% of primary outcomes were surrogate endpoints.

To promote the assessment of patient-important outcomes, patients' follow-up should be extended but this can be hampered by logistical issues (organization of phone call, medical consultation, etc.) which can considerably increase the costs of the study. As a result, we found that patients' follow-up was short since only 12% of trials assessed primary outcomes beyond 30 days from randomization. Patient-important outcomes were initially promoted to evaluate outcomes of chronic diseases [13, 15] for which patients' follow-up is easier to perform because the patient is cared for by the same medical team. This situation is quite different for critically ill patients who are often cared for by a different team after ICU discharge. The advent of post-ICU consultation [50] could foster a better assessment of patient-important outcomes by intensivists and researchers in the field.

Additionally, lengthy technical questionnaires are usually used to assess patient-reported outcomes (i.e., quality of life or functional status) after ICU discharge. This often leads to a high proportion of non-responders that renders interpretation more Difficult [51]. The question of the applicability to the ICU setting of the tools used is also raised by ICU experts: "Are existing instruments suitable for capturing important nuances of post-ICU sequelae or should disease-specific instruments be captured" [6].

The decisions intensivists make at the bedside aim at both saving lives and preserving—at best—their patients' prior quality of life. Medical research and especially RCTs should help them to better evaluate the efficacy of their interventions (drug administration, therapeutic strategy implementation or device use) on these relevant issues.

Our results indicate that outcomes of many RCTs remained too often centered on physiological criteria (oxygenation or hemodynamic stabilization for instance) or assessed mortality as sole outcome of importance for patients. This has two pitfalls: quality of life of survivors is not assessed, and given the noticeable improvement of vital prognosis in a number of ICU situations (ARDS for example), many interventional studies using mortality as primary outcome have been negative in recent years, mandating the use of alternative outcome measures, such as patient-important ones [48, 52, 53].

Conclusion

Our study shows that only a small number of primary outcomes measures in recent RCTs performed in the ICU are patient-important outcomes. To better address patient needs, researchers should take the crucial post-ICU period into account in the design of future RCTs. This is one of the challenges for future ICU research. This paradigm shift would be in the interest of patients.

Abbreviations

ICU: intensive care units; RCT: randomized controlled trial; PRISMA: Preferred Reporting Items for Systematic Reviews and Meta-Analysis; ARDS: acute respiratory distress syndrome; NIHSS: National Institute of Health Stroke Score; BNP: brain natriuretic peptide; NGAL: neutrophil gelatinase-associated lipocalin.

Authors' contributions

StG, JM, TB and FT performed the data extraction; SyG and ED performed the literature search; BP performed statistical analysis; StG, JM, J-DR, DD and FT wrote and reviewed the manuscript. All authors read and approved the final manuscript.

Author details

[1] Service de Réanimation Médico-Chirurgicale, Hôpital Louis Mourier, AP-HP, 178 rue des Renouillers, 92700 Colombes, France. [2] ECEVE, UMRS 1123, Sorbonne Paris Cité, Univ Paris Diderot, Paris, France. [3] ECEVE, U1123, CIC 1421, INSERM, Paris, France. [4] IAME, UMR 1137, INSERM, 75018 Paris, France. [5] IAME, UMR 1137, Sorbonne Paris Cité, Univ Paris Diderot, 75018 Paris, France. [6] Département de Biostatistiques, Santé Publique et Informatique Médicale, CIC 1421, Hôpital Pitié Salpétrière, AP-HP, Paris, France. [7] Unité de Recherche Clinique Paris Nord, Hôpital Bichat, AP-HP, Paris, France. [8] Université Pierre et Marie Curie, Sorbonne Universités, Paris, France.

Competing interests

The authors declare that they have no competing interests.

References

1. Guyatt G, Montori V, Devereaux PJ, Schünemann H, Bhandari M. Patients at the center: in our practice, and in our use of language. ACP J Club. 2004;140(1):A11–2.
2. Wittes J, Lakatos E, Probstfield J. Surrogate endpoints in clinical trials: cardiovascular diseases. Stat Med. 1989;8(4):415–25.

3. Pino C, Boutron I, Ravaud P. Outcomes in registered, ongoing randomized controlled trials of patient education. PLoS ONE. 2012;7(8):e42934.
4. Brower R, Matthay M, Moris A. Ventilation with lower tidal volumes as compared with traditional tidal volumes for acute lung injury and the acute respiratory distress syndrome. The Acute Respiratory Distress Syndrome Network. N Engl J Med. 2000;342(18):1301–8.
5. Guerin C, Reignier J, Richard J-C, Beuret P, Gacouin A, Boulain T, et al. Prone positioning in severe acute respiratory distress syndrome. N Engl J Med. 2013;368(23):2159–68.
6. Angus DC, Carlet J. 2002 Brussels Roundtable Participants. Surviving intensive care: a report from the 2002 Brussels Roundtable. Intensive Care Med. 2003;29(3):368–77.
7. Desai SV, Law TJ, Needham DM. Long-term complications of critical care. Crit Care Med. 2011;39(2):371–9.
8. Stevens RD, Dowdy DW, Michaels RK, Mendez-Tellez PA, Pronovost PJ, Needham DM. Neuromuscular dysfunction acquired in critical illness: a systematic review. Intensive Care Med. 2007;33(11):1876–91.
9. Van der Schaaf M, Beelen A, Dongelmans DA, Vroom MB, Nollet F. Poor functional recovery after a critical illness: a longitudinal study. J Rehabil Med. 2009;41(13):1041–8.
10. Chelluri L, Im KA, Belle SH, Schulz R, Rotondi AJ, Donahoe MP, et al. Long-term mortality and quality of life after prolonged mechanical ventilation. Crit Care Med. 2004;32(1):61–9.
11. Davydow DS, Gifford JM, Desai SV, Bienvenu OJ, Needham DM. Depression in general intensive care unit survivors: a systematic review. Intensive Care Med. 2009;35(5):796–809.
12. Wake S, Kitchiner D. Post-traumatic stress disorder after intensive care. BMJ. 2013;346:f3232.
13. Gandhi GY, Murad MH, Fujiyoshi A, Mullan RJ, Flynn DN, Elamin MB, et al. Patient-important outcomes in registered diabetes trials. JAMA. 2008;299(21):2543–9.
14. Moher D, Shamseer L, Clarke M, Ghersi D, Liberati A, Petticrew M, et al. Preferred reporting items for systematic review and meta-analysis protocols (PRISMA-P) 2015 statement. Syst Rev. 2015;4:1.
15. Boers M, Brooks P, Simon LS, Strand V, Tugwell P. OMERACT: an international initiative to improve outcome measurement in rheumatology. Clin Exp Rheumatol. 2005;23(5 Suppl 39):S10–3.
16. Higgins JP, Green S. Cochrane handbook for systematic reviews of interventions. London: The Cochrane Collaboration; 2008.
17. Altman DG. Practical statistics for medical research. 1st ed. London: Chapman and Hall; 1991. p. 611.
18. Needham DM, Dinglas VD, Bienvenu OJ, Colantuoni E, Wozniak AW, Rice TW, et al. One year outcomes in patients with acute lung injury randomised to initial trophic or full enteral feeding: prospective follow-up of EDEN randomised trial. BMJ. 2013;346:f1532.
19. Herridge MS, Cheung AM, Tansey CM, Matte-Martyn A, Diaz-Granados N, Al-Saidi F, et al. One-year outcomes in survivors of the acute respiratory distress syndrome. N Engl J Med. 2003;348(8):683–93.
20. Herridge MS, Tansey CM, Matté A, Tomlinson G, Diaz-Granados N, Cooper A, et al. Functional disability 5 years after acute respiratory distress syndrome. N Engl J Med. 2011;364(14):1293–304.
21. Davydow DS, Gifford JM, Desai SV, Needham DM, Bienvenu OJ. Posttraumatic stress disorder in general intensive care unit survivors: a systematic review. Gen Hosp Psychiatr. 2008;30(5):421–34.
22. Bienvenu OJ, Colantuoni E, Mendez-Tellez PA, Dinglas VD, Shanholtz C, Husain N, et al. Depressive symptoms and impaired physical function after acute lung injury: a 2-year longitudinal study. Am J Respir Crit Care Med. 2012;185(5):517–24.
23. Hopkins RO, Weaver LK, Collingridge D, Parkinson RB, Chan KJ, Orme JF. Two-year cognitive, emotional, and quality-of-life outcomes in acute respiratory distress syndrome. Am J Respir Crit Care Med. 2005;171(4):340–7.
24. Mikkelsen ME, Christie JD, Lanken PN, Biester RC, Thompson BT, Bellamy SL, et al. The adult respiratory distress syndrome cognitive outcomes study: long-term neuropsychological function in survivors of acute lung injury. Am J Respir Crit Care Med. 2012;185(12):1307–15.
25. Iwashyna TJ, Ely EW, Smith DM, Langa KM. Long-term cognitive impairment and functional disability among survivors of severe sepsis. JAMA. 2010;304(16):1787–94.
26. Elliott D, Davidson JE, Harvey MA, Bemis-Dougherty A, Hopkins RO, Iwashyna TJ, et al. Exploring the scope of post-intensive care syndrome therapy and care: engagement of non-critical care providers and survivors in a second stakeholders meeting. Crit Care Med. 2014;42:2518.
27. Cella D, Yount S, Rothrock N, Gershon R, Cook K, Reeve B, et al. The Patient-Reported Outcomes Measurement Information System (PROMIS): progress of an NIH Roadmap cooperative group during its first two years. Med Care. 2007;45(5 Suppl 1):S3–11.
28. Williamson PR, Altman DG, Blazeby JM, Clarke M, Devane D, Gargon E, et al. Developing core outcome sets for clinical trials: issues to consider. Trials. 2012;13:132.
29. Prinsen CAC, Vohra S, Rose MR, King-Jones S, Ishaque S, Bhaloo Z, et al. Core Outcome Measures in Effectiveness Trials (COMET) initiative: protocol for an international Delphi study to achieve consensus on how to select outcome measurement instruments for outcomes included in a "core outcome set". Trials. 2014;15:247.
30. Blackwood B, Ringrow S, Clarke M, Marshall J, Rose L, Williamson P, et al. Core Outcomes in Ventilation Trials (COVenT): protocol for a core outcome set using a Delphi survey with a nested randomised trial and observational cohort study. Trials. 2015;16:368.
31. Giraudeau B, Caille A, Le Gouge A, Ravaud P. Participant informed consent in cluster randomized trials: review. PLoS ONE. 2012;7(7):e40436.
32. Baron G, Perrodeau E, Boutron I, Ravaud P. Reporting of analyses from randomized controlled trials with multiple arms: a systematic review. BMC Med. 2013;11:84.
33. Tugwell PS, Maxwell LJ, Beaton DE, Busse JW, Christensen R, Conaghan PG, et al. Deliberative dialogue on developing consensus on measurement and presentation of patient important outcomes in systematic reviews: a preconference meeting at OMERACT 12. J Rheumatol. 2015;42(10):1931–3.
34. Redline S, Baker-Goodwin S, Bakker JP, Epstein M, Hanes S, Hanson M, et al. Patient partnerships transforming sleep medicine research and clinical care: perspectives from the sleep apnea patient-centered outcomes network. JCSM. 2016;12(7):1053–8.
35. Morgans AK, van Bommel ACM, Stowell C, Abrahm JL, Basch E, Bekelman JE, et al. Development of a standardized set of patient-centered outcomes for advanced prostate cancer: an international effort for a unified approach. Eur Urol. 2015;68(5):891–8.
36. Murad MH, Shah ND, Van Houten HK, Ziegenfuss JY, Deming JR, Beebe TJ, et al. Individuals with diabetes preferred that future trials use patient-important outcomes and provide pragmatic inferences. J Clin Epidemiol. 2011;64(7):743–8.
37. Young K. Doctors' understanding of rheumatoid disease does not align with patients' experiences. BMJ. 2013;346:f2901.
38. Petit-Zeman S, Firkins L, Scadding JW. The James Lind Alliance: tackling research mismatches. Lancet Lond Engl. 2010;376(9742):667–9.
39. Partridge N, Scadding J. The James Lind Alliance: patients and clinicians should jointly identify their priorities for clinical trials. Lancet Lond Engl. 2004;364(9449):1923–4.
40. Selby JV, Beal AC, Frank L. The Patient-Centered Outcomes Research Institute (PCORI) national priorities for research and initial research agenda. JAMA. 2012;307(15):1583–4.
41. Frank L, Basch E, Selby JV. Patient-Centered Outcomes Research Institute. The PCORI perspective on patient-centered outcomes research. JAMA. 2014;312(15):1513–4.
42. Frank L, Forsythe L, Ellis L, Schrandt S, Sheridan S, Gerson J, et al. Conceptual and practical foundations of patient engagement in research at the patient-centered outcomes research institute. Qual Life Res Int J Qual Life Asp Treat Care Rehabil. 2015;24(5):1033–41.
43. Newhouse R, Barksdale DJ, Miller JA. The patient-centered outcomes research institute: research done differently. Nurs Res. 2015;64(1):72–7.
44. Richards T, Montori VM, Godlee F, Lapsley P, Paul D. Let the patient revolution begin. BMJ. 2013;346:f2614.
45. Echt DS, Liebson PR, Mitchell LB, Peters RW, Obias-Manno D, Barker AH, et al. Mortality and morbidity in patients receiving encainide, flecainide, or placebo. The Cardiac Arrhythmia Suppression Trial. N Engl J Med. 1991;324(12):781–8.
46. Hébert PC, Wells G, Blajchman MA, Marshall J, Martin C, Pagliarello G, et al. A multicenter, randomized, controlled clinical trial of transfusion requirements in critical care. Transfusion Requirements in Critical Care Investigators, Canadian Critical Care Trials Group. N Engl J Med. 1999;340(6):409–17.

47. Takala J, Ruokonen E, Webster NR, Nielsen MS, Zandstra DF, Vundelinckx G, et al. Increased mortality associated with growth hormone treatment in critically ill adults. N Engl J Med. 1999;341(11):785–92.
48. Angus DC, Mira J-P, Vincent J-L. Improving clinical trials in the critically ill. Crit Care Med. 2010;38(2):527–32.
49. Clermont G, Angus DC, Linde-Zwirble WT, Griffin MF, Fine MJ, Pinsky MR. Does acute organ dysfunction predict patient-centered outcomes? Chest. 2002;121(6):1963–71.
50. Dettling-Ihnenfeldt DS, De Graaff AE, Nollet F, Van Der Schaaf M. Feasibility of Post-Intensive Care Unit Clinics: an observational cohort study of two different approaches. Min Anestesiol. 2015;81(8):865–75.
51. Tian ZM, Miranda DR. Quality of life after intensive care with the sickness impact profile. Intensive Care Med. 1995;21(5):422–8.
52. Ospina-Tascón GA, Büchele GL, Vincent J-L. Multicenter, randomized, controlled trials evaluating mortality in intensive care: doomed to fail? Crit Care Med. 2008;36(4):1311–22.
53. Aberegg SK, Richards DR, O'Brien JM. Delta inflation: a bias in the design of randomized controlled trials in critical care medicine. Crit Care Lond Engl. 2010;14(2):R77.

15

Acid–base status and its clinical implications in critically ill patients with cirrhosis, acute-on-chronic liver failure and without liver disease

Andreas Drolz[1,2*†], Thomas Horvatits[1,2†], Kevin Roedl[1,2], Karoline Rutter[1,2], Richard Brunner[1], Christian Zauner[1], Peter Schellongowski[3], Gottfried Heinz[4], Georg-Christian Funk[5], Michael Trauner[1], Bruno Schneeweiss[1] and Valentin Fuhrmann[1,2]

Abstract

Background: Acid–base disturbances are frequently observed in critically ill patients at the intensive care unit. To our knowledge, the acid–base profile of patients with acute-on-chronic liver failure (ACLF) has not been evaluated and compared to critically ill patients without acute or chronic liver disease.

Results: One hundred and seventy-eight critically ill patients with liver cirrhosis were compared to 178 matched controls in this post hoc analysis of prospectively collected data. Patients with and without liver cirrhosis showed hyperchloremic acidosis and coexisting hypoalbuminemic alkalosis. Cirrhotic patients, especially those with ACLF, showed a marked net metabolic acidosis owing to increased lactate and unmeasured anions. This metabolic acidosis was partly antagonized by associated respiratory alkalosis, yet with progression to ACLF resulted in acidemia, which was present in 62% of patients with ACLF grade III compared to 19% in cirrhosis patients without ACLF. Acidemia and metabolic acidosis were associated with 28-day mortality in cirrhosis. Patients with pH values < 7.1 showed a 100% mortality rate. Acidosis attributable to lactate and unmeasured anions was independently associated with mortality in liver cirrhosis.

Conclusions: Cirrhosis and especially ACLF are associated with metabolic acidosis and acidemia owing to lactate and unmeasured anions. Acidosis and acidemia, respectively, are associated with increased 28-day mortality in liver cirrhosis. Lactate and unmeasured anions are main contributors to metabolic imbalance in cirrhosis and ACLF.

Keywords: Acid–base, Cirrhosis, Acute-on-chronic liver failure, Mortality

Background

Derangements in acid–base balance are frequently observed in critically ill patients at the intensive care unit (ICU) and present in various patterns [1–4]. Severe acid–base disorders, especially metabolic acidosis, have been associated with increased mortality [5, 6]. As a consequence, acid–base status in critically ill patients with various disease entities has been extensively studied.

*Correspondence: a.drolz@uke.de
†Andreas Drolz and Thomas Horvatits contributed equally to the work
[2] Department of Intensive Care Medicine, University Medical Center, Hamburg-Eppendorf, Martinistraße 52, 20246 Hamburg, Germany
Full list of author information is available at the end of the article

Yet, only a few studies assessed the impact of underlying chronic liver disease on acid–base equilibrium in critical illness [7, 8]. While a balance of offsetting acidifying and alkalinizing metabolic acid–base disorders with a resulting equilibrated acid–base status has been described in stable cirrhosis [9], severe derangements with resulting net acidosis owing to hyperchloremic, dilutional and lactic acidosis were observed when cirrhosis was accompanied by critical illness [7, 8]. Acute liver failure (ALF) is characterized by a different acid–base pattern with dramatically increased lactate levels [10]. The acidifying effect of this increase in lactate was neutralized by hypoalbuminemia in non-paracetamol-induced ALF [11].

Despite advantages in intensive care medicine, which have led to an improved outcome over the last decade [12], mortality in cirrhotic patients admitted to ICU is still high [13–15]. Measurement and knowledge of specific acid–base patterns and their implications in critically ill patients with liver cirrhosis may help to improve patient management, especially in the ICU setting [16]. However, to our knowledge, the acid–base profile of critically ill cirrhotic patients with acute-on-chronic liver disease (ACLF) has not been compared to critically ill patients without acute or chronic liver disease. Most information on the acid–base status of critically ill patients with cirrhosis was obtained by comparing these patients with healthy controls [8]. Yet, part of metabolic disturbances in critically ill patients with liver cirrhosis may be attributable to critical illness per se, rather than to the presence of chronic liver disease.

The aim of this study was to assess acid–base patterns of critically ill patients with liver cirrhosis and ACLF, respectively, in comparison with critically ill patients without acute or chronic liver disease.

Methods

Patients

All patients admitted to 3 medical ICUs at the Medical University of Vienna between July 2012 and August 2014 were screened for inclusion in the study. For the present study, only patients who had arterial blood samples drawn within 4 h after ICU admission were eligible for inclusion. Patients with acute liver injury in the absence of chronic liver disease were excluded. One hundred and seventy-eight patients with liver cirrhosis were identified as eligible for inclusion. The control group of 178 critically ill patients without acute or chronic liver disease was selected by propensity score matching (PSM).

On admission, Simplified Acute Physiology Score II (SAPS II) [17], SOFA [18], infections and organ dysfunctions were documented.

All patients were screened for the presence of acute kidney injury (AKI) defined by urine output and serum creatinine according to the Kidney Disease: Improving Global Outcomes (KDIGO) Clinical Practice Guidelines for Acute Kidney Injury [19].

The presence of liver cirrhosis was defined by a combination of characteristic clinical (ascites, caput medusae, spider angiomata, etc.), laboratory and radiological findings (typical morphological changes of the liver, sings of portal hypertension, etc., in ultrasonography or computed tomography scanning), or via histology, if available. ACLF was identified and graded according to recommendations of the chronic liver failure (CLIF) consortium of the European Association for the Study of the Liver (EASL) [20]. CLIF-SOFA score [20] and CLIF-C ACLF score [21] were calculated. Septic shock was defined according to the recommendations of the Surviving Sepsis Campaign [22].

Twenty-eight-day mortality and 1-year mortality were assessed on site or by contacting the patient or the attending physician, respectively.

This study is based on a post hoc analysis of prospectively collected data [23]. The Ethics Committee of the Medical University of Vienna waived the need for informed consent due to the observational character of this study.

Sampling and blood analysis

On admission, arterial blood samples were collected from arterial or femoral artery and parameters for the assessment of acid–base status were instantly measured.

pH, partial pressure of carbon dioxide ($PaCO_2$), ionized calcium (Ca^{2+}) and lactate were measured with a blood gas analyzer (ABL 725; Radiometer, Copenhagen, Denmark). Samples of separated plasma were analyzed for concentrations of sodium (Na^+), potassium (K^+), chloride (Cl^-), magnesium (Mg^{2+}), inorganic phosphate (Pi), albumin (Alb), plasma creatinine, blood urea nitrogen (BUN), aspartate aminotransferase (AST) and alanine aminotransferase (ALT) by a fully automated analyzer (Hitachi 917; Roche Diagnostics GmbH, Mannheim, Germany). Na^+ and Cl^- were measured using ion-selective electrodes. Lactate was measured with an amperometric electrode.

Acid–base analysis

Arterial concentration of bicarbonate ($HCO3^-$) was calculated from measured pH and $PaCO_2$ values according to the Henderson–Hasselbalch equation [24, 25]. Base excess (BE) was calculated according to the formulae by Siggaard-Andersen [24–26].

Quantitative physical–chemical analysis was performed using Stewart's biophysical methods [27], modified by Figge and colleagues [28].

Apparent strong ion difference (SIDa) was calculated:

$$\text{SIDa} = \text{Na}^+ + \text{K}^+ + 2 \times \text{Mg}^{2+} + 2 \times \text{Ca}^{2+} - \text{Cl}^- - \text{lactate}$$

(SIDa in mEq/l; all concentrations in mmol/l)

Effective strong ion difference (SIDe) was calculated in order to account for the role of weak acids [29]:

$$\text{SIDe} = 1000 \times 2.46 \times 10^{-11} \times \frac{\text{PaCO}_2}{10^{-\text{pH}}} + \text{Alb} \times (0.123 \times \text{pH} - 0.631) + \text{Pi} \times (0.309 \times \text{pH} - 0.469)$$

(SIDe in mEq/l; $PaCO_2$ in mmHg, Alb in g/l and Pi in mmol/l)

The effect of unmeasured charges was quantified by the strong ion gap (SIG) [30]:

$$SIG = SIDa - SIDe$$

(all parameters in mEq/l)

Based on the concept that BE can be altered by plasma dilution/concentration reflected by sodium concentration (BE_{Na}), changes of chloride (BE_{Cl}), albumin (BE_{Alb}), lactate (BE_{Lac}) and unmeasured anions (BE_{UMA}), the respective components contributing to BE were calculated according to Gilfix et al. [31]. The detailed formulae for the BE subcomponents are shown in "Appendix."

Thus, total BE is calculated by the sum of the BE subcomponents:

$$BE = BE_{Na} + BE_{Cl} + BE_{Alb} + BE_{Lac} + BE_{UMA}$$

Reference values were obtained from a historical cohort of healthy volunteers, as published elsewhere [8]. Acidemia and alkalemia were defined by pH < 7.36 and > 7.44, respectively. $HCO3^-$ < 22 and > 26 mmol/l, respectively, defined metabolic acidosis and alkalosis [2]. Respiratory acidosis and alkalosis were identified by $PaCO_2$ > 45 and < 35 mmHg, respectively. $BE_{Na} < -5$ and > 5 mmol/l defined dilutional acidosis and alkalosis, respectively. Hyperchloremic acidosis and hypochloremic alkalosis were defined by $BE_{Cl} < -5$ and > 5 mmol/l, respectively. $BE_{Alb} > 5$ mmol/l identified hypoalbuminemic alkalosis. Lactic acidosis was defined by $BE_{Lac} < -1.1$ mmol/l (calculated BE_{Lac} for lactate at the upper limit of normal) and metabolic acidosis owing to unmeasured anions by $BE_{UMA} < -5$ mmol/l.

Statistical analysis

Data are presented as median and interquartile range (25–75% IQR), if not otherwise specified. PSM was used to minimize the confounding effect of severity of disease on acid–base status when comparing cirrhosis to non-cirrhosis patients. One-to-one PSM (1:1) was done by cirrhosis versus non-cirrhosis based on the following variables: SOFA score, need for mechanical ventilation and the presence of AKI. IBM SPSS 22 (with SPSS Python essentials and FUZZY extension command) was used for PSM. McNemar test was used for the comparison of binary and Wilcoxon's signed-rank test for the comparison of metric variables between cirrhosis and matched controls. Nonparametric one-way ANOVA (Kruskal–Wallis test) with Dunn's post hoc analysis was performed to assess differences in acid–base parameters between matched controls, cirrhosis patients without ACLF and ACLF patients. Within each group, comparisons were made using Chi-squared test or Mann–Whitney *U* test, as appropriate. Spearman's rank correlation was used to assess correlations between metric variables. A receiver operating curve (ROC) analysis was performed, and the area under the ROC curve (AUROC) was calculated to evaluate the prognostic value of different metric variables. Impact of acid–base disorders on mortality was assessed using Cox regression. A p value < 0.05 is considered statistically significant. Statistical analysis was conducted using IBM SPSS Statistics version 22.

Results

Patients' characteristics

One hundred and seventy-eight patients had liver cirrhosis, and 157 of these patients (88%) were admitted with ACLF. The remaining cirrhosis patients ($n=21$, 12%) were admitted to ICU due to isolated non-kidney organ failure ($n=9$), isolated cerebral failure ($n=4$), bleedings ($n=4$), infections ($n=3$) and after surgery ($n=1$); all of which did not fulfill criteria for ACLF. The control group consisted of 178 critically ill patients without acute or chronic liver disease. SAPS II score and SOFA score did not differ between patients with and without cirrhosis (Table 1).

Causes of liver cirrhosis were alcoholic liver disease ($n=96$, 54%), viral hepatitis ($n=31$, 17%), combined alcoholic viral ($n=7$, 4%), cryptogenic ($n=23$, 13%), primary biliary cholangitis ($n=5$, 3%) and others ($n=16$, 9%). Triggers for occurrence ACLF were infections/sepsis ($n=110$, 70%), bleeding ($n=23$, 15%) and others.

Clinical and laboratory features of critically ill patients with and without cirrhosis are shown in Table 1.

Acid–base disorders in critically ill patients with and without cirrhosis

Disturbances of acid–base balance were evident in the vast majority of our critically ill patients, irrespective of cirrhosis (Tables 2, 3). Critically ill patients (irrespective of cirrhosis) showed coexisting hyperchloremic acidosis and hypoalbuminemic alkalosis, mostly antagonizing each other in their contribution to total BE. In ACLF, we observed a marked metabolic acidosis owing to increased lactate levels, unmeasured anions and (to a lesser extent) dilutional acidosis. Both BE_{UMA} and SIG differed significantly between critically ill patients with ACLF and without liver disease, respectively, although the small difference in SIG may be clinically negligible (Table 2). In cirrhosis patients without ACLF, BE_{UMA} was significantly higher compared to patients with ACLF. The resulting metabolic acidosis in ACLF was partly compensated by coexisting respiratory alkalosis in its contribution to pH; however, increasing net metabolic acidosis is resulted in acidemia in patients with ACLF grade III (62%, Table 3). Metabolic differences between critically ill patients with and without cirrhosis tended to increase with the severity

Table 1 Baseline characteristics

Parameter	Propensity score-matched controls (*n* = 178)	Liver cirrhosis (*n* = 178)	*p* value
Age, years (IQR)	65 (55–75)	55 (48–62)	< 0.01
Male gender, *n* (%)	79 (44%)	82 (46%)	0.837
SOFA score (IQR)	12 (8–16)	13 (10–16)	0.084
SAPS II score (IQR)	59 (44–72)	62 (44–79	0.101
CLIF-SOFA score (IQR)	–	14 (11–16)	
ACLF grade			
No ACLF, *n* (%)		21 (12%)	
Grade I, *n* (%)	–	27 (15%)	
Grade II, *n* (%)	–	45 (25%)	
Grade III, *n* (%)	–	85 (48%)	
CLIF-C ACLF score (IQR)	–	56.5 (48.8–63.3)	
MELD score (IQR)	–	26 (20–35)	
Child–Pugh score (IQR)	–	11 (10–13)	
Acute kidney injury, *n* (%)	133 (75%)	138 (78%)	0.575
Vasopressor support, *n* (%)	154 (87%)	158 (89%)	0.596
Mechanical ventilation, *n* (%)	116 (65%)	101 (57%)	0.120
Laboratory parameters			
AST, U/l (IQR)	51 (30–116)	94 (54–204)	< 0.01
ALT, U/l (IQR)	32 (19–71)	43 (24–85)	0.096
Bilirubin, mg/dl (IQR)	1.0 (0.6–1.9)	5.4 (2.9–14.4)	< 0.01
INR (IQR)	1.2 (1.1–1.4)	1.8 (1.5–2.5)	< 0.01
Creatinine, mg/dl (IQR)	1.8 (1.2–2.7)	1.8 (1.1–3.1)	0.851
Outcome			
28-Day mortality, *n* (%)	54 (30%)	105 (59%)	< 0.01

IQR interquartile range, *SOFA* Sequential Organ Failure Assessment, *SAPS* Simplified Acute Physiology Score, *CLIF-SOFA* Chronic Liver Failure—Sequential Organ Failure Assessment, *ACLF* acute-on-chronic liver failure, *CLIF-C ACLF* CLIF consortium ACLF score, *MELD* Model of End-Stage Liver Disease, *AST* aspartate aminotransferase, *ALT* alanine aminotransferase, *INR* international normalized ratio

of disease, as indicated by SOFA score (Additional file 1: Figure S1).

Both SIG and BE_{UMA} were associated with renal impairment (Additional file 2: Figure S2). Overall ($n = 356$), SIG was significantly higher and BE_{UMA} significantly lower in patients presenting with AKI as compared to those without [8.4 (IQR 6.0–11.1) mmol/l vs. 5.4 (IQR 2.7–7.5) mmol/l and −2.0 (IQR −6.0 to 1.4) mmol/l vs. 2.8 (IQR −0.3 to 5.6) mmol/l; $p < 0.01$ for both].

Lactate levels were significantly elevated in critically ill patients with liver cirrhosis compared to those without [3.0 (IQR 1.7–6.1) mmol/l vs. 1.4 (IQR 1.0–2.7) mmol/l; $p < 0.01$]. Additionally, lactate levels were higher in patients receiving vasopressors compared to those without [2.3 (IQR 1.3–4.6) mmol/l vs. 1.2 (IQR 0.9–1.8) mmol/l; $p < 0.01$]. Lactate levels increased with SOFA score in cirrhotic and non-cirrhotic patients (Additional file 1: Figure S1). Accordingly, highest lactate levels were observed in patients with ACLF (Table 2). Lactate levels correlated with bilirubin ($r = 0.41$) and international normalized ratio (INR, $r = 0.46$), respectively, but also weakly with serum creatinine ($r = 0.17$); $p < 0.01$ for all.

Metabolic acid–base characteristics of critically ill patients with and without liver disease are illustrated in Fig. 1 and Additional file 1: Figure S1.

Acid–base equilibrium and outcome in patients with liver cirrhosis

In particular, metabolic acidosis and acidemia, respectively, were linked to 28-day mortality in cirrhosis (Fig. 2, Additional file 3: Table S1). Accordingly, arterial pH values < 7.1 on admission were associated with 100% and HCO_3^- values < 10 mmol/l with 89% 28-day mortality, respectively (Fig. 2).

Similarly, BE showed a strong association with 28-day mortality (Additional file 3: Table S1). Analysis of the BE subgroups revealed that the impact on mortality in cirrhosis was primarily caused by lactate and unmeasured anions (Table 4). This effect remained significant after correction for demographics, ACLF grade and the presence of infection/sepsis (Table 4). AUROCs for admission lactate/BE_{Lac} and BE_{UMA} in prediction of 28-day mortality in critical ill patients with liver cirrhosis were 0.744 (95% CI 0.671–0.816) and 0.692 (95% CI 0.613–0.770),

Table 2 Acid–base parameters of critically ill patients with and without liver disease

Parameter	Propensity score-matched controls ($n=178$)	Cirrhosis ($n=178$)		Overall p value (Kruskal–Wallis)	Significant differences pairwise (Dunn's post hoc)
		No ACLF ($n=21$)	ACLF ($n=157$)		
pH	7.36 (7.27 to 7.43)	7.44 (7.37 to 7.47)	7.35 (7.23 to 7.45)	<0.01	No ACLF versus ACLF $p<0.01$, matched controls versus no ACLF $p<0.01$
$PaCO_2$, mmHg	40.0 (33.1 to 49.0)	38.1 (30.0 to 44.2)	35.0 (28.5 to 44.6)	<0.01	Matched controls versus ACLF $p<0.01$
HCO_3^-	22.0 (19.0 to 25.3)	22.7 (20.3 to 24.0)	18.9 (14.7 to 24.0)	<0.01	No ACLF versus ACLF $p<0.01$, matched controls versus ACLF $p<0.01$
BE	−3.5 (−7.4 to 0.8)	−1.2 (−3.9 to 1.7)	−7.0 (−12.6 to −0.5)	<0.01	No ACLF versus ACLF $p<0.01$, matched controls versus ACLF $p<0.01$
BE_{Na}	−0.3 (−1.5 to 0.9)	−0.9 (−1.8 to 0.3)	−1.2 (−3.0 to 0.3)	<0.01	Matched controls versus ACLF $p<0.01$
BE_{Cl}	−5.7 (−8.3 to −2.7)	−5.2 (−8.5 to −1.4)	−4.5 (−7.3 to 0.7)	0.062	
BE_{Alb}	4.2 (2.9 to 5.3)	5.2 (3.9 to 6.3)	4.9 (3.8 to 6.2)	<0.01	Matched controls versus ACLF $p<0.01$
$BE_{lactate}$	−0.6 (−1.9 to −0.2)	−0.9 (−1.9 to −0.4)	−2.7 (−6.0 to −0.9)	<0.01	No ACLF versus ACLF $p<0.01$, matched controls versus ACLF $p<0.01$
BE_{UMA}	−0.3 (−3.7 to 2.7)	1.5 (−0.7 to 4.3)	−1.8 (−6.1 to 1.9)	<0.01	No ACLF versus ACLF $p<0.01$, matched controls versus ACLF $p<0.01$
SIDe, mEq/l	33 (30 to 37)	32 (30 to 37)	29 (25 to 34)	<0.01	No ACLF versus ACLF $p<0.05$, matched controls versus ACLF $p<0.01$
SIDa, mEq/l	41 (37 to 43)	40 (36 to 44)	39 (35 to 42)	<0.01	Matched controls versus ACLF $p<0.01$
SIG, mEq/l	7 (4 to 10)	7 (5 to 8)	8 (6 to 11)	<0.01	No ACLF versus ACLF $p<0.05$, matched controls versus ACLF $p<0.01$
Na	138 (134 to 142)	136 (133 to 140)	135 (129 to 140)	<0.01	Matched controls versus ACLF $p<0.01$
Cl	106 (102 to 109)	105 (99 to 108)	102 (96 to 108)	<0.01	Matched controls versus ACLF $p<0.01$
$Cl_{Na\ corrected}$	107 (104 to 109)	106 (102 to 110)	106 (100 to 108)	0.075	
Ca total	2.1 (2.0 to 2.2)	2.0 (1.9 to 2.1)	2.0 (1.9 to 2.2)	0.191	
Ca ionized	1.1 (1.1 to 1.2)	1.2 (1.1 to 1.2)	1.1 (1.0 to 1.2)	<0.01	No ACLF versus ACLF $p<0.05$, matched controls versus ACLF $p<0.01$
Mg	0.9 (0.7 to 1.0)	0.7 (0.7 to 0.9)	0.9 (0.7 to 1.0)	<0.05	No ACLF versus ACLF $p<0.05$
Albumin, g/l	28.5 (24.3 to 33.8)	25.8 (21.8 to 30.5)	25.6 (21.1 to 30.3)	<0.01	Matched controls versus ACLF $p<0.01$
Lactate	1.4 (1.0 to 2.7)	1.7 (1.2 to 2.7)	3.5 (1.7 to 6.8)	<0.01	No ACLF versus ACLF $p<0.01$, matched controls versus ACLF $p<0.01$

ACLF acute-on-chronic liver failure, *$PaCO_2$* partial pressure of arterial carbon dioxide, *HCO_3^-* bicarbonate, *BE* base excess, *SBE* standard base excess, *BE_{Na}* BE caused by free water effect, *BE_{Cl}* BE caused by changes in chloride, *BE_{Alb}* BE caused by albumin effect, *$BE_{lactate}$* BE attributable to lactate elevation, *BE_{UMA}* BE attributable to unmeasured anions, *SIDe* effective strong ion difference, *SIDa* apparent strong ion difference, *SIG* strong ion gap, *Na* sodium, *Cl* chloride, *Ca* calcium, all values are given in mmol/l with interquartile range (IQR), unless otherwise indicated

respectively ($p<0.001$ for both). Thus, the predictive potential of admission arterial lactate levels regarding 28-day mortality in critically ill cirrhosis patients at the ICU was comparable to SOFA score [AUROC 0.780 (95% CI 0.713–0.847)].

In our matched controls, we observed no significant effect of acidemia, alkalemia, lactic acidosis and net metabolic acidosis, respectively, on 28-day mortality. Yet, pH values differed significantly between non-cirrhosis 28-day survivors and non-survivors [7.37 (IQR

Table 3 Acid–base disorders stratified according to the presence of cirrhosis and ACLF

Metabolic disturbances on admission	Propensity score-matched controls ($n = 178$)	Cirrhosis ($n = 178$)				p value for overall cirrhosis versus matched controls	p value for the effect of ACLF category*
		Overall cirrhosis ($n = 178$)	ACLF category				
			No ACLF ($n = 21$)	ACLF grade 1 and 2 ($n = 72$)	ACLF grade III ($n = 85$)		
Acidemia	87 (49%)	86 (48%)	4 (19%)	29 (40%)	53 (62%)	1.00	< 0.01
Alkalemia	35 (20%)	52 (29%)	11 (52%)	21 (29%)	20 (24%)	< 0.05	< 0.05
Respiratory acidosis	64 (36%)	41 (23%)	3 (14%)	13 (18%)	25 (29%)	< 0.05	0.052
Respiratory alkalosis	55 (31%)	88 (49%)	10 (48%)	40 (56%)	38 (45%)	< 0.01	0.338
Metabolic acidosis	89 (50%)	112 (63%)	7 (33%)	45 (63%)	60 (71%)	< 0.05	< 0.01
Metabolic alkalosis	38 (21%)	33 (19%)	4 (19%)	16 (22%)	13 (15%)	0.596	0.365
Dilutional acidosis	1 (0.6%)	11 (6%)	0	4 (6%)	7 (8%)	< 0.01	0.205
Concentrational alkalosis	2 (1.1%)	6 (3%)	0	6 (8%)	0	0.289	0.136
Hyperchloremic acidosis	98 (55%)	78 (44%)	11 (52%)	32 (44%)	35 (41%)	< 0.05	0.399
Hypochloremic alkalosis	7 (4%)	15 (8%)	0	8 (11%)	7 (8%)	0.134	0.702
Hypoalbuminemic alkalosis	58 (33%)	86 (48%)	11 (52%)	36 (50%)	39 (46%)	< 0.01	0.516
Acidosis owing to unmeasured anions	32 (18%)	48 (27%)	1 (5%)	16 (22%)	31 (37%)	0.061	< 0.01
Lactic acidosis	65 (37%)	118 (66%)	7 (33%)	44 (61%)	67 (79%)	< 0.01	< 0.01

All values are given in number (n) and percent (%)

ACLF acute-on-chronic liver failure

*p value calculated by univariate ordinal logistic regression

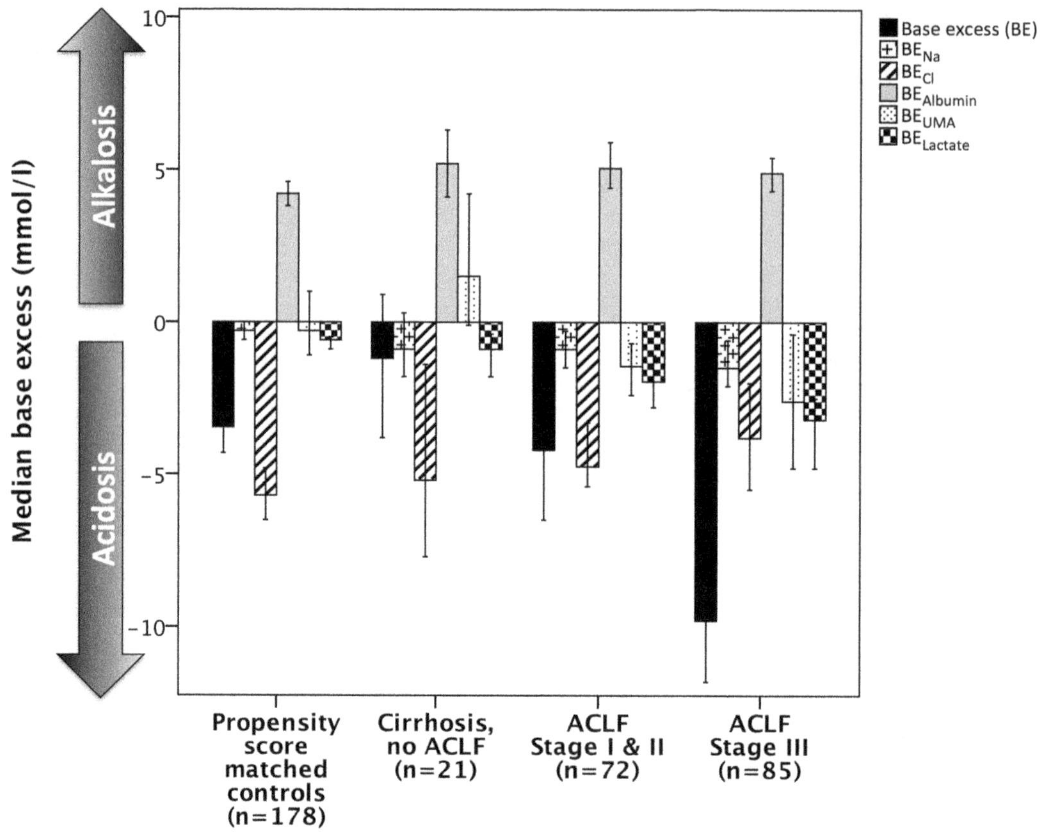

Fig. 1 Disequilibrium in acid–base status in critically ill patients with liver cirrhosis, acute-on-chronic liver failure (ACLF) and without chronic liver disease. Results displayed as median and 95% CI; associations of base excess and its subcomponents with ACLF stage in cirrhosis patients assessed by univariate ordinal regression: BE $p<0.001$, BE_{Na} $p=0.074$, BE_{Cl} $p=0.728$, BE_{Alb} $p=0.295$, BE_{Lac} $p<0.001$, BE_{UMA} $p<0.05$. Differences between cirrhosis and control patients are illustrated in Table 2

7.29–7.44) vs. 7.34 (IQR 7.22–7.34), $p<0.05$, Additional file 3: Table S1]. Acidosis attributable to unmeasured anions was associated with 28-day mortality in our propensity score-matched controls; however, BE_{UMA} did not differ significantly between non-cirrhotic 28-day survivors and non-survivors (Additional file 3: Table S1). Moreover, admission arterial lactate levels differed significantly between non-cirrhosis 28-day survivors and non-survivors [1.4 (IQR 0.9–2.4) mmol/l vs. 1.7 (IQR 1–4.1) mmol/l; $p<0.05$]. Yet, the association between metabolic derangement and outcome was more distinct in cirrhosis patients (Additional file 3: Table S1).

Discussion

Disturbances in acid–base equilibrium are common in critical illness [16]. In this study, we demonstrate that critically ill patients with cirrhosis and ACLF, respectively, differentiate considerably from patients without hepatic impairment in terms of acid–base balance.

In accordance with earlier reports, we observed in our cohort a marked hyperchloremic acidosis with coexisting hypoalbuminemic alkalosis [8, 9, 11]. This phenomenon, however, was not limited to patients with cirrhosis and should therefore not be considered an exclusive acid–base pattern of liver disease. Instead, this seems to be a characteristic pattern of critical illness per se [3]. Yet, hypoalbuminemia and resulting alkalosis were most pronounced in patients with ACLF. However, the main distinguishing metabolic acid–base characteristic between critically ill patients with and without cirrhosis was a marked metabolic acidosis attributable to an increased lactate (and unmeasured anions). In cirrhosis, coexisting respiratory alkalosis partly compensated for metabolic acidosis, thereby resulting in almost normal pH values. However, respiratory alkalosis failed to compensate for net metabolic acidosis in patients with ACLF.

Increased lactate levels in critically ill patients can result from both increased production (e.g., tissue malperfusion, impaired cellular oxygen metabolism during sepsis, hypermetabolic states) and reduced lactate clearance (e.g., loss of functioning hepatocytes in acute hepatic injury or chronic liver disease) [32–34]. The liver

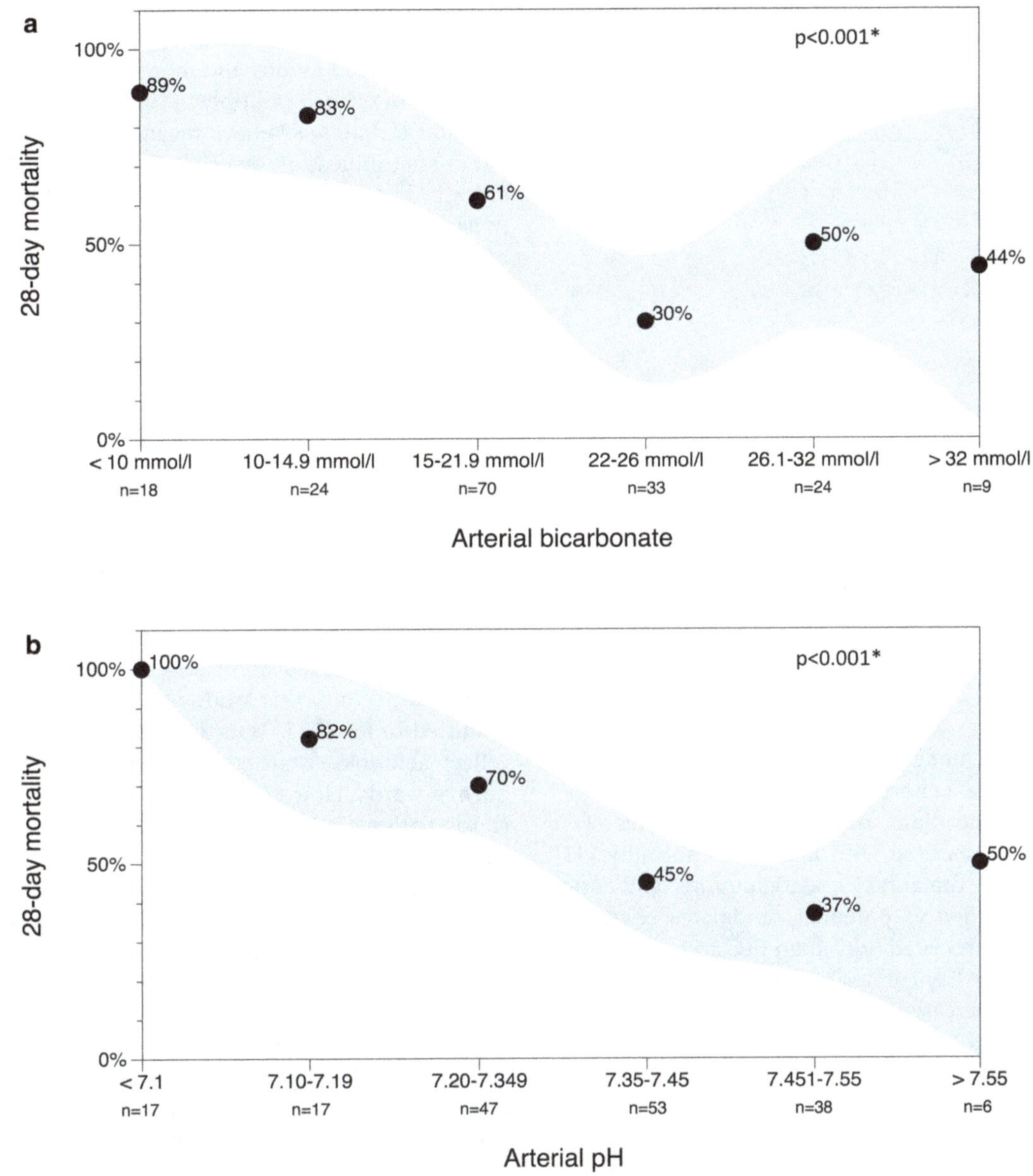

Fig. 2 Association of bicarbonate (**a**) and pH (**b**) with 28-day mortality in critically ill patients with liver cirrhosis. Black dots: observed 28-day mortality rate; gray area: 95% confidence interval. **p* values calculated by Chi-square test

not only is a crucial player in the disposal of lactate, but may also become a net producer of lactate, especially during hepatic parenchymal hypoxia. Although lactic acidosis has been described in the literature in critical ill patients with cirrhosis [7, 8], this is the first study investigating the association of metabolic disturbances with ACLF compared to a matched cohort of critically ill patients without liver disease. Indeed, the extent of lactic acidosis was directly associated with ACLF grade. Accordingly, lactic acidosis was present in almost 80% of all patients with ACLF grade III. Moreover, lactate levels were correlated with INR and bilirubin, thereby suggesting that lactate levels are directly related to liver function. Vasopressor support and severity of disease (as reflected by SOFA score) were also significantly associated with increased lactate levels. In sum, our data suggest that a combination of hepatic impairment and tissue hypoxia may contribute to lactic acidosis in critically ill patients with liver cirrhosis.

Great effort has been put in revealing the nature of unmeasured anions in critical illness [2, 35–38]. Still, source and clinical implications of unmeasured anions

Table 4 Cox regression model for risk factors for mortality in critically ill patients with liver cirrhosis

Parameter	Hazard ratio (95% CI)	
	Univariate	Multivariate
Age	1.02 (1.00–1.04)*	1.02 (1.00–1.04)*
Sex (male gender)	0.75 (0.51–1.11)	0.77 (0.51–1.15)
Liver disease		
ACLF grade 1 versus no ACLF	1.80 (0.63–5.19)	1.36 (0.47–4.01)
ACLF grade 2 versus no ACLF	2.02 (0.76–5.37)	1.44 (0.53–3.94)
ACLF grade 3 versus no ACLF	5.52 (2.22–13.74)**	3.68 (1.42–9.52)**
Sepsis/infection	1.69 (1.09–2.61)*	1.21 (0.76–1.92)
Base excess		
BE_{Na}	0.96 (0.90–1.03)	0.96 (0.89–1.04)
BE_{Cl}	1.00 (0.98–1.03)	0.97 (0.93–1.00)
BE_{Alb}	0.91 (0.81–1.02)	0.89 (0.79–1.00)
BE_{UMA}	0.95 (0.93–0.97)**	0.96 (0.92–0.99)*
$BE_{lactate}$	0.88 (0.85–0.92)**	0.92 (0.88–0.97)**

ACLF acute-on-chronic liver failure, BE_{Na} BE caused by free water effect, BE_{Cl} BE caused by changes in chloride, BE_{Alb} BE caused by albumin effect, $BE_{lactate}$ BE attributable to lactate elevation, BE_{UMA} BE attributable to unmeasured anions

*p value < 0.05; **p value < 0.01

are incompletely understood [39, 40]. Recently, it was shown in a large cohort of critically ill patients that increased concentrations of unmeasured anions were independently associated with increased mortality [41]. Citrate, acetate, fumarate, α-ketoglutarate and urate have been identified as potential candidates contributing to acidosis associated with high SIG in hemorrhagic shock [36]. Apart from states of shock, renal failure has been linked to increased levels of unmeasured anions in several studies [8, 42, 43]. As compared to non-ACLF cirrhosis patients, the presence of ACLF was associated with an increase in unmeasured anions, as reflected by BE_{UMA} and SIG. Both variables were strongly associated with acute kidney injury. Patients with liver cirrhosis are especially susceptible to renal failure [44–47], and renal impairment constitutes a central criterion for ACLF [20]. In sum, our findings indicate that impairment of renal function, rather than "hepatic failure," may be responsible for the increase in levels of unmeasured anions observed in patients with ACLF.

In the present study, metabolic acidosis and acidemia, respectively, were associated with increased 28-day mortality in liver cirrhosis. Accordingly, 28-day mortality rate was 91% in cirrhosis patients with arterial pH values <7.2 and 86% in those with arterial HCO_3^- values < 15 mmol/l. Lactic acidosis and acidosis attributable to unmeasured anions were identified as main contributors to acid–base imbalance in critically ill patients with liver cirrhosis. Earlier studies have challenged the prognostic value of unmeasured anions or lactate in critically ill patients [40]. Yet, the relationship between lactate levels, unmeasured anions and mortality and poor outcome has been described multiply in the literature [7, 8, 32, 33, 48], and lactate levels have recently been suggested as a parameter, indicating severity of disease in patients with chronic liver disease [49]. In our critically ill cirrhosis patients, we observed a dramatic independent impact of both lactate and BE_{UMA} on 28-day mortality. Thus, acid–base status in critically ill patients with cirrhosis and ACLF, respectively, is an early and independent predictor of outcome (Fig. 2). By contrast, acid–base status was of poor prognostic value in our propensity score-matched controls. This may be attributable to the fact that our control patients were matched to critically ill cirrhosis patients, thereby resulting in the exclusion of less severely ill non-cirrhosis patients with better acid–base profiles and lower mortality rates.

This study has strengths and limitations. First, this is a post hoc analysis; however, our study comprises structured acid–base analyses from a large cohort of critically ill patients stratified according to the presence of liver cirrhosis. Second, this study was performed in patients admitted to the ICU. Thus, our findings may not entirely reflect acid–base status of cirrhotic patients treated at normal wards. However, our study also incorporates cirrhosis patients without ACLF and patients of all ACLF categories. Third, there are pros and cons of propensity score matching. In this study, we have decided to use propensity score-matched controls in order to minimize the confounding effect of severity of disease on acid–base balance. Although we were able to achieve good comparability, inherent differences between cirrhotic and non-cirrhotic patients affecting acid base balance cannot be entirely abolished by matching procedures. Moreover, the loss of heterogeneity (by selection of the most severely ill patients) hampers survival analyses in the control group. Fourth, residual confounding is, as always, a matter of concern and cannot be entirely excluded. Future studies should confirm these results and focus on therapeutic implications for patients with liver disease at the ICU.

Conclusions

In conclusion, we could demonstrate that hyperchloremic acidosis and hypoalbuminemic alkalosis coexist in critically ill patients, including those with liver cirrhosis. In cirrhosis, but particularly in ACLF, net metabolic acidosis was caused by lactate and unmeasured anions. Lactate was linked to liver function and vasopressor use, whereas unmeasured anions were strongly related to acute kidney injury. Metabolic differences between cirrhosis and non-cirrhosis critically ill patients increase with the severity of disease, resulting in pronounced acidemia in cirrhosis patients with ACLF. Acidemia and metabolic acidosis, respectively, were associated with poor outcome in cirrhosis patients. Lactate and BE_{UMA} were identified as independent predictors of 28-day mortality in critically ill patients with liver cirrhosis and ACLF.

Additional files

Additional file 1: Figure S1. Acid–base disturbances and their relation to severity of disease in critically ill patients with and without liver cirrhosis. Overall following parameter differed significantly between cirrhosis and non-cirrhosis patients (Wilcoxon's signed-rank test): BE ($p < 0.01$), lactate ($p < 0.001$), BE_{UMA} ($p < 0.05$), SIG ($p < 0.01$) and $PaCO_2$ ($p < 0.01$), but not pH ($p = 0.624$). *p values between regression slopes were obtained from linear regression models with interaction terms

Additional file 2: Figure S2. Base excess attributable to unmeasured anions (BE_{UMA}) and strong ion gap (SIG) are associated with acute kidney injury in critically ill patients with and without cirrhosis. BE_{UMA} ($p < 0.05$) and SIG ($p < 0.01$) differed significantly between patients with and without cirrhosis, but correlated significantly with stage of acute kidney injury in both groups ($p < 0.001$). The association of BE_{UMA} and SIG, respectively, with acute kidney injury did not differ between patients with and without cirrhosis ($p = 0.994$ and 0.824)

Additional file 3: Table S1.

Abbreviations
ICU: intensive care unit; ALF: acute liver failure; ACLF: acute-on-chronic liver failure; PSM: propensity score matching; SAPS II: Simplified Acute Physiology Score II; SOFA: Sequential Organ Failure Assessment; AKI: acute kidney injury; KDIGO: Kidney Disease: Improving Global Outcomes; CLIF: chronic liver failure; EASL: European Association for the Study of the Liver; CLIF-SOFA: Chronic Liver Failure Sequential Organ Failure Assessment; CLIF-C ACLF: chronic liver failure consortium acute-on-chronic liver failure score; $PaCO_2$: partial pressure of arterial carbon dioxide; Ca^{2+}: total calcium; K^+: potassium; Cl^-: chloride; Mg^{2+}: magnesium; Pi: inorganic phosphate; Alb: albumin; BUN: blood urea nitrogen; AST: aspartate aminotransferase; ALT: alanine aminotransferase; $HCO3^-$: bicarbonate; BE: base excess; SID_a: apparent strong ion difference; SID_e: effective strong ion difference; SIG: strong ion gap; UMA: unmeasured anions; BE_{Na}: base excess attributable to sodium; BE_{Cl}: base excess attributable to chloride; BE_{Alb}: base excess attributable to albumin; BE_{Lac}: base excess attributable to lactate; BE_{UMA}: base excess attributable to unmeasured anions; IQR: interquartile range; ROC: receiver operating characteristic; AUROC: area under the receiver operating characteristic curve.

Authors' contributions
AD, TH, BS and VF participated in conception and design of the study. KRo, KRu, RB, CZ, PS and GH contributed to acquisition and interpretation of data. AD, TH and VF performed the statistical analysis. AD and TH drafted the manuscript. GCF, MT, BS and VF critically read and revised the manuscript for important intellectual content. All authors read and approved the final manuscript.

Author details
[1] Division of Gastroenterology and Hepatology, Department of Internal Medicine III, Medical University of Vienna, Vienna, Austria. [2] Department of Intensive Care Medicine, University Medical Center, Hamburg-Eppendorf, Martinistraße 52, 20246 Hamburg, Germany. [3] Division of Oncology and Infectious Diseases, Department of Internal Medicine I, Medical University of Vienna, Vienna, Austria. [4] Division of Cardiology, Department of Internal Medicine II, Medical University of Vienna, Vienna, Austria. [5] Department of Respiratory and Critical Care Medicine, and Ludwig Boltzmann Institute for COPD, Otto-Wagner Hospital, Vienna, Austria.

Acknowledgements
Not applicable.

Competing interests
The authors declare that there are no competing interests.

Funding
No funding.

Appendix
BE subcomponents reflecting the contributions of sodium (BE_{Na}), chloride (BE_{Cl}), albumin (BE_{Na}), lactate (BE_{Lac}) and unmeasured anions (BE_{UMA}), according to Gilfix et al. [31]:

(A) Na^+ was used to assess BE caused by free water effect (dilution)

$$BE_{Na} = 0.3 \times \left(Na^+ - Na^+_{normal}\right)$$
$$\left(Na^+_{normal} = 139\ mmol/l\right)$$

(B) After correction Cl^- for changes in free water ($Cl^-_{Na\ corrected}$)

$$Cl^-_{Na\ corrected} = Cl^- \times \frac{Na^+_{normal}}{Na^+}$$

BE attributable to chloride (BE_{Cl}) was calculated:

$$BE_{Cl} = Cl^-_{normal} - Cl^-_{Na\ corrected}$$
$$\left(Cl^-_{normal} = 101\ mmol/l\right)$$

(C) BE attributable to albumin was calculated as follows [28]:

$$BE_{Alb} = (0.148 \times pH - 0.818) \times (Alb_{normal} - Alb_{observed})$$
$$\left(Alb_{normal} = 44.4\ g/l\right)$$

(D) BE due to lactate was calculated:

$$BE_{Lac} = lactate_{normal} - lactate_{observed}$$
$$(lactate_{normal} = 0.8\ mmol/l)$$

(E) Changes in BE not related to the aforementioned factors correspond to UMA, which are quantified as follows:

$$BE_{UMA} = BE - (BE_{Na} + BE_{Cl} + BE_{Alb} + BE_{Lac})$$

References
1. Kassirer JP. Serious acid–base disorders. N Engl J Med. 1974;291:773–6.
2. Kellum JA. Determinants of blood pH in health and disease. Crit Care. 2000;4:6–14.
3. Noritomi DT, Soriano FG, Kellum JA, Cappi SB, Biselli PJC, Libório AB, Park M. Metabolic acidosis in patients with severe sepsis and septic shock: a longitudinal quantitative study. Crit Care Med. 2009;37:2733–9.
4. Mæhle K, Haug B, Flaatten H, Nielsen E. Metabolic alkalosis is the most common acid–base disorder in ICU patients. Crit Care. 2014;18:420.

5. Neyra JA, Canepa-Escaro F, Li X, Manllo J, Adams-Huet B, Yee J, Yessayan L. Acute Kidney Injury in Critical Illness Study Group: association of hyperchloremia with hospital mortality in critically ill septic patients. Crit Care Med. 2015;43:1938–44.
6. Smith I, Kumar P, Molloy S, Rhodes A, Newman PJ, Grounds RM, Bennett ED. Base excess and lactate as prognostic indicators for patients admitted to intensive care. Intensive Care Med. 2001;27:74–83.
7. Moreau R, Hadengue A, Soupison T, Kirstetter P, Mamzer MF, Vanjak D, Vauquelin P, Assous M, Sicot C. Septic shock in patients with cirrhosis: hemodynamic and metabolic characteristics and intensive care unit outcome. Crit Care Med. 1992;20:746–50.
8. Funk G-C, Doberer D, Kneidinger N, Lindner G, Holzinger U, Schneeweiss B. Acid–base disturbances in critically ill patients with cirrhosis. Liver Int. 2007;27:901–9.
9. Funk G-C, Doberer D, Osterreicher C, Peck-Radosavljevic M, Schmid M, Schneeweiss B. Equilibrium of acidifying and alkalinizing metabolic acid–base disorders in cirrhosis. Liver Int. 2005;25:505–12.
10. Bihari D, Gimson AE, Lindridge J, Williams R. Lactic acidosis in fulminant hepatic failure. Some aspects of pathogenesis and prognosis. J Hepatol. 1985;1:405–16.
11. Funk G-C, Doberer D, Fuhrmann V, Holzinger U, Kitzberger R, Kneidinger N, Lindner G, Schneeweiss B. The acidifying effect of lactate is neutralized by the alkalinizing effect of hypoalbuminemia in non-paracetamol-induced acute liver failure. J Hepatol. 2006;45:387–92.
12. McPhail MJW, Shawcross DL, Abeles RD, Chang A, Patel V, Lee G-H, Abdulla M, Sizer E, Willars C, Auzinger G, Bernal W, Wendon JA. Increased survival for patients with cirrhosis and organ failure in liver intensive care and validation of the chronic liver failure-sequential organ failure scoring system. Clin Gastroenterol Hepatol. 2015;13(7):1353–60.
13. Weil D, Levesque E, McPhail M, Cavallazzi R, Theocharidou E, Cholongitas E, Galbois A, Pan HC, Karvellas CJ, Sauneuf B, Robert R, Fichet J, Piton G, Thevenot T, Capellier G, Di Martino V. METAREACIR Group: prognosis of cirrhotic patients admitted to intensive care unit: a meta-analysis. Ann Intensive Care. 2017;7:33.
14. Warren A, Soulsby CR, Puxty A, Campbell J, Shaw M, Quasim T, Kinsella J, McPeake J. Long-term outcome of patients with liver cirrhosis admitted to a general intensive care unit. Ann Intensive Care. 2017;7:37.
15. Piton G, Chaignat C, Giabicani M, Cervoni J-P, Tamion F, Weiss E, Paugam-Burtz C, Capellier G, Di Martino V. Prognosis of cirrhotic patients admitted to the general ICU. Ann Intensive Care. 2016;6:94.
16. Scheiner B, Lindner G, Reiberger T, Schneeweiss B, Trauner M, Zauner C, Funk G-C. Acid–base disorders in liver disease. J Hepatol. 2017;67:1062–73.
17. Le Gall JR, Lemeshow S, Saulnier F. A new Simplified Acute Physiology Score (SAPS II) based on a European/North American multicenter study. JAMA. 1993;270:2957–63.
18. Vincent JL, Moreno R, Takala J, Willatts S, De Mendonça A, Bruining H, Reinhart CK, Suter PM, Thijs LG. The SOFA (Sepsis-related Organ Failure Assessment) score to describe organ dysfunction/failure. On behalf of the Working Group on sepsis-related problems of the European Society of Intensive Care Medicine. Intensive Care Med. 1996;22:707–10.
19. Kidney Disease Improving Global Outcomes KDIGO Acute Kidney. Injury Work Group: KDIGO clinical practice guideline for acute kidney injury. Kidney Int Suppl. 2012;2012(2):1–138.
20. Moreau R, Jalan R, Gines P, Pavesi M, Angeli P, Cordoba J, Durand F, Gustot T, Saliba F, Domenicali M, Gerbes A, Wendon J, Alessandria C, Laleman W, Zeuzem S, Trebicka J, Bernardi M, Arroyo V. CANONIC Study Investigators of the EASL–CLIF Consortium: acute-on-chronic liver failure is a distinct syndrome that develops in patients with acute decompensation of cirrhosis. Gastroenterology. 2013;144:1426–37.
21. Jalan R, Saliba F, Pavesi M, Amorós À, Moreau R, Gines P, Levesque E, Durand F, Angeli P, Caraceni P, Hopf C, Alessandria C, Rodriguez E, Solis-Muñoz P, Laleman W, Trebicka J, Zeuzem S, Gustot T, Mookerjee R, Elkrief L, Soriano G, Cordoba J, Morando F, Gerbes A, Agarwal B, Samuel D, Bernardi M, Arroyo V. CANONIC Study Investigators of the EASL–CLIF Consortium: development and validation of a prognostic score to predict mortality in patients with acute-on-chronic liver failure. J Hepatol. 2014;61:1038–47.
22. Dellinger RP, Levy MM, Carlet JM, Bion J, Parker MM, Jaeschke R, Reinhart K, Angus DC, Brun-Buisson C, Beale R, Calandra T, Dhainaut J-F, Gerlach H, Harvey M, Marini JJ, Marshall J, Ranieri M, Ramsay G, Sevransky J, Thompson BT, Townsend S, Vender JS, Zimmerman JL, Vincent J-L. Surviving Sepsis Campaign: international guidelines for management of severe sepsis and septic shock: 2008. Intensive Care Med. 2008;34:17–60.
23. Drolz A, Horvatits T, Roedl K, Rutter K, Staufer K, Kneidinger N, Holzinger U, Zauner C, Schellongowski P, Heinz G, Perkmann T, Kluge S, Trauner M, Fuhrmann V. Coagulation parameters and major bleeding in critically ill patients with cirrhosis. Hepatology. 2016;64:556–68.
24. Siggaard-Andersen O, Fogh-Andersen N. Base excess or buffer base (strong ion difference) as measure of a non-respiratory acid–base disturbance. Acta Anaesthesiol Scand Suppl. 1995;107:123–8.
25. Siggaard-Andersen O, Gøthgen IH, Wimberley PD, Fogh-Andersen N. The oxygen status of the arterial blood revised: relevant oxygen parameters for monitoring the arterial oxygen availability. Scand J Clin Lab Invest Suppl. 1990;203:17–28.
26. Siggaard-Andersen O. The van Slyke equation. Scand J Clin Lab Invest Suppl. 1977;146:15–20.
27. Stewart PA. Modern quantitative acid–base chemistry. Can J Physiol Pharmacol. 1983;61:1444–61.
28. Figge J, Rossing TH, Fencl V. The role of serum proteins in acid–base equilibria. J Lab Clin Med. 1991;117:453–67.
29. Fencl V, Jabor A, Kazda A, Figge J. Diagnosis of metabolic acid–base disturbances in critically ill patients. Am J Respir Crit Care Med. 2000;162:2246–51.
30. Kellum JA. Closing the gap on unmeasured anions. Crit Care. 2003;7:219–20.
31. Gilfix BM, Bique M, Magder S. A physical chemical approach to the analysis of acid–base balance in the clinical setting. J Crit Care. 1993;8:187–97.
32. Mizock BA. Controversies in lactic acidosis. Implications in critically ill patients. JAMA. 1987;258:497–501.
33. Oster JR, Perez GO. Acid–base disturbances in liver disease. J Hepatol. 1986;2:299–306.
34. Mallat J, Lemyze M, Meddour M, Pepy F, Gasan G, Barrailler S, Durville E, Temime J, Vangrunderbeeck N, Tronchon L, Vallet B, Thevenin D. Ratios of central venous-to-arterial carbon dioxide content or tension to arteriovenous oxygen content are better markers of global anaerobic metabolism than lactate in septic shock patients. Ann Intensive Care. 2016;6:10.
35. Forni LG, McKinnon W, Lord GA, Treacher DF, Peron J-MR, Hilton PJ. Circulating anions usually associated with the Krebs cycle in patients with metabolic acidosis. Crit Care. 2005;9:R591–5.
36. Bruegger D, Kemming GI, Jacob M, Meisner FG, Wojtczyk CJ, Packert KB, Keipert PE, Faithfull NS, Habler OP, Becker BF, Rehm M. Causes of metabolic acidosis in canine hemorrhagic shock: role of unmeasured ions. Crit Care. 2007;11:R130.
37. Kneidinger N, Lindner G, Fuhrmann V, Doberer D, Dunkler D, Schneeweiss B, Funk GC. Acute phase proteins do not account for unmeasured anions in critical illness. Eur J Clin Invest. 2007;37:820–5.
38. Mizock BA, Belyaev S, Mecher C. Unexplained metabolic acidosis in critically ill patients: the role of pyroglutamic acid. Intensive Care Med. 2004;30:502–5.
39. Balasubramanyan N, Havens PL, Hoffman GM. Unmeasured anions identified by the Fencl–Stewart method predict mortality better than base excess, anion gap, and lactate in patients in the pediatric intensive care unit. Crit Care Med. 1999;27:1577–81.
40. Rocktaeschel J, Morimatsu H, Uchino S, Bellomo R. Unmeasured anions in critically ill patients: can they predict mortality? Crit Care Med. 2003;31:2131–6.
41. Masevicius FD, Rubatto Birri PN, Risso Vazquez A, Zechner FE, Motta MF, Valenzuela Espinoza ED, Welsh S, Guerra Arias EF, Furche MA, Berdaguer FD, Dubin A. Relationship of at admission lactate, unmeasured anions, and chloride to the outcome of critically ill patients. Crit Care Med. 2017;45:e1233–9.
42. Naka T, Bellomo R. Bench-to-bedside review: treating acid–base abnormalities in the intensive care unit—the role of renal replacement therapy. Crit Care. 2004;8:108–14.

43. Naka T, Bellomo R, Morimatsu H, Rocktaschel J, Wan L, Gow P, Angus P. Acid–base balance during continuous veno-venous hemofiltration: the impact of severe hepatic failure. Int J Artif Organs. 2006;29:668–74.
44. Nadim MK, Durand F, Kellum JA, Levitsky J, O'Leary JG, Karvellas CJ, Bajaj JS, Davenport A, Jalan R, Angeli P, Caldwell SH, Fernández J, Francoz C, Garcia-Tsao G, Gines P, Ison MG, Kramer DJ, Mehta RL, Moreau R, Mulligan D, Olson JC, Pomfret EA, Senzolo M, Steadman RH, Subramanian RM, Vincent J-L, Genyk YS. Management of the critically ill patient with cirrhosis: a multidisciplinary perspective. J Hepatol. 2016;64:717–35.
45. Angeli P, Gines P, Wong F, Bernardi M, Boyer TD, Gerbes A, Moreau R, Jalan R, Sarin SK, Piano S, Moore K, Lee SS, Durand F, Salerno F, Caraceni P, Kim WR, Arroyo V, Garcia-Tsao G. Diagnosis and management of acute kidney injury in patients with cirrhosis: revised consensus recommendations of the International Club of Ascites. Int J Hepatol. 2015;62:968–74.
46. Arroyo V, Ginès P, Gerbes AL, Dudley FJ, Gentilini P, Laffi G, Reynolds TB, Ring-Larsen H, Schölmerich J. Definition and diagnostic criteria of refractory ascites and hepatorenal syndrome in cirrhosis. Hepatology. 1996;23:164–76.
47. Drolz A, Horvatits T, Roedl K, Rutter K, Staufer K, Haider DG, Zauner C, Heinz G, Schellongowski P, Kluge S, Trauner M, Fuhrmann V. Outcome and features of acute kidney injury complicating hypoxic hepatitis at the medical intensive care unit. Ann Intensive Care. 2016;6:61.
48. Dell'Anna AM, Sandroni C, Lamanna I, Belloni I, Donadello K, Creteur J, Vincent J-L, Taccone FS. Prognostic implications of blood lactate concentrations after cardiac arrest: a retrospective study. Ann Intensive Care. 2017;7:101.
49. Edmark C, McPhail MJW, Bell M, Whitehouse T, Wendon J, Christopher KB. LiFe: a liver injury score to predict outcome in critically ill patients. Intensive Care Med. 2016;42:361–9.

In-hospital and day-120 survival of critically ill solid cancer patients after discharge of the intensive care units: results of a retrospective multicenter study

François Vincent[1*], Marcio Soares[2,3], Djamel Mokart[4], Virginie Lemiale[5], Fabrice Bruneel[6], Marouane Boubaya[7], Frédéric Gonzalez[8], Yves Cohen[8], Elie Azoulay[5,9], Michaël Darmon[5] and on behalf of the GrrrOH: Groupe de recherche respiratoire en réanimation en Onco-Hématologie (Group for respiratory research in intensive care in Onco-Hematology, http://www.grrroh.com/)

Abstract

Objectives: To assess outcomes at hospital discharge and day-120 after intensive care unit (ICU) discharge among patients with solid cancer admitted to ICU and to identify characteristics associated with in-hospital and day-120 after ICU discharge mortalities.

Design: International, multicenter, retrospective study.

Setting: Five ICUs in France and Brazil, two located in cancer centers, two in university affiliated and one in general hospitals.

Patients: Consecutive patients aged > 18 years, with underlying solid cancers (known before admission to the ICU or diagnosed during the stay in the ICU), admitted to the participating ICUs and discharged alive from the ICU from January 2006 to December 2011 were included in this study. Patients admitted after scheduled surgery or to secure procedure were excluded. Variables of interest were in-hospital and day-120 post-ICU mortality among patients discharged alive from the ICU.

Interventions: None.

Measurements and results: A total of 1053 patients aged 63 years (54–71) (median [IQR]) were included. Most of the patients were of the male gender (66.8%). The in-ICU, in-hospital, and four-month post-ICU discharge mortalities were, respectively, 41.3, 60.7, and 65.8%. Among patients discharged alive from the ICU, in multivariate analysis, factors

*Correspondence: frncsvncnt@aol.com
[1] Medical-Surgical Intensive Care Unit, Le Raincy-Montfermeil General Hospital, 10, rue du Général Leclerc, 93370 Montfermeil, France
Full list of author information is available at the end of the article

associated with four months post-ICU discharge mortality were type of cancer (OR from 0.25 to 0.52 when compared to lung cancers), systemic extension of the disease (OR 2.54; 95% CI 1.87–3.45), need for invasive mechanical ventilation (OR 2.54; 95% CI 1.80–3.59), for vasopressors (OR 2.35; 95% CI 1.66–3.29), or renal replacement therapy (OR 1.54; 95% CI 0.99–2.38). A predictive score, "Oncoscore," was built performing fairly in predicting 4 months post-ICU discharge outcome (AUC 0.74; 95% CI 0.71–0.77).

Conclusion: Despite the high day-120 mortality following the ICU discharge, our study reports a meaningful medium-term survival rate after the ICU discharge of solid cancer patients. Of utmost importance, the "Oncoscore" must be validated in prospective studies and cannot be used, in its form without external validation, for individual decision making. Prospective studies to answer questions not provided by this study are needed, including only patients with solid cancers admitted in the ICU for medical reasons or after emergency surgery.

Keywords: Follow-up study, Intensive care unit, Post-intensive, Prognosis, Score, Solid cancers

Background

Survival of patients with cancer has substantially increased in recent decades in developed countries, which, consequently, has led to increasing number of hospitalizations in the intensive care unit (ICU) [1, 2]. A retrospective study showed that among 118,541 patients, 5.2% (95% confidence interval [95% CI] 5.0–5.3%) were admitted to an ICU within 2 years following cancer diagnosis [3]. Despite this, data regarding in-hospital mortality and mainly post-ICU outcome of such patients remain scarce. In a literature review of adult patients with solid cancers admitted to the ICU from January 2000 to April 2014, Puxty et al. [4] identified 48 studies, among which in-ICU mortality was reported in 32 studies, in-hospital mortality reported in 25 studies, and mortality at 1, 3, and 6 months, respectively, reported in only 4, 5, and 7 studies. One of the most obvious reasons is that studies on cancer patients hospitalized in the ICU are still ongoing, and even the most recent ones continue to mix patients with hematological malignancies and those with solid cancers under the generic term "cancer patients" [5, 6]. However, there is evidence for several years that the prognosis of solid cancer patients is totally different depending on the type of cancer, whether hematological or solid [7]. One of the most recent and best documented studies is probably that of Ha et al. [8]. Its main interest lies in the fact that the population studied (unplanned admissions) was similar to ours.

The primary objective of our study was to assess hospital mortality of critically ill patients with solid cancers. The secondary objectives were to assess post-ICU day-120 mortality, to assess risk factors for poor outcomes in this population, and to develop a prediction score, named "Oncoscore," regarding post-ICU day-120 mortality.

Patients and methods

Patients and centers

This retrospective cohort study was performed in five ICUs (two cancer institute ICUs [Instituto Nacional de Câncer, Rio de Janeiro and Paoli-Calmettes Institute, Marseille], two university-affiliated hospital ICUs [Saint-Louis Hospital, Paris and Avicenne Hospital, Bobigny], and one general hospital ICU [Versailles Hospital, Le Chesnay]). Consecutive patients aged > 18 years, with underlying solid cancers (known before admission to the ICU or diagnosed during the stay in the ICU), admitted to the participating centers from January 2006 to December 2011 and discharged alive from the ICU were included in this study. Cancer patients admitted following a scheduled surgery [9], those admitted to secure a procedure, or patients with prostate cancer (to avoid the debate on the overdiagnosis of this cancer) [10] were excluded from this study. Thus, only consecutive patients with solid cancers admitted for a medical reason or after emergency surgery were included. To analyze the vital status 4 months following ICU discharge, day 1 was considered as the day of ICU discharge.

In case of multiple admissions in the ICU, only the first one was considered.

According to the French law (L.1121-1 paragraph 1 and R1121-2, Public Health Code), informed consent was unnecessary for anonymous data extraction and analysis from patients' medical files. This retrospective study was approved by the Ethics Commission of the French Intensive Care Society (CE SRLF16-49).

Data collection and definitions

Variables collected within the first 24 h of ICU admission included age, gender, type of cancer, cancer extension (localized or with distant metastases ["systemic extension"]), cancer status (controlled or remission, uncontrolled or new diagnosis, uncontrolled or disease progression), primary reason for ICU admission, hospital days before ICU admission, simplified acute physiology score (SAPS II) [11], sequential organ failure assessment (SOFA) score [12], need for IMV, use of any vasopressors, and need for renal replacement therapy (RRT). During the ICU stay, details regarding the need for IMV, vasopressors, RRT, occurrence of neutropenia (neutrophils < 0.5 G/L), and do not resuscitate (DNR) codes were collected daily. The ICU length of stay (LOS), hospital LOS, vital status at the ICU and hospital discharges, and vital status 4 months following ICU discharges were collected for each patient.

Statistical analysis

Results are reported as medians and quartiles (interquartile range, IQR) or numbers (%). Categorical variables were compared using the Chi-square test or Fisher's exact test, as appropriate, and continuous variables were compared using the nonparametric Wilcoxon test or the Mann–Whitney test.

Logistic regression analyses were performed to identify the variables statistically significantly associated with hospital mortality and day-120 post-ICU discharge mortality, as measured by the estimated odds ratio (OR) with 95% CIs. Variables yielding P values < 0.20 in the univariate analyses or considered clinically relevant were entered in a forward stepwise logistic regression model. Non-log-linear continuous variables were dichotomized. The covariates were entered in the model with critical entry and removal P values of 0.20 and 0.1, respectively. Multi-collinearity and interactions were tested. The Hosmer–Lemeshow test was used to check goodness-of-fit of the logistic regression.

A score, named "Oncoscore," was then built based upon independent factors associated with post-ICU day-120 outcome. To assess its performance in distinguishing post-ICU day-120 outcome, we plotted the receiver operating characteristic (ROC) curves of the proportion of true positives against the proportion of false positives. Two cutoff values were then selected (sensitive and specific cutoff) to define subgroups. Survival curves were then constructed according to the Kaplan–Meier method. Comparison across prediction class was performed using log-rank test.

All tests were two sided, and P values < 0.05 were considered statistically significant. Statistical tests were performed using SPSS 13 software package (IBM, Armonk, NY, USA).

Results

A total of 1248 patients with solid cancers were screened during the study period. Of those, 195 had missing data and were excluded. Thus, 1053 were included in the study. The characteristics of the included patients are reported in Table 1.

Six hundred and ninety one (65.6%) were males with a median age of 63 years (range 54–71). Initial severity scores according to the SOFA and SAPS II scores were 6 (3–10) and 48 (36–62), respectively. The primary underlying malignancies were lung cancers in 202 (19.2%), colorectal cancer in 178 (16.9%), breast cancer in 129 (12.5%), and head and neck cancer in 125 (11.9%). Cancer was considered to be in partial or complete remission in 332 (31.5%) and was diagnosed during the ICU stay in 71 (6.7%). Overall, 561 (53.3%) had systemic extension (presence of distant metastasis) of their disease. Acute condition leading to ICU admission was considered as related to cancer status in 350 (33.3%).

The primary reasons for ICU admission were sepsis or septic shock in 405 (38.5%), acute respiratory failure in 275 (26.1%), and coma in 80 (7.6%). Seven hundred and twenty one (68.5%) required mechanical ventilation, 529 (50.2%) required vasopressors, and 168 (16.0%) required RRT. Cancer chemotherapy was required during ICU stay in 40 (3.8%), and 70 (6.6%) experienced neutropenia during their ICU stay.

Hospital outcome

Survival after the ICU discharge was, respectively, for in-hospital 413/618 (66.8%) and for 120-days 360/618 (58.2%) (Additional file 1: Fig. S1). Factors independently associated with in-hospital mortality are reported in Table 2. After adjustment, lung cancers (when compared to other underlying malignancies), systemic extension of the disease (OR 2.64; 95% CI 1.95–3.57), and organ support (namely need for renal replacement therapy [RRT], vasopressors, or IMV (OR 1.65 [95% CI 1.08–2.53], OR 2.55 [95% CI 1.84–3.55] and OR 2.81 [95% CI 2.00–3.95]), respectively) were associated with poor outcome.

During the ICU stay, decisions to forgo life-sustaining therapies were taken for 362 patients (34.4%). They were not selected in the first multivariable model. However, when these decisions were forced in the final model, these variables did not change this later.

Day-120 after the ICUs discharge outcome

Overall, of the 618 ICU survivors, 258 (41.7%) died before day 120 (Additional file 1: Fig. S1 and Additional file 2: Fig. S2). Factors independently associated with poor day-120 outcome are reported in Table 2 and were found to be consistent with factors associated with hospital outcome. Of note, lung cancers remained associated with poor 4-month mortality in ICU survivors (Additional file 2: Fig. S2). By doing the analysis by center, no "center-effect" appeared.

"Oncoscore"

"Oncoscore" ranges from 0 to 11 (Table 3). In the studied population, the median "Oncoscore" was 6 (range 3–7). The overall model area under the ROC curve in predicting day-120 outcome was fair (0.74; 95% CI 0.71–0.77) (Additional file 3: Fig. S3). Two cutoff values were

Table 1 Patients characteristics per hospital outcome

Variable	Hospital decedents ($n=639$)	Hospital survivors ($n=414$)	*P* value
Male gender	404 (63.2%)	287 (69.3%)	0.05
Age (years)	63 [55–71]	63 [53–71]	0.29
Type of malignancy			
Lung	157 (24.6%)	45 (10.9%)	< 0.001
Colorectal	90 (14.1%)	88 (21.3%)	
Breast	68 (10.6%)	61 (14.7%)	
Head and neck	79 (12.4%)	46 (11.1%)	
Others	245 (38.4%)	174 (42.0%)	
Diagnosis to ICU (months)	3 [1–14]	6 [1–36]	
Cancer status			0.002
Complete remission	99 (15.5%)	90 (21.8%)	–
Partial remission	92 (14.4%)	51 (12.4%)	0.004
Diagnosis during ICU stay	52 (13.0%)	19 (7.5%)	0.04
Distant metastases	384 (60.1%)	177 (42.8%)	< 0.001
Severity at ICU admission			
SAPS II	54 [42–72]	39 [30–50]	< 0.001
SOFA	8 [5–12]	4 [2–7]	< 0.001
Treatments during ICU stay			
Invasive mechanical ventilation	518 (81.3%)	203 (49.0%)	< 0.001
Vasopressors and/or inotropic drug	403 (63.1%)	126 (30.5%)	< 0.001
Renal replacement therapy	127 (19.9%)	41 (10.0%)	< 0.001
Cancer chemotherapy	27 (4.4%)	13 (3.3%)	0.48
Neutropenia during ICU stay	52 (8.2%)	18 (4.4%)	0.02

Table 2 Independent predictors of in-hospital mortality after discharged alive from the ICUs (conditional forward logistic regression)

Variable	Odds ratio	95% CI	*P* value
Systemic extension of the disease	2.54	1.87–3.45	< 0.001
Underlying tumor			
Lung cancers	Ref.	–	–
Colonic cancer	0.29	0.17–0.48	< 0.001
Breast cancer	0.25	0.14–0.43	< 0.001
Head and neck	0.52	0.29–0.93	0.03
Other	0.52	0.33–0.82	0.004
Renal replacement therapy during ICU	1.54	0.99–2.38	0.05
Vasopressors	2.35	1.66–3.29	< 0.0001
Mechanical ventilation	2.54	1.80–3.59	< 0.0001

Hosmer–Lemeshow goodness-of-fit: $k^2=1.90$; $P=0.98$. C-stat: 0.70

CI confidence interval, *Ref.* reference

assessed, including a sensitive cutoff (score of 4, sensitivity 0.84) and a specific cutoff (score of 8; specificity 0.92). According to these cutoff values, day-120 mortality rates were 40% ($n=111$), 70% ($n=363$), and 87% ($n=216$) in patients with "Oncoscore" < 4, between 4 and 7, and ≥ 8, respectively (Fig. 2).

Discussion

Studies that specifically focus on patients with solid cancers in the ICU are scarce, especially those which considered after-ICU survival [4]. Most of them are unicentric or based on databases and primarily focused on patients with lung cancers. In addition, they often only concern one type of cancer and mix patients admitted for scheduled surgery surveillance and those admitted after urgent surgery or for medical reasons that have absolutely no same prognosis in the short, medium, or long term. The largest to date retrospectively analyzed the unplanned admissions of 12,290 patients with solid cancers in 80 ICUs in the Netherlands over a 4-year period [5]. About 59.3% of all admissions were surgical (albeit unplanned), and these had a mortality (9.0 vs. 8.9% in the ICU and 17.4 vs. 14.6% in the hospital) like that of patients with no cancer diagnosis. Medical patients with cancer, however, had higher mortalities (30.4 vs. 16.2% in the ICU and 44.6 vs. 23.7% in the hospital). There was also a difference in outcomes for medical patients per cancer diagnosis; respiratory tract cancers were associated with an OR of 2.15

Table 3 Calculation of the Oncoscore

Characteristics	Points
Type of cancer	
Lung	2
Breast or colorectal	0
Others	1
Presence of distant metastasis	
No	0
Yes	2
Type of organ support received in the intensive care unit	
Invasive mechanical ventilation	3
Vasoactive and/or inotropic drug(s) (whatever the type)	2
Renal replacement therapy (whatever the type)	2

for ICU death, and upper gastrointestinal cancers were associated with an OR of 1.42. Among 35,308 Medicare beneficiaries who survived the ICU stay, the 6-month mortality was influenced by the existence of solid tumors without metastasis (adjusted hazard ratio [AHR] 1.15; 95% CI 1.08–1.23) [13]. The most important comorbidity, which determined the 6-month mortality after ICU discharge, was solid metastatic cancer (AHR 3.31; 95% CI 3.06–3.51). To the best of our knowledge, only three studies have questioned about the quality of life (QOL) of oncology patients after ICU discharge [14–16]. Only eight studies (six concerning patients with lung cancers) have reported the rates of patients who could receive anticancer treatment after a stay in the ICU [17–24].

The influence of ICU stay on the nature of subsequent antineoplastic therapy was evaluated in three studies, with change rates between 31 and 34% in relation to the project defined before the stay in the ICU [20, 23, 24].

Our findings report some data on a poorly studied subject. Contrary to what is observed in patients with hematological malignancies, our findings suggest that cancer characteristics (type and remote location) influence the in-hospital and four-month survival [25]. Other elements seem specific to patients with solid cancers. The first one is the primary reason for admission, which, in our study, is sepsis or septic shock, while acute respiratory failure is the first one in large sets of hematology patients admitted to the ICU [26]. Second, our findings suggest that cancer characteristics influence the short- and medium-term survival in contrast to hematology patients [4, 27, 28]. This contrasts with the fact that other characteristics of cancer such as status previous specific treatment and age of diagnosis do not seem to influence the 4-month mortality. For this reason, these two parameters should substantially influence ICU triage decisions in patients with solid cancers as suggested by the "Oncoscore." Third, few patients leaving the ICU alive died in the wards (3.3%). Moreover, the 4-month survival rate of 34.2% of all patients, among them, 360/618 (58.2%) who were discharged alive from the intensive care unit which was our variable of interest, is quite acceptable (Figs. 1, 2). These results, however, deserve to be modulated by not taking into account patients with lung cancers. Fourth, although some studies demonstrated a case–volume relationship in critically ill patients with hematological malignancies, it was not observed in our results [29]. Although it is, to our knowledge, the first to describe the medium-term outcome of "homogeneous" critically ill oncology patients (excluding those hospitalized in the ICU for scheduled surgery surveillance, i.e., planned admissions), our study has many limitations. First, it is a retrospective, multicenter, and international study. Though standard definitions were used, biases related to differences in data collection between the centers cannot be ruled out. Second, the choice of 4 months follow-up after the ICU discharge is debatable. Third, like most of the studies performed on this subject, the retrospective observational design does not describe data regarding patients who were not referred to the ICU, possibly introducing a significant selection bias. Fourth, we reported only crude mortality. A variable of interest among patients emerging alive from the ICU and hospital should probably be the possibility of reinstating optimal oncological treatment course. Fifth, we were not able to collect the Eastern Cooperative Oncology Group performance status (ECOG PS) score, or other one, on admission or on discharge of the ICU [30]; however, numerous studies on critically ill oncology patients suggest that this is one of the key determinants of short-term and medium-term survivals [4, 31]. Sixth, our data are simply quantitative and not qualitative. Seventh, it should be underlined that Oncoscore cannot be used to support individual decision making with respect to defining adequate goals of therapy in any form. We just postulated that the clinical and therapeutic data observed in the ICU could influence survival at 4 months after the ICU discharge. It should probably be adjusted regularly to reflect the advances in oncology. Finally, we believed that the prognosis of oncologic patients admitted in the ICU remains to be described and that improvement pathways are needed, as in patients with malignant hematological diseases [32]. Prospective studies to answer questions not provided by our one including only patients with solid cancers admitted in the ICU for medical reasons or after emergency surgery are urgently needed [8].

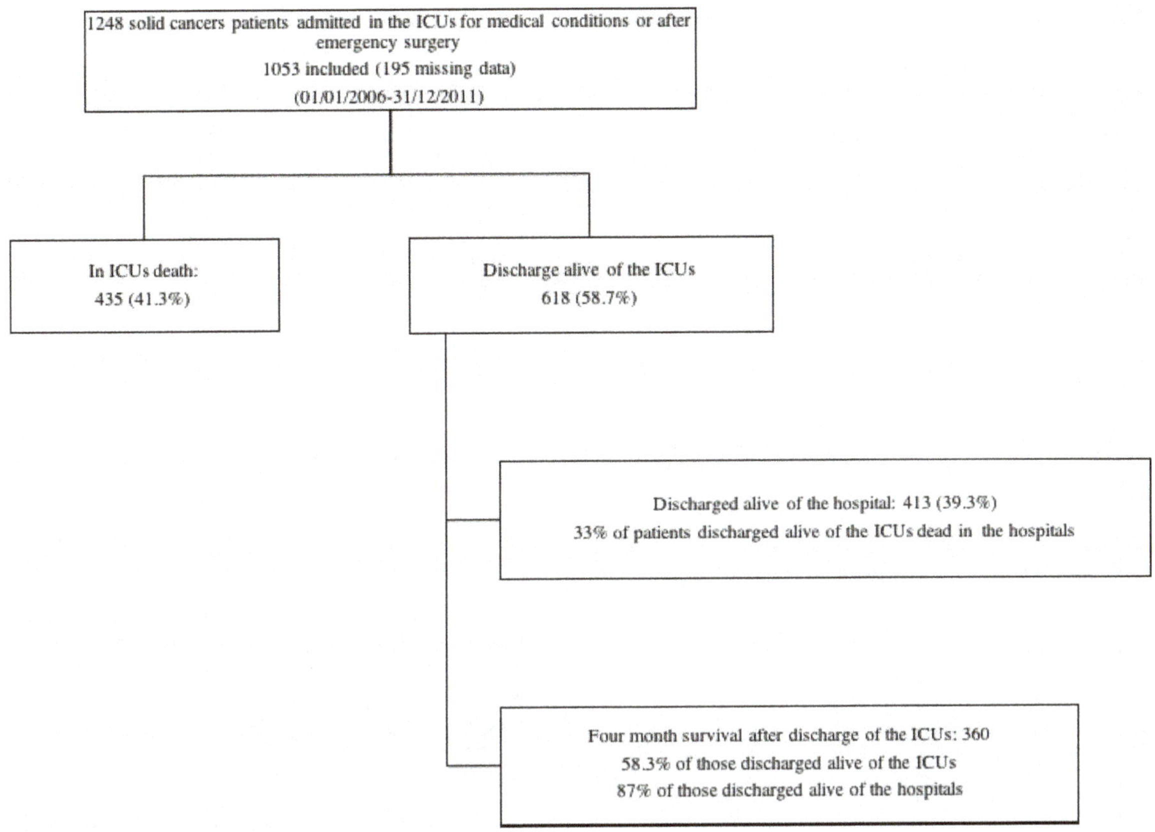

Fig. 1 Four-month follow-up, after ICU discharge, of the 1053 patients included in the study

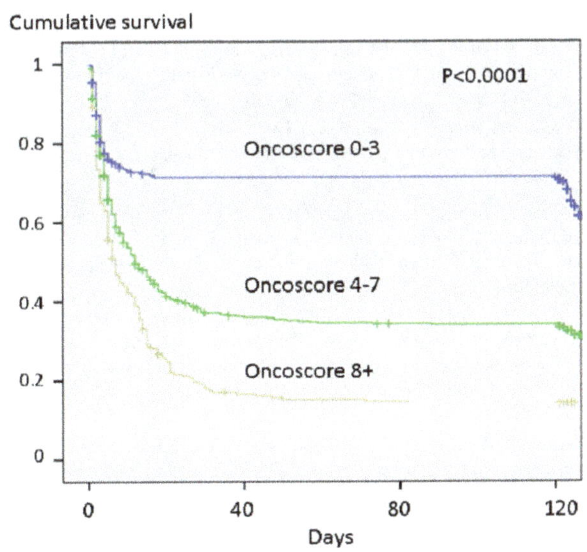

Fig. 2 Cumulative 4 months after ICU discharge survival per the value of the Oncoscore (the overall model area under ROC curve in predicting day-120 post-ICU outcome was fair [0.74; 95% CI 0.71–0.77]. A score of 4 was found to be sensitive of poor outcome [sensitivity 0.84], while a score of 8 was specific [specificity 0.92]).

Conclusion

The challenge for intensivists is to identify which patients with solid cancers would benefit from ICU cares. Our data, although reporting a high mortality in the ICU and in the hospital, show that the medium-term survival of these patients is quite acceptable, especially for patients with cancers other than lung cancers. The Oncoscore must be validated in a prospective cohort.

Abbreviations

AUC: area under the curve; CE SRLF: Ethics Commission of the French Intensive Care Society; ECOG PS: Eastern Cooperative Oncology Group performance status; HR: hazard ratio; ICU: intensive care unit; OR: odds ratio; QOL: quality of life; ROC curve: receiver operating characteristic curve; 95% CI: 95% interval of confidence.

Authors' contributions

FV, MS, EA, and MD were involved in conception and design. MS, DM, FV, VL, FB, and FG were involved in provision of study materials or patients. MD, FV, MS, MB, and EA were involved in data analysis and interpretation. All authors were involved in manuscript writing. All authors are accountable for all aspects of the work. All authors read and approved the final manuscript.

Author details
[1] Medical-Surgical Intensive Care Unit, Le Raincy-Montfermeil General Hospital, 10, rue du Général Leclerc, 93370 Montfermeil, France. [2] D'Or Institute for Research and Education, Rio de Janeiro, Brazil. [3] Programa de Pós-Graduação em Oncologia, Instituto Nacional de Câncer, Rio de Janeiro, Brazil. [4] Anesthesiology and Intensive Care Unit, Paoli Calmette Institute, Marseille, France. [5] Medical Intensive Care Unit, Saint-Louis University Hospital, AP-HP, Paris, France. [6] Medical-Surgical Intensive Care Unit, Mignot Hospital, Le Chesnay, France. [7] Clinical Research Unit, Avicenne University Hospital, AP-HP, Bobigny, France. [8] Medical-Surgical Intensive Care Unit, Avicenne University Hospital, AP-HP, Bobigny, France. [9] ECSTRA Team, Biostatistics and Clinical Epidemiology, UMR 1153 (Center of Epidemiology and Biostatistics, Sorbonne Paris Cité, CRESS), INSERM, Paris Diderot Sorbonne University, Paris, France.

Acknowledgements
An external validation of the statistical study was carried out by Professor Vincent LEVY (Clinical Research Unit, Avicenne University Hospital, AP-HP, Bobigny, France).

Competing interests
The authors declare that they have no competing interests.

References

1. Wigmore T, Farquhar-Smith P. Outcomes for critically ill cancer patients in the ICU: current trends and prediction. Int Anesthesiol Clin. 2016;54:e62–75.
2. Miller KD, Siegel RL, Lin CC, Mariotto AB, Kramer JL, Rowland JH, Stein KD, Alteri R, Jemal A. Cancer treatment and survivorship statistics, 2016. CA Cancer J Clin. 2016;66:271–89.
3. Puxty K, McLoone P, Quasim T, Sloan B, Kinsella J, Morrison DS. Risk of critical illness among patients with solid cancers: a population-based observational study. JAMA Oncol. 2015;1:1078–85.
4. Puxty K, McLoone P, Quasim T, Kinsella J, Morrison D. Survival in solid cancer patients following intensive care unit admission. Intensive Care Med. 2014;40:1409–28.
5. Bos MM, Verburg IW, Dumaij I, Stouthard J, Nortier JW, Richel D, van der Zwan EP, de Keizer NF, de Jonge E. Intensive care admission of cancer patients: a comparative analysis. Cancer Med. 2015;4:966–76.
6. Torres VB, Vassalo J, Silva UV, Caruso P, Torelly AP, Silva E, Teles JM, Knibel M, Rezende E, Netto JJ, Piras C, Azevedo LC, Bozza FA, Spector N, Salluh JI, Soares M. Outcomes in critically ill patients with cancer-related complications. PLoS ONE. 2016;11:e0164537.
7. Staudinger T, Stoiser B, Mullner M, Locker GJ, Laczika K, Knapp S, Burgmann H, Wilfing A, Kofler J, Thalhammer F, Frass M. Outcome and prognostic factors in critically ill cancer patients admitted to the intensive care unit. Crit Care Med. 2000;28:1322–8.
8. Ha FJ, Weickhardt AJ, Parakh S, Vincent AD, Glassford NJ, Warrillow S, Jones D. Survival and functional outcomes of patients with metastatic solid organ cancer admitted to the intensive care unit of a tertiary centre. Crit Care Resusc. 2017;19:159–66.
9. Soares M, Caruso P, Silva E, Teles JM, Lobo SM, Friedman G, Dal Pizzol F, Mello PV, Bozza FA, Silva UV, Torelly AP, Knibel MF, Rezende E, Netto JJ, Piras C, Castro A, Ferreira BS, Rea-Neto A, Olmedo PB, Salluh JI. Characteristics and outcomes of patients with cancer requiring admission to intensive care units: a prospective multicenter study. Crit Care Med. 2010;38:9–15.
10. Attard G, Parker C, Eeles RA, Schroder F, Tomlins SA, Tannock I, Drake CG, de Bono JS. Prostate cancer. Lancet. 2016;387:70–82.
11. Le Gall JR, Lemeshow S, Saulnier F. A new Simplified Acute Physiology Score (SAPS II) based on a European/North American multicenter study. JAMA. 1993;270:2957–63.
12. Vincent JL, Moreno R, Takala J, Willatts S, De Mendonca A, Bruining H, Reinhart CK, Suter PM, Thijs LG. The SOFA (Sepsis-related Organ Failure Assessment) score to describe organ dysfunction/failure. On behalf of the Working Group on Sepsis-Related Problems of the European Society of Intensive Care Medicine. Intensive Care Med. 1996;22:707–10.
13. Wunsch H, Guerra C, Barnato AE, Angus DC, Li G, Linde-Zwirble WT. Three-year outcomes for medicare beneficiaries who survive intensive care. JAMA. 2010;303:849–56.
14. Cense HA, Hulscher JB, de Boer AG, Dongelmans DA, Tilanus HW, Obertop H, Sprangers MA, van Lanschot JJ. Effects of prolonged intensive care unit stay on quality of life and long-term survival after transthoracic esophageal resection. Crit Care Med. 2006;34:354–62.
15. Oeyen SG, Benoit DD, Annemans L, Depuydt PO, Van Belle SJ, Troisi RI, Noens LA, Pattyn P, Decruyenaere JM. Long-term outcomes and quality of life in critically ill patients with hematological or solid malignancies: a single center study. Intensive Care Med. 2013;39:889–98.
16. Normilio-Silva K, de Figueiredo AC, Pedroso-de-Lima AC, Tunes-da-Silva G, Nunes da Silva A, Delgado Dias Levites A, de-Simone AT, Lopes Safra P, Zancani R, Tonini PC, Vasconcelos de Andrade ESU, Buosi Silva T, Martins Giorgi J, Eluf-Neto J, Costa A, Abrahao Hajjar L, Biasi Cavalcanti A. Long-term survival, quality of life, and quality-adjusted survival in critically ill patients with cancer. Crit Care Med. 2016;44:1327–37.
17. Roques S, Parrot A, Lavole A, Ancel PY, Gounant V, Djibre M, Fartoukh M. Six-month prognosis of patients with lung cancer admitted to the intensive care unit. Intensive Care Med. 2009;35:2044–50.
18. Andrejak C, Terzi N, Thielen S, Bergot E, Zalcman G, Charbonneau P, Jounieaux V. Admission of advanced lung cancer patients to intensive care unit: a retrospective study of 76 patients. BMC Cancer. 2011;11:159.
19. Bonomi MR, Smith CB, Mhango G, Wisnivesky JP. Outcomes of elderly patients with stage IIIB-IV non-small cell lung cancer admitted to the intensive care unit. Lung Cancer. 2012;77:600–4.
20. Soares M, Toffart AC, Timsit JF, Burghi G, Irrazabal C, Pattison N, Tobar E, Almeida BF, Silva UV, Azevedo LC, Rabbat A, Lamer C, Parrot A, Souza-Dantas VC, Wallet F, Blot F, Bourdin G, Piras C, Delemazure J, Durand M, Tejera D, Salluh JI, Azoulay E, Lung Cancer in Critical Care Study I. Intensive care in patients with lung cancer: a multinational study. Ann Oncol. 2014;25:1829–35.
21. Kim YJ, Kim MJ, Cho YJ, Park JS, Kim JW, Chang H, Lee JO, Lee KW, Kim JH, Yoon HI, Bang SM, Lee JH, Lee CT, Lee JS. Who should be admitted to the intensive care unit? The outcome of intensive care unit admission in stage IIIB-IV lung cancer patients. Med Oncol. 2014;31:847.
22. Razazi K, Parrot A, Khalil A, Djibre M, Gounant V, Assouad J, Carette MF, Fartoukh M, Cadranel J. Severe haemoptysis in patients with nonsmall cell lung carcinoma. Eur Respir J. 2015;45:756–64.
23. Camus MF, Ameye L, Berghmans T, Paesmans M, Sculier JP, Meert AP. Rate and patterns of ICU admission among colorectal cancer patients: a single-center experience. Support Care Cancer. 2015;23:1779–85.
24. Auclin E, Charles-Nelson A, Abbar B, Guerot E, Oudard S, Hauw-Berlemont C, Thibault C, Monnier A, Diehl JL, Katsahian S, Fagon JY, Taieb J, Aissaoui N. Outcomes in elderly patients admitted to the intensive care unit with solid tumors. Ann Intensive Care. 2017;7:26.
25. Tavares M, Lemiale V, Mokart D, Pene F, Lengline E, Kouatchet A, Mayaux J, Vincent F, Nyunga M, Bruneel F, Rabbat A, Lebert C, Perez P, Meert AP, Benoit D, Darmon M, Azoulay E. Determinants of 1-year survival in critically ill acute leukemia patients: a GRRR-OH study. Leuk Lymphoma. 2017;1:1–9.
26. Azoulay E, Pene F, Darmon M, Lengline E, Benoit D, Soares M, Vincent F, Bruneel F, Perez P, Lemiale V, Mokart D, Groupe de Recherche Respiratoire en Reanimation O-H. Managing critically ill hematology patients: time to think differently. Blood Rev. 2015;29(6):359–67.
27. Azoulay E, Adrie C, De Lassence A, Pochard F, Moreau D, Thiery G, Cheval C, Moine P, Garrouste-Orgeas M, Alberti C, Cohen Y, Timsit JF. Determinants of postintensive care unit mortality: a prospective multicenter study. Crit Care Med. 2003;31:428–32.
28. Heo SJ, Kim G, Lee CK, Chung KS, Choi HJ, Sohn J, Lee S. Prediction of short- and long-term survival for advanced cancer patients after ICU

admission. Support Care Cancer. 2015;23:1647–55.
29. Zuber B, Tran TC, Aegerter P, Grimaldi D, Charpentier J, Guidet B, Mira JP, Pene F. Impact of case volume on survival of septic shock in patients with malignancies. Crit Care Med. 2012;40:55–62.
30. Oken MM, Creech RH, Tormey DC, Horton J, Davis TE, McFadden ET, Carbone PP. Toxicity and response criteria of the Eastern Cooperative Oncology Group. Am J Clin Oncol. 1982;5:649–55.
31. Christodoulou C, Rizos M, Galani E, Rellos K, Skarlos DV, Michalopoulos A. Performance status (PS): a simple predictor of short-term outcome of cancer patients with solid tumors admitted to the intensive care unit (ICU). Anticancer Res. 2007;27:2945–8.
32. Azoulay E, Schellongowski P, Darmon M, Bauer PR, Benoit D, Depuydt P, Divatia JV, Lemiale V, van Vliet M, Meert AP, Mokart D, Pastores SM, Perner A, Pene F, Pickkers P, Puxty KA, Vincent F, Salluh J, Soubani AO, Antonelli M, Staudinger T, von Bergwelt-Baildon M, Soares M. The intensive care medicine research agenda on critically ill oncology and hematology patients. Intensive Care Med. 2017;43:1366–82.

17

Acute kidney injury epidemiology, risk factors, and outcomes in critically ill patients 16–25 years of age treated in an adult intensive care unit

Dana Y. Fuhrman[1*], Sandra Kane-Gill[2], Stuart L. Goldstein[3], Priyanka Priyanka[4] and John A. Kellum[4]

Abstract

Background: Most studies of acute kidney injury (AKI) have focused on older adults, and little is known about AKI in young adults (16–25 years) that are cared for in an adult intensive care unit (ICU). We analyzed data from a large single-center ICU database and defined AKI using the Kidney Disease Improving Global Outcomes criteria. We stratified patients 16–55 years of age into four age groups for comparison and used multivariable logistic regression to identify associations of potential susceptibilities and exposures with AKI and mortality.

Results: AKI developed in 52.6% ($n = 8270$) of the entire cohort and in 39.8% of the young adult age group (16–25 years). The AUCs for the age categories were similar at 0.754, 0.769, 0.772, and 0.770 for the 16–25-, 26–35-, 36–45-, and 45–55-year age groups, respectively. For the youngest age group, diabetes (OR 1.89; 95% CI 1.09–3.29), surgical reason for admission (OR 1.79; 95% CI 1.44–2.23), severity of illness (OR 1.02; 95% CI 1.02–1.03), hypotension (OR 1.13; 95% CI 1.04–1.24), and certain medications (vancomycin and calcineurin inhibitors) were all independently associated with AKI. AKI was a significant predictor for longer length of stay, ICU mortality, and mortality after discharge.

Conclusions: AKI is a common event for young adults admitted to an adult tertiary care center ICU with an associated increased length of stay and risk of mortality. Potentially modifiable risk factors for AKI including medications were identified for all stratified age groups.

Keywords: Young adult, Acute kidney injury (AKI), Critically ill

Background

An association of acute kidney injury (AKI) and adverse outcomes including length of hospital stay, progression to chronic kidney disease (CKD), and mortality is consistently shown in multiple patient populations [1–6]. In critically ill patients the rates of AKI vary based on the population studied and definition of AKI used, with reported rates of 8–89% for children [7–11] and 7–25% for adults [12–15]. Recently, investigators in the Assessment of Worldwide Acute Kidney Injury, Renal Angina, and Epidemiology (AWARE) study explored the association of AKI with morbidity and mortality in patients 3 months to 25 years of age admitted to a pediatric intensive care unit (ICU) [5]. However, no prior study has investigated specifically the incidence and implications of AKI in the young adult critically ill patient population treated in an adult ICU, a patient group that is growing in adult critical care practices [16].

Given the complexity and diversity of the critical care patient population, it can be challenging to identify and address the numerous risk factors for AKI encountered in the ICU. Since we continue to have no direct pharmacologic therapies for AKI, prevention is of paramount importance. An understanding of the potentially modifiable risk factors that may be unique to different patient groups within the ICU is critical to the prevention of

*Correspondence: dana.fuhrman@chp.edu
[1] Children's Hospital of Pittsburgh, 4401 Penn Avenue, Children's Hospital Drive, Faculty Pavilion Suite 2000, Pittsburgh, PA 15224, USA
Full list of author information is available at the end of the article

AKI. As a result of an increasing number of individuals with childhood chronic illnesses surviving into adulthood [17], there is a need to understand the potentially unique modifiable risk factors for AKI in the 16–25-year-old or young adult ICU population. Little is known about the potential comorbid conditions that may exist in this age group, possibly impacting their AKI incidence and outcomes. As a result of certain comorbid conditions prior to entering the ICU, patients may have a greater exposure to nephrotoxic pharmacologic agents thereby potentially increasing their risk of AKI. Hui-Stickle et al. [18] demonstrated that nephrotoxic medications were the most common cause of acute renal failure for older children and adolescents, while ischemia was the most common etiology in patients 5 years of age or less. There have been no previous studies to date exploring the susceptibilities, exposures, and outcomes of AKI specifically in young adult ICU patients cared for outside of a children's hospital. Thus, we sought to determine if the incidence, risks, and associated outcomes for AKI varied by age across a population of 16–55-year-old ICU patients treated in an adult hospital ICU.

Methods

Study population

After obtaining institutional review board approval, data were obtained from the High-Density Intensive Care (HiDenIC) database, which includes clinical variables on all patients admitted to the University of Pittsburgh, a tertiary care academic medical center, from July 2000–September 2008. The HiDenIC database includes data on adult patients admitted to one of eight ICUs (medical, cardiac, transplant, surgical, neurological, and trauma). Exclusion criteria were applied including: (1) history of hemodialysis or renal transplant, (2) baseline creatinine > 3.5 mg/dl, (3) liver transplant during the index hospitalization, (4) insufficient information to determine AKI status, and (5) unknown age (Fig. 1). We defined the young adult population as those individuals 16–25 years of age. The remaining cohort was stratified into 10-year age increments including: 26–35 years, 36–45 years, and 46–55 years.

Clinical variables

The risk factors included the analysis are significant predictors of AKI in previous studies [19, 20]. The potential risk factors include sex, race, reference creatinine, estimated glomerular filtration rate (eGFR) derived from the reference creatinine [21], comorbid conditions defined by ICD-9 codes (cardiac disease, CKD, diabetes, fluid overload, history of hypertension, malignancies), admission type (medical or surgical), and moderate anemia (defined by The World Health Organization [22]). Fluid balance was calculated by subtracting total intake from output divided by the admission weight (kg) × 100 in the first 24 h of ICU admission [23]. We defined fluid overload as a fluid balance > 5%. Severity of illness was evaluated with the Acute Physiology and Chronic Healthy

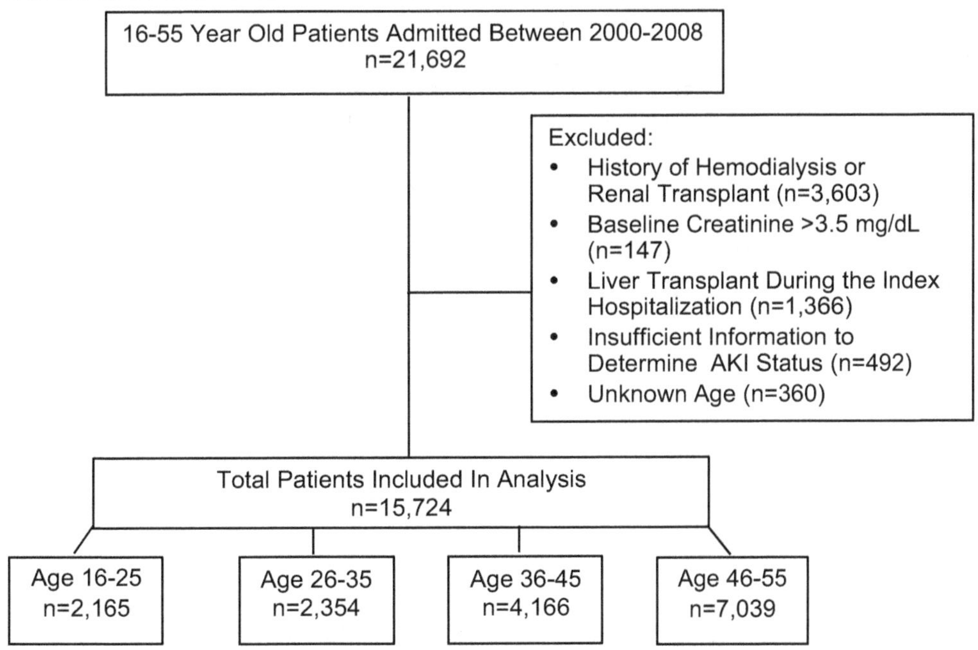

Fig. 1 Flow diagram of the study cohort

Evaluation (APACHE) III score [24]. In the first 24 h of ICU admission, the need for vasopressors, mechanical ventilation as well as concern for sepsis (the ordering of blood cultures and antibiotics within 24 h of each other) was also included. Additionally, we evaluated exposure to potentially nephrotoxic medications within the first 24 h of ICU admission, including angiotensin-converting enzyme inhibitors, angiotensin II receptor blockers, vancomycin, aminoglycosides, antibiotics other than vancomycin or aminoglycosides (including piperacillin/tazobactam, cephalosporins, quinolones, macrolides, sulfonamides, and carbapenems), calcineurin inhibitors, nonsteroidal anti-inflammatory drug (NSAID) medications, acyclovir, mannitol, and phenytoin.

Outcomes

We defined AKI according to the Kidney Disease Improving Global Outcomes (KDIGO) criteria [4]. Any patient meeting the criteria for KDIGO stage 1 or more based on either serum creatinine or urine output during their ICU stay was deemed to have AKI. We defined the reference creatinine as the baseline creatinine when available (lowest value between the most recent hospital creatinine value up to 1 year prior the index hospital admission and the creatinine recorded in the first 24 h of hospital admission) or the lowest value between the creatinine recorded in the first 24 h of hospital admission, first 24 h of ICU admission, and (for patients without a history of CKD) the creatinine derived from the Modification of Diet in Renal Disease (MDRD) equation for creatinine using an eGFR of 75 ml/min/1.73 m^2 [25, 26]. The reference creatinine was used to determine creatinine changes for defining AKI. We evaluated for each age strata rates of AKI, need for renal replacement therapy (RRT), recovery from RRT, ICU length of stay, hospital length of stay, ICU mortality, hospital mortality, 90-day mortality, and 1-year mortality.

Statistical analysis

Categorical variables were summarized as number and percentage, and continuous variables were summarized as median with interquartile range. Given the large number of patients in the study, statistical differences alone are unlikely to be meaningful. Therefore, we set 10% as a clinically meaningful difference between age groups. Age per 5 years was included as a risk factor for each age group to account for differences within the age groups. To determine the susceptibilities and exposures associated with AKI, multivariable logistic regression was performed whereby: (1) the cohort was stratified by age group (each of 10 years, starting from age 16–25) and (2) with age group as a main effect and accounting for interactions between age group and all other risk factors. Age-stratified models were built using the following steps: (1) adding each risk factor to age as a continuous variable and using the Wald statistic to determine their significance, (2) the individual size of all variables in step 1 was tested with the Wald statistic as they were added to a multivariable logistic regression model, (3) variables with $p \geq 0.05$ were taken out of the model and a reduced model was fit, and (4) lastly to compare nested models in steps 2 and 3 the likelihood ratio test was used to determine a final model. For the interaction models, in order to find a main effects model, age group was used as a main effect and steps 1 through 4 were repeated. With age retained in the models regardless of significance level, all possible interactions were added one at a time and their significance was determined with the Wald statistic. STATA's "roctab" function was used to assess the area under the receiver operating characteristic curve (AUC) for each age-stratified model. In addition, the "rocreg" function that uses bootstrap (1000 replications) for inference was also used to assess nonparametric ROC estimation under the presence of covariates. Model selection for ICU mortality, hospital mortality, mortality at 90 days after ICU admission, and mortality 1 year after ICU admission across age groups was done using the stepwise selection methodology described above to identify the best model for mortality prediction. Goodness of fit was assessed using Hosmer–Lemeshow [27]. Statistical analyses were performed using STATA software (version SE 14.0, StataCorp LP) and SAS 9.4 with statistical significance set at $p < 0.05$.

Results

After applying the exclusion criteria, 15,724 patients were included in the analysis. The reference creatinine was determined from a documented baseline creatinine in 5543 patients and estimated in 10,181 patients. AKI occurred in 8270 (52.6%) patients. The characteristics of individuals that developed AKI are shown in Table 1. In the 16–25-year-old age group, 39.8% of the patients developed AKI. In all age groups stage I AKI occurred with the greatest frequency. Although stage 3 AKI occurred with the lowest frequency in the 16–25-year-old age group, it occurred in 15% of patients. Only a few variables met our criteria of 10% as a clinically meaningful difference between age groups. Cardiac disease, hypertension, multiple comorbidities, vasopressor use and NSAID use were more common in older adults (Table 1). The distributions for the remainder of the variables were similar between groups.

Sepsis and vancomycin use were found to be highly associated with AKI in the overall cohort as well as for each individual age group. Given that sepsis was defined as the ordering of blood cultures and antibiotics within

Table 1 Patient characteristics by age group (years) with acute kidney injury

Characteristic	16–25 N = 862	26–35 N = 1098	36–45 N = 2189	46–55 N = 4121	All N = 8270
% of age group with AKI	39.8	46.6	52.5	58.5	52.6
Age (years), Median (Q1–Q3)	22 (19–24)	31 (28–33)	41 (39–44)	51 (48–53)	45 (36–51)
Males *N* (%)	573 (66.5)	670 (61.2)	1304 (60)	2500 (61)	5047 (61)
Race *N* (%)					
White	597 (69)	790 (72)	1654 (76)	3127 (76)	6168 (76)
Black	132 (15)	131 (12)	226 (10)	409 (10)	898 (11)
Other	133 (15)	177 (16)	309 (14)	585 (14)	1204 (15)
Reference creatinine (mg/dl), median (Q1–Q3)	0.9 (0.7–1.1)	0.9 (0.7–1.1)	0.9 (0.7–1.1)	0.9 (0.7–1.1)	0.9 (0.7–1.1)
eGFR (ml/min/1.73 m^2), median (Q1–Q3)	121.2 (92.8–133)	111.4 (81.9–123.1)	95.7 (79.4–113.9)	86.2 (76.9–104.8)	96.5 (78.6–113.2)
Fluid balance > 5%	111 (12.9)	161 (14.7)	285 (13.1)	485 (11.8)	1042 (12.6)
Cardiac disease *N* (%)	41 (5)	95 (9)	225 (10)	666 (16)	1027 (12)
Chronic kidney disease *N* (%)	16 (2)	26 (2)	135 (6)	218 (5)	395 (5)
Diabetes *N* (%)	50 (6)	102 (9)	227 (10)	741 (18)	1120 (14)
History of hypertension *N* (%)	59 (7)	135 (12)	459 (21)	1274 (31)	1927 (23)
Malignancy *N* (%)	7 (0.8)	15 (1)	62 (2.8)	156 (3.8)	240 (3)
Multiple comorbidities *N* (%)	142 (17)	290 (26)	803 (37)	1889 (46)	3124 (38)
Mechanical ventilation *N* (%)	580 (67)	684 (62)	1340 (61)	2413 (59)	5017 (61)
Surgical admission *N* (%)	504 (65)	601 (60)	1128 (57)	2216 (59)	4449 (59)
Suspected sepsis *N* (%)	122 (14)	198 (18)	395 (18)	698 (17)	1413 (17)
APACHE III score, median (Q1–Q3)	54 (36–72)	53 (34–73)	52 (35–74)	57 (38–80)	55 (37–76)
Vasopressor use *N* (%)	149 (17)	224 (20)	521 (24)	1125 (27)	2019 (24)
Moderate anemia *N* (%)	227 (26)	315 (29)	577 (26)	1259 (31)	2378 (29)
Maximum KDIGO *N* (%)					
Stage 1	400 (46)	444 (41)	738 (34)	1241 (30)	2823 (34)
Stage 2	335 (39)	433 (39)	906 (41)	1783 (43)	3457 (42)
Stage 3	127 (15)	221 (20)	545 (25)	1097 (27)	1990 (24)
Medication exposure *N* (%)					
ACE inhibitor/ARB	21(2)	27 (2)	93 (4)	269 (7)	410 (5)
Vancomycin	124 (14)	203 (18)	373 (17)	669 (16)	1369 (17)
Aminoglycoside	31 (3.6)	44 (4)	87 (4)	157 (4)	319 (4)
Other Antibiotics	62 (7)	82 (7)	137 (6)	258 (6)	539 (6)
Calcineurin inhibitor	58 (7)	94 (9)	153 (7)	264 (6)	569 (7)
NSAID	40 (5)	90 (8)	269 (12)	716 (17)	1115 (14)
Acyclovir	18 (2)	29 (2.6)	462 (2.1)	67 (1.6)	160 (2)
Mannitol	28 (3)	26 (2)	32 (1.5)	30 (0.7)	116 (1)
Phenytoin	32 (3.7)	24 (2)	47 (2)	82 (2)	185 (2)

AKI acute kidney injury, *eGFR* estimated glomerular filtration rate, *APACHE* Acute Physiology and Chronic Healthy Evaluation, *KDIGO* Kidney Disease Improving Global Outcomes, *ACE* angiotensin-converting enzyme, *ARB* angiotensin II receptor blocker, *NSAID* nonsteroidal anti-inflammatory drug

24 h of each other and vancomycin was the most common antibiotic prescribed, not surprisingly sepsis was highly colinear with vancomycin. Therefore, sepsis was not included in the final individual logistic regression models built for each age group (Table 2). The area under the curve (AUC) for each of the four age groups was similar indicating a comparable ability to predict AKI across the different age strata at 0.754, 0.769, 0.772, and 0.770 for the 16–25-, 26–35-, 36–45-, and 46–55-year-old age groups, respectively. In order to gain more precise estimates, the AUC was re-fitted using bootstrapping and similar AUC values were also determined across the four age strata. Diabetes, APACHE III score, and vancomycin were significantly positively associated with AKI across all age groups. Specifically, for the young adults (ages 16–25), age, race, diabetes, surgical admission, APACHE III score, hypotensive index, vancomycin, calcineurin inhibitor, NSAID, and other nephrotoxic medication

Table 2 Multivariable logistic regression of risk factors for individuals with acute kidney injury compared to those without acute kidney injury by age categories (years)

Characteristic	16–25 OR (95% CI *p* value)	26–35 OR (95% CI *p* value)	36–45 OR (95% CI *p* value)	46–55 OR (95% CI *p* value)
Age per 5 years	1.39 (1.14–1.69, < 0.01)	1.21 (1.02–1.43, 0.02)	–	–
Black	1.41 (1.04–1.91, 0.02)	–	–	–
Other race	–	–	–	–
Diabetes	1.89 (1.09–3.29, 0.02)	1.86 (1.20–2.89, < 0.01)	1.52 (1.14–2.02, 0.01)	1.55 (1.28–1.85, 0.01)
Fluid balance > 5%	–	–	–	–
Malignancy	–	–	–	–
Hypertension	–	–	–	–
Cardiac disease	–	3.75 (2.23–6.29, < 0.01)	2.00 (1.47–2.72, < 0.01)	1.36 (1.12–1.64, 0.01)
Chronic kidney disease	–	–	–	–
Surgical admission	1.79 (1.44–2.23, < 0.01)	1.39 (1.14–1.71, < 0.01)	1.23 (1.05–1.72, < 0.01)	–
Vasopressor use	–	1.48 (1.04–2.12, 0.03)	1.34 (1.05–1.65, 0.01)	1.41 (1.19–1.69, < 0.01)
Mechanical ventilation	–	1.39 (1.09–2.12, < 0.01)	1.38 (1.16–1.31, < 0.01)	1.53 (1.33–1.73, < 0.01)
Moderate anemia	–	–	–	–
APACHE III score	1.02 (1.02–1.03, < 0.01)	1.02 (1.02–1.26, < 0.01)	1.03 (1.02–1.04, < 0.01)	1.03 (1.03–1.03, < 0.01)
eGFR	–	–	0.98 (0.98–0.99, < 0.01)	0.98 (0.98–0.99, < 0.01)
Hypotensive Index	1.13 (1.04–1.24, < 0.01)	–	–	1.04 (1.01–1.07, 0.01)
ACE inhibitor/ARB	–	–	–	–
Vancomycin	1.46 (1.00–2.13, 0.04)	1.56 (1.13–1.39, < 0.01)	1.39 (1.08–1.77, 0.01)	1.45 (1.18–1.77, < 0.01)
Other antibiotics	–	–	–	–
Calcineurin inhibitor	2.72 (1.45–5.12, < 0.01)	–	2.45 (1.59–3.75, < 0.01)	–
NSAID	0.51 (0.32–0.82, < 0.01)	0.68 (0.49–0.80, 0.02)	0.78 (0.63–0.96, 0.01)	0.92 (0.80–1.07, 0.03)
Other nephrotoxic medications	1.60 (1.03–2.49, 0.03)	–		–
AUC (Q1–Q3)	0.754 (0.732–0.776)	0.769 (0.749–0.789)	0.772 (0.757–0.787)	0.770 (0.758–0.781)

OR odds ratio, *CI* confidence interval, *APACHE* Acute Physiology and Chronic Healthy Evaluation, *eGFR* estimated glomerular filtration rate, *ACE* angiotensin-converting enzyme, *ARB* angiotensin II receptor blocker, *NSAID* nonsteroidal anti-inflammatory drug, *ROC* receiver operator curve

use were all significantly associated with AKI (Table 2). Included in the category of other nephrotoxic medications were acyclovir, mannitol, and phenytoin. However, when each of these drugs was included individually in the model, there was no significant association with AKI.

Statistically significant interactions between age groups and the potential risk factors were determined (Table 3). Despite a similar ability to predict AKI across the four age strata, certain risk factors were significantly different with respect to age group. The risk factors that had significant interactions with age were cardiac disease, surgical admission, eGFR, calcineurin inhibitor, NSAID, and other nephrotoxic medication use.

Table 4 shows outcomes of the patients with AKI in each of the four age strata. In the young adult patients, even though only a small number of patients received RRT ($n = 46$), 47.8% of patients that received RRT while hospitalized had no recovery from RRT at 90 days. In the 640 patients in the overall patient cohort that received RRT, 59.4% had no recovery from RRT at 90 days. The ICU and hospital length of stay were similar between age groups. Hospital, ICU, 90-day, and 1-year mortality were greater in the older adult groups. AKI was a significant predictor of hospital mortality, ICU mortality, mortality at 90 days and mortality at 1 year in the young adult patients (Table 5). Tables 6 and 7 show the significant role that AKI contributed toward predicting hospital and 1 year post-discharge mortality in the 16–25-year-old age group. Patients with AKI had an increased risk of 1 year post-discharge mortality in all age groups (Fig. 2). Among the variables included in the multivariable logistic regression, it was the APACHE III score, a diagnosis of malignancy, and a diagnosis of AKI during the time of ICU admission only that significantly contributed toward predicting mortality 1 year after discharge (Table 7).

Discussion

Even in young adult patients, AKI occurred in 39.8%. Similar to the AWARE study, a strength of this investigation is that we defined AKI using both the KDIGO serum creatinine and urine output criteria, given that defining AKI using serum creatinine has been shown to decrease the sensitivity for AKI detection [5]. Our rate of AKI in the young adult patient cohort falls between the

Table 3 Multivariable logistic regression of interactions between age groups and risk factors associated with AKI

Interaction of age group with	χ^2 (*df*)	*p* value*
Race	5.19 (6)	0.52
Diabetes	4.31 (3)	0.22
Cardiac disease	17.55 (3)	< 0.01
Chronic kidney disease	4.67 (3)	0.19
Surgical admission	18.42 (3)	< 0.01
Vasopressor use	1.73 (3)	0.62
Mechanical ventilation	4.57 (3)	0.20
Moderate anemia	2.02 (3)	0.56
APACHE III score	7.07 (3)	0.06
eGFR	16.5 (3)	< 0.01
Hypotensive Index	2.25 (3)	0.52
Vancomycin	1.06 (3)	0.78
Calcineurin inhibitor	12.84 (3)	< 0.01
NSAID	3.30 (3)	< 0.01
Other nephrotoxic medications	8.08 (3)	0.04

AKI acute kidney injury, *APACHE* Acute Physiology and Chronic Healthy Evaluation, *eGFR* estimated glomerular filtration rate, *NSAID* nonsteroidal anti-inflammatory drug

*Each *p* value comes from a different multivariable logistic regression with age group, 15 risk factors and one interaction

rates reported by AWARE (26.9%) and the Acute Kidney Injury-Epidemiologic Prospective Investigation (AKI-EPI) published in 2015 (57.3%) [5, 28].

Importantly, we show AKI to be a significant predictor of hospital and ICU mortality as well as mortality after discharge in young adult critically ill patients, treated in an adult ICU. Similarly, including both ICU and non-ICU patients less than 18 years of age, Sutherland et al. show a significant association of AKI (defined using the KDIGO criteria) with ICU mortality and hospital length of stay. However, in contrast to our findings, they describe no significant association of AKI with mortality outside of the ICU [6]. Along with differences in patient age, the inclusion of patients with non-ICU AKI in their study may explain the discrepant results when compared to ours, which show AKI to be a significant predictor of hospital and 1 year post-discharge mortality in the 16–25-year-old age group.

Given the poor outcomes associated with AKI in this study as well as prior studies, it is imperative that those caring for critically ill patients identify and address the risk factors that are unique to specific patient groups. The results of this analysis suggest that there are potentially modifiable risk factors for AKI in critically ill young adults. The use of medications such as vancomycin and calcineurin inhibitors was found to be significantly associated with AKI in patients 16–25 years of age. When grouped together, mannitol, acyclovir, and phenytoin were uniquely associated with AKI in the 16–25-year-old cohort. Due to the low rate of use of these medications in our overall patient cohort, we cannot make any determination about AKI risk of each medication individually.

Table 4 Outcomes of patients with acute kidney injury for each of the four age categories (years)

Outcome	Age 16–25	Age 26–35	Age 36–45	Age 46–55	All
Need for RRT *N* (%)	46 (5.3)	77 (7)	172 (7.9)	345 (8.4)	640 (7.7)
No recovery from RRT at 90 Days *N* (%)	22 (47.8)	37 (48.1)	92 (53.5)	229 (66.4)	380 (59.4)
ICU length of stay (days), mean (SD)	9.6 (10.7)	10.3 (15.1)	8.7 (11.6)	8.8 (12.9)	9 (12.7)
Hospital length of stay (days), mean (SD)	20.1 (22.2)	21.7 (25.4)	19.5 (24.1)	19.5 (24.2)	19.9 (24.1)
ICU mortality *N* (%)	51 (5.9)	80 (7.3)	245 (11.2)	486 (11.8)	862 (10.4)
Hospital mortality *N* (%)	64 (7.4)	107 (9.7)	319 (14.6)	674 (16.4)	1164 (14.1)
90-Day mortality *N* (%)	67 (7.8)	123 (11.2)	390 (17.8)	860 (20.9)	1440 (17.4)
1-Year mortality *N* (%)	90 (10.4)	180 (16.4)	498 (22.8)	1145 (27.8)	1913 (23.1)

RRT renal replacement therapy, *ICU* intensive care unit, *SD* standard deviation

Table 5 Multivariable logistic regression of outcomes related to acute kidney injury by age categories (years)

Outcome	Age 16–25 OR (95% CI *p* value)	Age 26–35 OR (95% CI *p* value)	Age 36–45 OR (95% CI *p* value)	Age 46–55 OR (95% CI *p* value)	All OR (95% CI *p* value)
Hospital mortality	2.48 (1.25–4.90, < 0.01)	8.63 (1.04–71.70, 0.04)	21.73 (4.02–117.44, < 0.01)	4.88 (2.55–9.34, < 0.01)	2.03 (1.69–2.43, < 0.01)
ICU mortality	2.78 (1.30–5.94, < 0.01)	1.024 (0.58–1.82, 0.934)	1.67 (1.11–2.51, 0.01)	1.48 (1.12–1.97, 0.07)	3.74 (2.09–6.68, < 0.01
Mortality at 90 days	2.04 (1.09–3.82, 0.03)	1.313 (0.84–2.06, 0.233)	2.31 (1.70–3.14, < 0.01)	1.63 (1.34–1.98, < 0.01)	1.78 (1.53–2.07, < 0.01)
Mortality at 1 year	2.25 (1.14–4.45, 0.02)	2.50 (1.50–4.15, < 0.01)	1.98 (1.45–2.70, < 0.01)	1.90 (1.54–2.36, < 0.01)	2.03 (1.74–2.39, < 0.01)

OR odds ratio, *CI* confidence interval, *ICU* Intensive Care Unit

Table 6 Multivariable logistic regression of risk factors for hospital mortality by age categories (years)

Outcome	Age 16–25 OR (95% CI *p* value)	Age 26–35 OR (95% CI *p* value)	Age 36–45 OR (95% CI *p* value)	Age 46–55 OR (95% CI *p* value)	All OR (95% CI *p* value)
Age per 5 years	0.73 (0.43–1.23, 0.23)	1.26 (0.88–1.80, 0.20)	1.51 (1.19–1.93, < 0.01)	1.23 (1.04–1.44, 0.01)	1.14 (1.09–1.18, < 0.01)
AKI	2.48 (1.25–4.90, < 0.01)	1.65 (0.98–2.79, 0.05)	2.06 (1.44–2.95, < 0.01)	2.00 (1.56–2.56, < 0.01)	2.03 (1.69–2.43, < 0.01)
APACHE III score	1.03 (1.01–1.03, < 0.01)	1.03 (1.02–1.03, < 0.01)	1.03 (1.02–1.03, < 0.01)	1.03 (1.02–1.03, < 0.01)	1.03 (1.03–1.04, < 0.01
Hypotensive Index	1.01 (1.01–1.02, < 0.01)	1.00 (0.99–1.01, 0.12)	1.00 (1.00–1.01, < 0.01)	1.00 (1.00–1.00, < 0.01)	1.01 (1.01–1.01, < 0.01)
Vasopressors	3.28 (1.60–6.75, < 0.01)	3.98 (2.46–6.43, < 0.01)	2.46 (1.79–3.38, < 0.01)	1.97 (1.61–2.42, < 0.01)	2.30 (2.0–2.7, < 0.01)
Surgical Admission	0.63 (0.35–1.15, < 0.01)	0.66 (0.43–1.01, 0.05)	0.54 (0.41–0.71, < 0.01)	0.60 (0.49–0.72, < 0.01)	0.60 (0.51–0.68, < 0.01)
Moderate anemia	1.12 (0.60–2.11, 0.72)	0.81 (0.51–1.3, 0.39)	0.87 (0.64–1.19, 0.41)	0.86 (0.70–1.05, 0.14)	0.87 (0.75–1.01, 0.07)
Hypertension	0.76 (0.21–2.69, 0.67)	0.85 (0.42–1.72, 0.65)	0.89 (0.61–1.30, 0.57)	0.94 (0.74–1.18, 0.59)	0.89 (0.74–1.07, 0.20)
Malignancy	5.23 (1.47–18.61, 0.01)	2.55 (1.09–5.94, 0.02)	1.80 (1.10–2.96, 0.01)	1.52 (1.12–2.05, 0.00)	1.68 (1.32–2.14, < 0.01)
Chronic liver disease	0.61 (0.06–6.01, 0.67)	1.37 (0.57–3.25, 0.47)	1.49 (0.93–2.4, 0.09)	1.56 (1.17–2.08, 0.00)	1.47 (1.16–1.85, < 0.01)
Multiple comorbidities	1.27 (0.51–3.17, 0.60)	1.58 (0.87–2.88, 0.13)	1.18 (0.80–1.73, 0.38)	0.82 (0.63–1.06, 0.13)	1.02 (0.84–1.24, 0.84)
AUC (Q1–Q3)	0.895 (0.854–0.932)	0.8942 (0.868–0.920)	0.8855 (0.868–0.902)	0.853 (0.838–0.867)	0.875 (0.865–0.884)

RRT renal replacement therapy, *ICU* intensive care unit, *SD* standard deviation

Table 7 Multivariable logistic regression of risk factors for 1-year mortality by age categories (years)

Outcome	Age 16–25 OR (95% CI *p* value)	Age 26–35 OR (95% CI *p* value)	Age 36–45 OR (95% CI *p* value)	Age 46–55 OR (95% CI *p* value)	All OR (95% CI *p* value)
Age	1.04 (0.94–1.16, 0.47)	1.03 (0.96–1.10, 0.34)	1.04 (0.99–1.09, 0.06)	1.04 (1.01–1.07, 0.01)	1.04 (1.03–1.04, < 0.01)
AKI	2.25 (1.14–4.45, 0.02)	2.50 (1.50–4.15, < 0.01)	1.98 (1.45–2.70, < 0.01)	1.90 (1.54–2.36, < 0.01)	2.03 (1.74–2.39, < 0.01)
Race[a]	0.63 (0.23–1.73, 0.37)	0.53 (0.25–1.11, 0.09)	0.62 (0.39–0.99, 0.05)	0.745 (0.55–1.02, 0.07)	0.67 (0.53–0.84, < 0.01)
APACHE III score	1.02 (1.01–1.03, < 0.01)	1.02 (1.02–1.03, < 0.01)	1.02 (1.02–1.03, < 0.01)	1.02 (1.02–1.03, < 0.01)	2.04 (1.73 –2.39, < 0.01)
BMI	0.98 (0.94–1.01, 0.20)	1.01 (0.99–1.03, 0.56)	0.99 (0.98–1.01, 0.46)	0.99 (0.98–0.99, 0.02)	0.99 (0.99–0.99, 0.02)
Hypotensive Index	1.01 (1.00–1.02, 0.06)	1.00 (0.99–1.01, 0.44)	1.01 (1.00–1.01, < 0.01)	1.00 (1.00–1.01, 0.01)	1.00 (1.00–1.01, < 0.01)
Vasopressors	1.99 (0.94–4.20, 0.07)	2.41 (1.54 –3.81, < 0.01)	1.62 (1.20–2.18, < 0.01)	1.35 (1.11–1.64, < 0.01)	1.54 (1.33–1.80, < 0.01)
Surgical admission	0.80 (0.44–1.46, 0.47)	0.52 (0.36–0.77, < 0.01)	0.53 (0.42– 0.69, < 0.01)	0.52 (0.44–0.62, < 0.01)	0.54 (0.47–0.61, < 0.01)
Hypertension	1.17 (0.42–3.27, 0.77)	0.80 (0.42–1.52, 0.50)	0.85 (0.61–1.19, 0.35)	0.85 (0.69–1.05, 0.13)	0.82 (0.69–0.97, 0.02)
Malignancy	17.84 (4.66–68.35, < 0.01)	2.43 (1.08–5.45, 0.03)	1.08 (0.62–1.88, 0.08)	2.04 (1.48–2.80, < 0.01)	1.91 (1.49–2.46, < 0.01)
Chronic liver disease	2.65 (0.77 –8.92, 0.12)	0.90 (0.43–1.88, 0.76)	1.26 (0.83 –1.92, 0.27)	1.70 (1.30–2.20, < 0.01)	1.48 (1.21–1.82, < 0.01)
History of COPD	13.96 (0.73– 268.49, 0.08)	1.31 (0.40–4.46, 0.66)	1.21 (0.68 –2.17, 0.52)	1.41 (1.06–1.89, 0.02)	1.30 (1.01–1.68, 0.04)
Multiple comorbidities	2.00 (0.87–4.61, 0.10)	3.22 (1.88–5.54, < 0.01)	2.07 (1.45 –2.95, < 0.01)	1.06 (0.84–1.36, 0.61)	1.53 (1.28–1.83, < 0.01)
AUC (Q1–Q3)	0.862 (0.816–0.907)	0.848 (0.818–0.878)	0.816 (0.794–0.837)	0.799 (0.783–0.814)	0.823 (0.812–0.834)

AKI acute kidney injury, *APACHE* Acute Physiology and Chronic Healthy Evaluation, *BMI* Body Mass Index, *COPD* chronic obstructive pulmonary disease

[a] Black compared to white

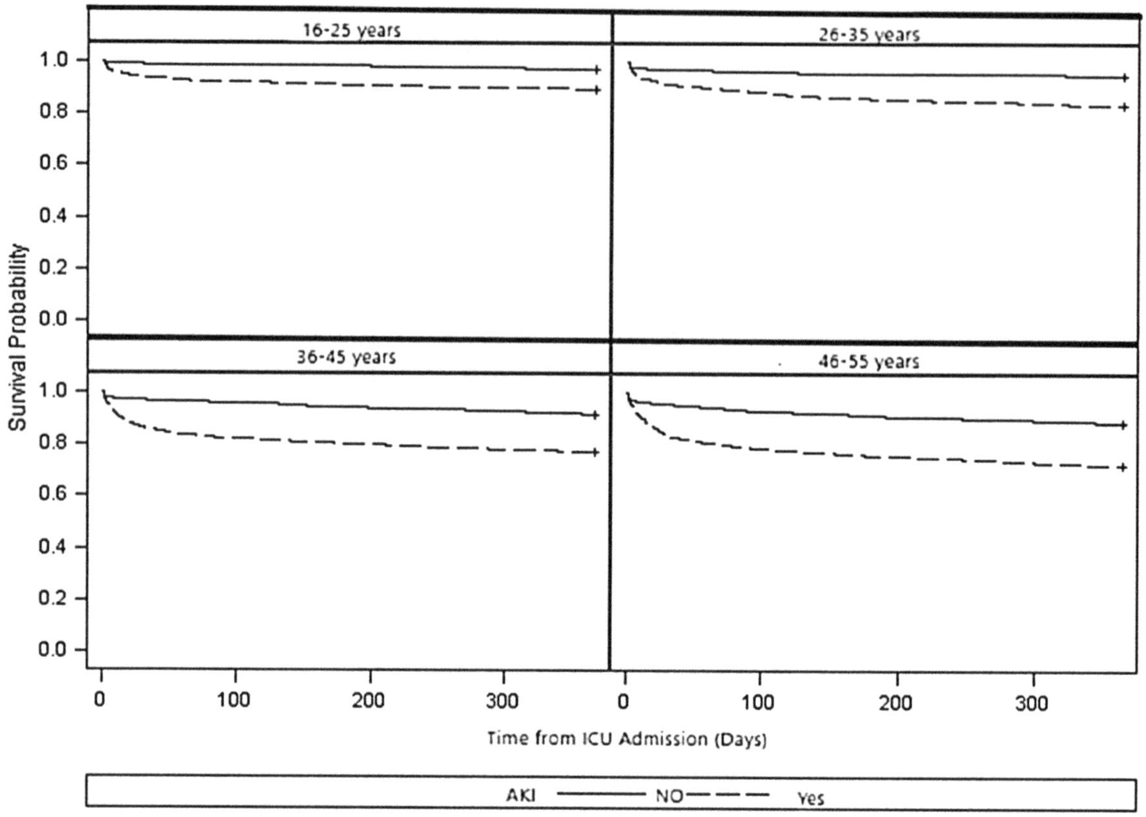

Fig. 2 Kaplan–Meier survival curves for 1-year mortality after ICU discharge

The significant association of nephrotoxic medications and AKI in the 16–25-year-old age group suggests the need for future studies exploring the effect of different drug combinations in young adults on AKI development. At the bedside, frequent evaluations for transitioning medications to less nephrotoxic alternatives along with the use of therapeutic drug monitoring when available should be initiated.

The multivariable logistic regression demonstrates a "protective effect" of NSAID use on AKI risk across all of the age groups. NSAIDs are frequently withheld from patients in the ICU due to the concern of nephrotoxicity [29]. We speculate that our study results are due to a possible healthy user bias whereby patients without CKD and/or less comorbid conditions may have been more likely to receive NSAIDs during their ICU stay than patients with an elevated creatinine values and more comorbidities. However, given that increased NSAID use was not found to be positively associated with AKI in this critically ill patient cohort, intermittent NSAID use in patients without underlying renal disease who are euvolemic should be considered for analgesia given the low risk of renal side effects, as discussed in previous investigations [30, 31]. This may be particular important given recent attention to opiate use in the critically ill.

In this study, which did not include patients over 55 years of age, we show a similar ability to predict AKI when comparing the four age strata. Also using the HiDenIC database, but including ICU patients 55 years and older, Kane-Gill et al. [20] demonstrated that the ability of similar variables used in our study to predict AKI decreases with age. Specifically, they report that for patients greater than or equal to 75 years of age an AUC for predicting AKI of 0.673 [20]. This is in contrast to the higher AUC values determined in this study for younger adults, which demonstrates the superior ability to predict and, therefore, potentially prevent AKI in patients less than 55 years of age. Notably, the risk factors between those age 16–55 in our study and those > 75 in the previously published study varied with different drugs, history of hypertension, and sepsis in the older adult group [20].

Our models for mortality were also quite robust with all AUCs of at least 0.80 and some approaching 0.90 (Tables 6, 7). While our intent was not to develop a risk prediction model for mortality with AKI, and our models are likely overtrained, these results are far better than most reports in the literature [32]. Use of younger patients and stratification by age group may have led to significantly better predicative value. While the AUC values appear to increase with decreasing age, the confidence intervals overlap. Future studies are needed to validate these models in independent populations.

Our study has important limitations. The identified risk factors for AKI may be surrogates of other variables. For example, the association of calcineurin inhibitor use and AKI may reflect the association of AKI with transplant status. Notably, surgical as opposed to medical admission was an increasingly powerful risk factor for AKI in younger patients, especially those 16–25 years of age. However, it could not be determined from the database if surgeries were elective versus emergent. APACHE III scores and the MDRD equation for estimating GFR have not been validated in patients less than 18 years of age. Importantly, the MDRD equation was derived from patients with CKD, and its use in patients with critical illness is unclear. All of the young adults in this study were treated in adult intensive care units at a single institution. Given the single-center nature of this study, the comorbidities of a young adult patient group treated at other institutions may be different from our cohort of patients. Therefore, the results should be validated at other centers.

Conclusions

Using the KDIGO criteria for both serum creatinine and urine output to define AKI, 39.8% of patients between the ages of 16–25 met AKI criteria during admission to an adult tertiary care center, indicating that AKI is a common event in this patient group. The diagnosis of AKI during hospital admission independently contributed toward increased hospital mortality, increased ICU mortality and increased mortality 90 days and 1 year after hospital discharge in the young adult patients. Potentially modifiable risk factors for AKI were identified, most notably nephrotoxic medication exposure. Risk factors identified in this younger population varied from published data in older adults (> 75 years old).

Abbreviations

AKI: acute kidney injury; CKD: chronic kidney disease; AWARE: Assessment of Worldwide Acute Kidney Injury, Renal Angina, and Epidemiology; ICU: intensive care unit; HiDenIC: High-Density Intensive Care; eGFR: estimated glomerular filtration rate; APACHE: Acute Physiology and Chronic Health Evaluation; NSAID: nonsteroidal anti-inflammatory drug; KDIGO: Kidney Disease Improving Global Outcomes.

Authors' contributions

DYF, JAK, and SLG contributed to study concept and design; DYF, JAK, and PP analyzed the data; DYF, JAK, SLK-G, and SLG interpreted the data; DYF and PP performed statistical analysis; JAK helped in procurement of funding. Each author contributed important intellectual content during manuscript drafting or revision and accepted accountability for the overall work by ensuring that questions pertaining to the accuracy or integrity of any portion of the work are appropriately investigated and resolved. All authors read and approved the final manuscript.

Author details

[1] Children's Hospital of Pittsburgh, 4401 Penn Avenue, Children's Hospital Drive, Faculty Pavilion Suite 2000, Pittsburgh, PA 15224, USA. [2] School of Pharmacy, University of Pittsburgh, 638 Salk Hall, 3501 Terrace Street, Pittsburgh, PA 15261, USA. [3] Center for Acute Care Nephrology, Cincinnati Children's Hospital Medical Center, 3333 Burnet Avenue, Cincinnati, OH 45229, USA. [4] The Center for Critical Care Nephrology, 3347 Forbes Avenue, Ste 220, Pittsburgh, PA 15213, USA.

Acknowledgements

None.

Competing interests

The authors declare that they have no competing interests.

Funding

This work was funded by the University of Pittsburgh Medical Center and the University of Pittsburgh; and additional support was provided by R01DK083961 from the National Institute of Diabetes, and Digestive, and Kidney Diseases (NIDDK) to JAK. The content of this paper is solely the responsibility of the authors and does not necessarily represent the official views of the NIDDK or National Institutes of Health.

References

1. Uchino S, Kellum JA, Bellomo R, et al. Acute renal failure in critically ill patients: a multinational, multicenter study. JAMA. 2005;294(7):813–8.
2. Liano F, Pascual J. Epidemiology of acute renal failure: a prospective, multicenter, community-based study. Madrid Acute Renal Failure Study Group. Kidney Int. 1996;50(3):811–8.
3. Ali T, Khan I, Simpson W, et al. Incidence and outcomes in acute kidney injury: a comprehensive population-based study. J Am Soc Nephrol. 2007;18(4):1292–8.
4. Kidney Disease: Improving Global Outcomes (KDIGO) Work Group. KDIGO clinical practice guildeline for acute kidney injury. Kidney Int Suppl. 2012;2:1–138.
5. Kaddourah A, Basu RK, Bagshaw SM, Goldstein SL, Investigators A. Epidemiology of acute kidney injury in critically ill children and young adults. N Engl J Med. 2017;376(1):11–20.
6. Sutherland SM, Byrnes JJ, Kothari M, et al. AKI in hospitalized children: comparing the pRIFLE, AKIN, and KDIGO definitions. Clin J Am Soc Nephrol. 2015;10(4):554–61.
7. Bailey D, Phan V, Litalien C, et al. Risk factors of acute renal failure in critically ill children: a prospective descriptive epidemiological study. Pediatr Crit Care Med. 2007;8(1):29–35.
8. Schneider J, Khemani R, Grushkin C, Bart R. Serum creatinine as stratified in the RIFLE score for acute kidney injury is associated with mortality and length of stay for children in the pediatric intensive care unit. Crit Care Med. 2010;38(3):933–9.
9. Zappitelli M, Parikh CR, Akcan-Arikan A, Washburn KK, Moffett BS, Goldstein SL. Ascertainment and epidemiology of acute kidney injury varies with definition interpretation. Clin J Am Soc Nephrol. 2008;3(4):948–54.
10. Akcan-Arikan A, Zappitelli M, Loftis LL, Washburn KK, Jefferson LS, Goldstein SL. Modified RIFLE criteria in critically ill children with acute kidney injury. Kidney Int. 2007;71(10):1028–35.
11. Basu RK, Zappitelli M, Brunner L, et al. Derivation and validation of the renal angina index to improve the prediction of acute kidney injury in critically ill children. Kidney Int. 2014;85(3):659–67.
12. Groeneveld AB, Tran DD, van der Meulen J, Nauta JJ, Thijs LG. Acute renal failure in the medical intensive care unit: predisposing, complicating factors and outcome. Nephron. 1991;59(4):602–10.

13. de Mendonca A, Vincent JL, Suter PM, et al. Acute renal failure in the ICU: risk factors and outcome evaluated by the SOFA score. Intensive Care Med. 2000;26(7):915–21.
14. Brivet FG, Kleinknecht DJ, Loirat P, Landais PJ. Acute renal failure in intensive care units–causes, outcome, and prognostic factors of hospital mortality; a prospective, multicenter study. French Study Group on Acute Renal Failure. Crit Care Med. 1996;24(2):192–8.
15. Wilkins RG, Faragher EB. Acute renal failure in an intensive care unit: incidence, prediction and outcome. Anaesthesia. 1983;38(7):628–34.
16. Edwards JD, Houtrow AJ, Vasilevskis EE, Dudley RA, Okumura MJ. Multi-institutional profile of adults admitted to pediatric intensive care units. JAMA Pediatr. 2013;167(5):436–43.
17. Janse AJ, Uiterwaal CS, Gemke RJ, Kimpen JL, Sinnema G. A difference in perception of quality of life in chronically ill children was found between parents and pediatricians. J Clin Epidemiol. 2005;58(5):495–502.
18. Hui-Stickle S, Brewer ED, Goldstein SL. Pediatric ARF epidemiology at a tertiary care center from 1999 to 2001. Am J Kidney Dis. 2005;45(1):96–101.
19. Cartin-Ceba R, Kashiouris M, Plataki M, Kor DJ, Gajic O, Casey ET. Risk factors for development of acute kidney injury in critically ill patients: a systematic review and meta-analysis of observational studies. Crit Care Res Pract. 2012;2012:691013.
20. Kane-Gill SL, Sileanu FE, Murugan R, Trietley GS, Handler SM, Kellum JA. Risk factors for acute kidney injury in older adults with critical illness: a retrospective cohort study. Am J Kidney Dis. 2015;65(6):860–9.
21. Levey AS, Stevens LA, Schmid CH, et al. A new equation to estimate glomerular filtration rate. Ann Intern Med. 2009;150(9):604–12.
22. WHO. World Health Organization: Haemoglobin concentrations for the diagnosis of anaemia and assessment of severity. http://www.who.int/vmnis/indicators/haemoglobin.pdf (2011). Accessed 5 April 2016.
23. Sutherland SM, Zappitelli M, Alexander SR, et al. Fluid overload and mortality in children receiving continuous renal replacement therapy: the prospective pediatric continuous renal replacement therapy registry. Am J Kidney Dis. 2010;55(2):316–25.
24. Knaus WA, Wagner DP, Draper EA, et al. The APACHE III prognostic system. Risk prediction of hospital mortality for critically ill hospitalized adults. Chest. 1991;100(6):1619–36.
25. Hoste EA, Clermont G, Kersten A, et al. RIFLE criteria for acute kidney injury are associated with hospital mortality in critically ill patients: a cohort analysis. Crit Care. 2006;10(3):R73.
26. Zavada J, Hoste E, Cartin-Ceba R, et al. A comparison of three methods to estimate baseline creatinine for RIFLE classification. Nephrol Dial Transpl. 2010;25(12):3911–8.
27. DaL Hosmer S. Applied logistic regression. 2nd ed. New York: Wiley; 2000.
28. Hoste EA, Bagshaw SM, Bellomo R, et al. Epidemiology of acute kidney injury in critically ill patients: the multinational AKI-EPI study. Intensive Care Med. 2015;41(8):1411–23.
29. Whelton A. Nephrotoxicity of nonsteroidal anti-inflammatory drugs: physiologic foundations and clinical implications. Am J Med. 1999;106(5B):13S–24S.
30. Mann JF, Goerig M, Brune K, Luft FC. Ibuprofen as an over-the-counter drug: is there a risk for renal injury? Clin Nephrol. 1993;39(1):1–6.
31. Musu M, Finco G, Antonucci R, et al. Acute nephrotoxicity of NSAID from the foetus to the adult. Eur Rev Med Pharmacol Sci. 2011;15(12):1461–72.
32. Uchino S, Bellomo R, Morimatsu H, et al. External validation of severity scoring systems for acute renal failure using a multinational database. Crit Care Med. 2005;33(9):1961–7.

18

Epidemiology, causes, evolution and outcome in a single-center cohort of 1116 critically ill patients with hypoxic hepatitis

Astrid Van den broecke[1,3*†], Laura Van Coile[1†], Alexander Decruyenaere[1,2], Kirsten Colpaert[1,3], Dominique Benoit[1,3], Hans Van Vlierberghe[1,4] and Johan Decruyenaere[1,3]

Abstract

Background: Hypoxic hepatitis (HH) is a type of acute hepatic injury that is histologically characterized by centrilobular liver cell necrosis and that is caused by insufficient oxygen delivery to the hepatocytes. Typical for HH is the sudden and significant increase of aspartate aminotransferase (AST) in response to cardiac, circulatory or respiratory failure. The aim of this study is to investigate its epidemiology, causes, evolution and outcome.

Methods: The screened population consisted of all adults admitted to the intensive care unit (ICU) at the Ghent University Hospital between January 1, 2007 and September 21, 2015. HH was defined as peak AST > 5 times the upper limit of normal (ULN) after exclusion of other causes of liver injury. Thirty-five variables were retrospectively collected and used in descriptive analysis, time series plots and Kaplan–Meier survival curves with multi-group log-rank tests.

Results: HH was observed in 4.0% of the ICU admissions at our center. The study cohort comprised 1116 patients. Causes of HH were cardiac failure (49.1%), septic shock (29.8%), hypovolemic shock (9.4%), acute respiratory failure (6.4%), acute on chronic respiratory failure (3.3%), pulmonary embolism (1.4%) and hyperthermia (0.5%). The 28-day mortality associated with HH was 45.0%. Mortality rates differed significantly ($P = 0.007$) among the causes, ranging from 33.3% in the hyperthermia subgroup to 52.9 and 56.2% in the septic shock and pulmonary embolism subgroups, respectively. The magnitude of AST increase was also significantly correlated ($P < 0.001$) with mortality: 33.2, 44.4 and 55.4% for peak AST 5–10× ULN, 10–20× ULN and > 20× ULN, respectively.

Conclusion: This study surpasses by far the largest cohort of critically ill patients with HH. HH is more common than previously thought with an ICU incidence of 4.0%, and it is associated with a high all-cause mortality of 45.0% at 28 days. The main causes of HH are cardiac failure and septic shock, which include more than 3/4 of all episodes. Clinicians should search actively for any underlying hemodynamic or respiratory instability even in patients with moderately increased AST levels.

Keywords: Critical care medicine, Critically ill, Epidemiology, Hypoxic hepatitis, Intensive care medicine, Ischemic hepatitis, Liver failure, Mortality, Outcome, Shock liver

Background

Hypoxic hepatitis (HH), also referred to as "ischemic hepatitis" or "shock liver," is a type of acute hepatic injury that is histologically characterized by centrilobular liver cell necrosis and that is caused by insufficient oxygen delivery to the hepatocytes [1]. Typical for this form of liver cell necrosis is the sudden and significant increase of aspartate aminotransferase (AST) in response to cardiac, circulatory or respiratory failure [1]. Although often missed, HH is a fairly common cause of hepatic dysfunction in an intensive care unit (ICU) with a pooled incidence of 2.5% from a recent meta-analysis of 1782

*Correspondence: Astrid.Vandenbroecke@UGent.be
†Astrid Van den broecke and Laura Van Coile have contributed equally to this study and are the joint first authors
[3] Department of Intensive Care Medicine, Ghent University Hospital, De Pintelaan 185, 9000 Ghent, Belgium
Full list of author information is available at the end of the article

patients [2]. Its incidence varies widely among published studies, ranging from 0.16 to 12%, depending upon institution, population studied and definition used [1–8]. However, a high associated mortality of approximately 50% has been consistently observed in all studies [2–6, 8].

The major causes of HH are septic shock, respiratory failure and cardiogenic shock [1, 2]. Possible pathophysiological mechanisms include (1) ischemia due to reduced blood supply (forward failure) or due to right heart failure (backward failure) with venous congestion, (2) hypoxemia due to reduced blood oxygenation and (3) increased oxygen consumption due to elevated metabolic demand (e.g., in severe hyperthermia or septic shock) [1, 9]. Patients with comorbidities are more likely to develop HH, as they have an increased vulnerability even to minor hemodynamic or respiratory insults, such as short periods of hypotension or hypoxemia. These comorbidities contribute substantially to the high mortality associated with HH [4, 7, 8].

HH is reflected by a typical pattern of liver enzyme alterations. It presents with a sudden and significant increase of AST, alanine aminotransferase (ALT) and lactate dehydrogenase (LDH), reaching their peak levels around 24 h after ICU admission [4] and declining steadily to baseline within 10–15 days [1]. Initially, AST exceeds ALT, but as ALT declines more slowly, a reversal of the AST/ALT ratio is observed within 3 days after the peak [5, 6, 8, 10]. Although this biochemical pattern is highly suggestive of HH, it is not pathognomonic and warrants further evaluation [1]. Other common causes of significant increases in aminotransferase levels are drug-induced liver injury (e.g., acetaminophen toxicity) and acute viral hepatitis. However, studies have shown that a sudden and significant increase of AST is caused by HH in more than 50% of the cases [11, 12]. Furthermore, HH is frequently associated with a prolonged prothrombin time and accompanied by additional evidence of end-organ hypoperfusion, such as impaired renal function and increased lactate level [3–6]. A rapid rise and subsequent fall in aminotransferase levels with reversal of the initial AST/ALT ratio, a prolongation of prothrombin time and an increase in serum creatinine level comprise a triad of biochemical abnormalities that can suggest the diagnosis of HH, as proposed by Raurich et al. [6].

Currently, only limited data from small retrospective studies are available, making HH an understudied disease. The largest cohort described to date was recently published and included 565 patients [8]. The aim of this study is to investigate in detail the epidemiology, causes, evolution and outcome of HH in a large single-center cohort. More insight in HH may improve awareness and facilitate earlier diagnosis.

Methods

Study cohort and data collection

The screened population consisted of all consecutive adults ($\geq$ 18 years, n = 29,874) who were admitted to the surgical, cardiac or medical ICU at the Ghent University Hospital between January 1, 2007 and September 21, 2015. HH was defined as a significant but transient increase in AST level above 5 times the upper limit of normal (ULN) after exclusion of other potential causes of liver injury. Different AST cutoff values for defining HH are used in the literature [2]. As HH has been histologically proven to occur even in patients with moderately elevated AST levels (at AST levels of 252 and 300 IU/L in the cohort of Cohen et al. [13] and Bynum et al. [14], respectively), a cutoff of at least 5 times the ULN was used in this study, i.e., 155 and 185 U/L for females and males, respectively. The 4012 identified patients whose AST level exceeded our cutoff value were evaluated for the presence of HH by three independent experts based on the pattern of liver enzyme alterations, the daily clinical notes and the discharge summaries. The sine qua non was the exposure to a hemodynamic or respiratory insult preceding the AST increase and the exclusion of other potential causes of liver injury. A flow diagram of the exclusion criteria is shown in Fig. 1. Reasons for exclusion were (1) acute liver failure, (2) chronic liver failure, (3) other conditions associated with abnormal liver tests such as cholangitis and pancreatitis, (4) liver surgery, (5) surgery near the liver, (6) hepatic vessel injury or thrombosis, (7) rhabdomyolysis, (8) an unclear increase of creatine kinase (CK), (9) post-anesthesia without overt evidence of an acute cardiac or respiratory event perioperatively, (10) missing data and (11) duplicate patients. (In patients having developed multiple episodes of HH during the study period, only the first episode is eligible for analysis.) Rhabdomyolysis was defined as serum CK exceeding 5 times the ULN (i.e., 850 and 974 U/L for females and males, respectively) with a CK-MB/CK ratio below 6% [6]. Patients with elevated CK levels but with unknown CK-MB value were excluded due to the uncertain CK increase. This study was approved by the Ethics Committee of the Ghent University Hospital (project numbers 2015/0796-0797). Due to the retrospective nature of this study, the need for informed consent was waived.

Routinely available biochemical parameters were recorded, including AST (U/L), ALT (U/L), LDH (U/L), bilirubin (mg/dL), alkaline phosphatase (AP) (U/L), gamma-glutamyl transpeptidase (U/L), lipase (U/L), international normalized ratio (INR), platelet count (10^3/μL), white blood cell count (10^3/μL), hemoglobin (g/dL), CK (U/L), creatinine (mg/dL), urea (mg/dL) and lactate (mg/dL). Values at specific time points were estimated

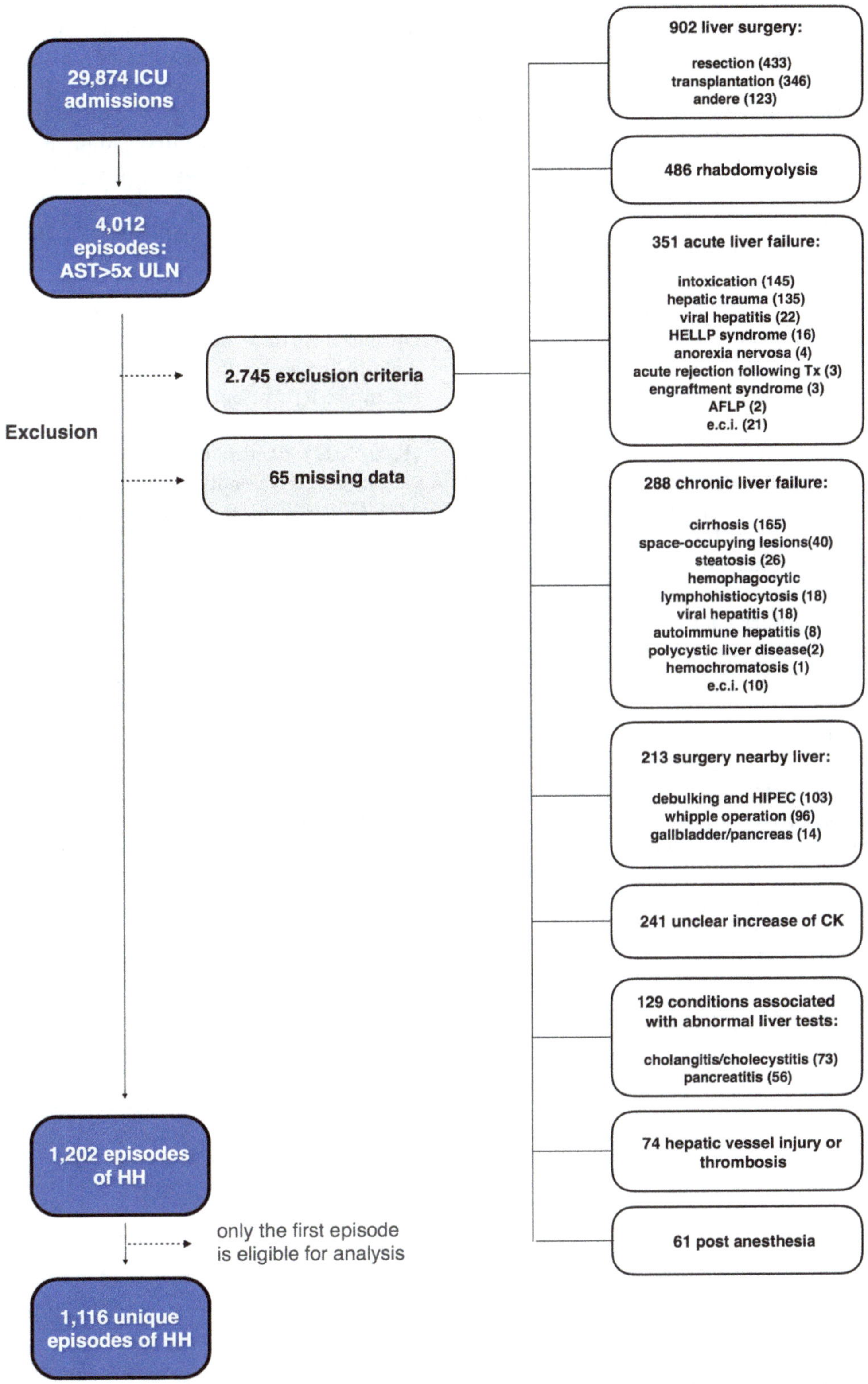

Fig. 1 Flow diagram of the exclusion criteria. *AFLP* acute fatty liver of pregnancy, *AST* aspartate aminotransferase, *CK* creatine kinase, *e.c.i* e causa ignota, *HELLP* hemolysis, elevated liver enzymes and low platelet count, *HH* hypoxic hepatitis, *HIPEC* hyperthermic intraperitioneal chemotherapy, *ICU* intensive care unit

using linear interpolation between consecutive recorded values. Parameters related to patient characteristics included sex, age, body mass index (BMI) and comorbidities (diabetes mellitus, cardiac function and chronic respiratory disease). Parameters related to the episode of HH included cause, severity of illness scores [acute physiology II score (APS-II) and the simplified acute physiology II score (SAPS-II)], supportive therapy (inotropic agents, vasopressor agents, mechanical ventilation, intra-aortic balloon pump (IABP) and need for dialysis), ICU and hospital length of stay, duration of the HH episode, and ICU and in-hospital mortality at 28 days. The peak of HH was defined as the point in time (T-ASTmax) when AST reached its peak value (ASTmax). In this study, the time origin was set to T-ASTmax (designated as time 0) and all recorded values are expressed in time relative to T-ASTmax for optimal comparison. Severity of illness scores were recorded over a time span of 24 h around T-ASTmax. Three categories for severity of HH were used: "5–10× ULN", "10–20× ULN" and "> 20× ULN". Seven underlying causes of HH were defined: cardiac failure, septic shock, hypovolemic shock, pulmonary embolism, acute respiratory failure, acute on chronic respiratory failure and hyperthermia.

Statistical analysis

Categorical data are reported as counts and percentages. Continuous data are reported as the median with the first (Q1) and third (Q3) quartiles. For categorical variables, comparisons between groups are performed using the Pearson's Chi square test for contingency. For continuous variables, a permutation test based on difference in medians between groups is used. A Tukey-like approach with permutation resampling is applied to adjust *P* values for multiple pairwise comparisons. All statistical tests are performed as two-sided tests at a significance level of 0.05. The time trend of laboratory variables is graphically assessed using time series plots and stacked bar charts. Kaplan–Meier survival curves until 28 days after T-ASTmax and multi-group log-rank tests are used to compare the all-cause mortality between groups. Statistical analysis is performed using R version 3.3.2 [15].

Results

Patient and episode characteristics

During the study period, 29,874 adult patients with a male-to-female ratio of approximately 3:2 were admitted to the ICU at our center, of whom 4012 patients had peak AST levels exceeding 5 times the ULN. In 30.0% (1202/4012) of the cases, the elevation of AST was caused by HH, resulting in an overall ICU incidence of 4.0% (1202/29,874). As only the first episode was eligible for analysis in patients with multiple episodes of HH during the study period, the final study cohort comprised 1116 patients.

The all-cause mortality of patients admitted to the ICU at our center during the study period was 7.7% (2302/29,874). Among these non-survivors, 19.8% (455/2302) had developed HH during their ICU stay. The all-cause mortality associated with HH was 45.0% (502/1116) at 28 days, of which 90.6% occurred during ICU stay. The survival curves by cause of HH are presented in Fig. 2.

In our study cohort, the median age was 66.0 (Q1–Q3 55.0–74.0) years with a male-to-female ratio of 3:2. The median SAPS-II score at T-ASTmax was 66.0 (Q1–Q3

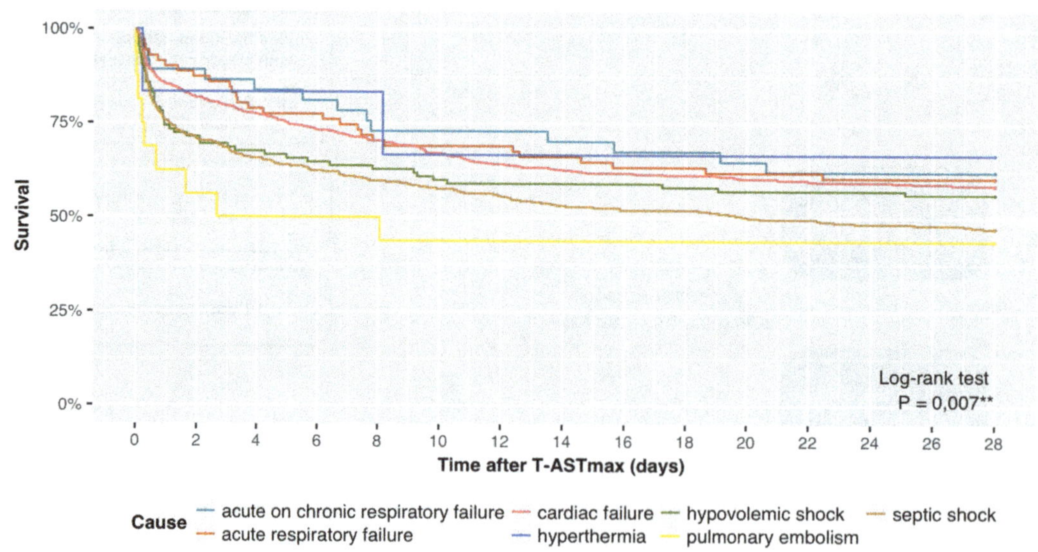

Fig. 2 Survival curves by cause of hypoxic hepatitis. T-ASTmax is designated as the time 0. *T-ASTmax* time point of maximum AST value

43.0–81.0). 74.9% of patients required mechanical ventilation. Vasopressor and inotropic agents were used in 60.8 and 43.2%, respectively, and 9.5% were on dialysis at T-ASTmax. The causes of HH, in decreasing order of frequency, were cardiac failure (49.1%), septic shock (29.8%), hypovolemic shock (9.4%), acute respiratory failure (6.4%), acute on chronic respiratory failure (3.3%), pulmonary embolism (1.4%) and hyperthermia (0.5%). An episode of HH (length of time that AST levels are exceeding 5 times the ULN) had a median duration of 54.3 (Q1–Q3 26.4–94.2) h, during which the median recovery time (duration from peak AST to levels below 5 times the ULN) was 34.7 (Q1–Q3 14.6–67.2) h.

Survivors had significantly lower severity of illness scores (median SAPS-II score of 54.0 vs. 76.0, $P < 0.001$ and median APS-II score 25.0 vs. 30.0, $P = 0.005$) as compared to non-survivors. They were less likely to have septic shock (25.6 vs. 35.1%, $P = 0.003$). Peak AST levels above 20 times ULN were less commonly seen in survivors (33.4 vs. 50.8%, $P < 0.001$). More characteristics, classified according to survival status, are presented in Table 1.

The three ASTmax subgroups ("5–10× ULN" vs. "10–20× ULN" vs. "> 20× ULN") were also compared with each other. The causes of HH were equally represented within each subgroup. Patients with higher peak AST levels had higher severity of illness scores (median SAPS-II score of 57.0 vs. 60.0 vs. 73.0, $P < 0.001$; median APS-II score of 24.0 vs. 26.5 vs. 32.0, $P < 0.001$) and a higher need for supportive therapy, such as inotropic agents (38.5 vs. 37.9 vs. 50.2%, $P < 0.001$), vasopressor agents (50.9 vs. 59.4 vs. 70.0%, $P < 0.001$), dialysis (4.8 vs. 8.4 vs. 14.1%, $P < 0.001$) and IABP (13.7 vs. 20.7% vs. 18.9%, $P = 0.041$). In addition, higher peak AST levels were associated with higher 28-day mortality rates (33.2 vs. 44.4 vs. 55.4%, $P < 0.001$). More characteristics, classified according to severity of HH and to cause of HH, are presented in Tables 2 and 3, respectively.

Trend of liver tests

The time trend of the liver tests is illustrated in Fig. 3. Once the AST level exceeded 5 times the ULN (designated as start of HH), it reached a median peak level of 521.2 (Q1–Q3 269.1–1581.6) U/L within a median of 16.3 (Q1–Q3 7.9–26.8) h. Subsequently, AST started to decline, dropping below 5 times the ULN after a median time of 34.7 (Q1–Q3 14.6–67.2) h and normalizing after a median time of 6.4 (Q1–Q3 3.9–10.9) days in survivors.

ALT and LDH peaked at median values of 332.0 (Q1–Q3 149.4–953.6) U/L and 1180.6 (Q1–Q3 684.1–2770.8) U/L within a median time of 22.0 (Q1–Q3 9.7–43.0) and 21.4 (Q1–Q3 10.0–43.6) h after start of HH, respectively. In survivors, LDH returned to baseline (< 233 U/L) within a median of 5.1 (Q1–Q3 1.3–15.9) days after its peak. ALT declined more slowly, returning to baseline (< 31 and < 40 U/L for females and males, respectively) within 8.6 (Q1–Q3 3.9–16.5) days after its peak. When considering all patients, including those with AST already exceeding 5 times the ULN at ICU admission, ALT and LDH peaked at T-ASTmax in the majority of patients (65.5 and 53.1%, respectively) and to a lesser extent after T-ASTmax (26.2 and 29.8%, respectively).

The median relative increase of AST, ALT and LDH at T-ASTmax was 15.0, 8.7 and 4.7 times their ULN, respectively. LDH exceeded both AST and ALT at all time points in more than 80% of patients. The median AST/ALT ratio was 1.6 at the start of HH, increased to 1.8 at T-ASTmax and subsequently declined, reversing within a median of 32.5 h after T-ASTmax.

In addition, Fig. 3 illustrates that the median INR, creatinine and bilirubin levels also peaked at T-ASTmax, albeit to a much less extent, with median bilirubin level never exceeding the ULN. This is also illustrated in Fig. 4. Both in survivors and non-survivors, the proportion of patients with bilirubin level above the ULN increased mildly at T-ASTmax and then gradually decreased again. The proportion of survivors with bilirubin above 3 times the ULN was limited and increased slightly later during ICU stay. Likewise, AP remained stable during HH, except for a mild increase later during ICU stay, as illustrated in Figs. 3 and 4.

The pattern of liver enzyme alterations described above was found in all ASTmax subgroups (see Appendix Figs. 5, 6, 7). Median values of other laboratory tests at start of HH and at T-ASTmax are presented in Table 4.

28-day mortality

HH was associated with high mortality rates, especially early in its course. 18.5% died within 24 h after T-ASTmax. After this first day, the hazard declined dramatically, but remained quite high, resulting in 40.2 and 45.0% all-cause mortality at 14 and 28 days, respectively. 90.6% of deaths occurred during ICU stay.

Twenty-eight-day mortality rates differed significantly among the causes of HH ($P = 0.007$). The high number of early deaths in the pulmonary embolism, septic shock and hypovolemic shock subgroups mainly accounted for the early mortality associated with HH. 37.5, 24.3, 25.7% of these patients died within 24 h after T-ASTmax. The mortality rate in the pulmonary embolism subgroup exceeded at all times those of other subgroups and ultimately resulted in 56.2% mortality at 28 days. The septic shock and hypovolemic shock subgroups had a 28-day mortality of 52.9 and 43.8%, respectively. While the early mortality in the cardiac failure subgroup was less pronounced, yet still considerable as 14.8% of these patients

Table 1 Characteristics of patients with HH classified by in-hospital 28-day mortality

Variable	Patients: Total (*n* = 1116)	In-hospital 28-day mortality: No (*n* = 614)	In-hospital 28-day mortality: Yes (*n* = 502)	*P*
Sex[a]				
Male	61.3% (684)	62.2% (382)	60.2% (302)	0.483
Age[b] (year)	66.0 (55.0–74.0)	63.0 (53.0–73.0)	68.0 (58.0–76.8)	*< 0.001*
BMI[b] (kg/m^2)	25.4 (22.9–28.9)	25.4 (23.0–28.5)	25.4 (22.9–29.4)	0.774
Cause[a]				
Cardiac failure	49.1% (548)	52.3% (321)	45.2% (227)	0.103
Septic shock	29.8% (333)	25.6% (157)	35.1% (176)	*0.003*
Hypovolemic shock	9.4% (105)	9.6% (59)	9.2% (46)	0.999
Acute respiratory failure	6.4% (71)	7.0% (43)	5.6% (28)	0.927
Acute on chronic respiratory failure	3.3% (37)	3.7% (23)	2.8% (14)	0.956
Pulmonary embolism	1.4% (16)	1.1% (7)	1.8% (9)	0.945
Hyperthermia	0.5% (6)	0.7% (4)	0.4% (2)	0.995
Comorbidities				
Echocardio[a]				
Overall				0.406
Normal	40.0% (446)	42.0% (258)	37.5% (188)	–
LV dysfunction	25.1% (280)	23.5% (144)	27.1% (136)	–
Missing	22.2% (248)	22.5% (151)	23.3% (117)	–
LV and RV dysfunction	8.0% (89)	8.0% (49)	8.0% (40)	–
RV dysfunction	4.7% (53)	5.2% (32)	4.2% (21)	–
DM[a]	18.7% (209)	17.4% (107)	20.3% (102)	0.218
Chronic respiratory failure[a]	11.4% (127)	10.7% (66)	12.2% (61)	0.287
SOI scores[c]				
APS-II[b]	28.0 (21.0–34.0)	25.0 (18.0–32.0)	30.0 (24.0–35.2)	*0.005*
SAPS-II[b]	66.0 (46.0–81.0)	54.0 (36.0–71.0)	76.0 (58.0–89.0)	*< 0.001*
ASTmax[a]				
5–10× ULN	35.4% (395)	43.0% (264)	26.1% (131)	*< 0.001*
10–20× ULN	23.4% (261)	23.6% (145)	23.1% (116)	0.985
> 20× ULN	41.2% (460)	33.4% (205)	50.8% (255)	*< 0.001*
Supportive therapy[c]				
Ventilation[a]	74.9% (836)	66.4% (408)	85.3% (428)	*< 0.001*
Medication				
Inotropic agents[a]	43.2% (482)	39.3% (241)	48.0% (241)	*0.003*
Vasopressor agents[a]	60.8% (678)	51.1% (314)	72.5% (364)	*< 0.001*
Dialysis[a]	9.5% (106)	6.8% (42)	12.7% (64)	*< 0.001*
IABP[a]	17.5% (195)	19.5% (120)	14.9% (75)	*0.044*
LOS				
ICU[b] (day)	4.4 (1.2–11.7)	6.4 (2.7–17.7)	1.8 (0.4–7.1)	*< 0.001*
Hospital[b] (day)	12.1 (3.0–28.9)	25.7 (13.9–48.1)	2.1 (0.4–8.1)	*< 0.001*
Duration				
Episode of HH[b] (h)	54.3 (26.4–94.2)	53.4 (23.9–94.2)	56.7 (30.7–94.1)	0.527
Recovery of HH[b] (h)	34.7 (14.6–67.2)	35.5 (14.1–68.0)	32.6 (16.2–61.4)	0.393
28-day mortality				
ICU[a]	40.8% (455)	0.0% (0)	90.6% (455)	*< 0.001*
In-hospital[a]	45.0% (502)	0.0% (0)	100.0% (502)	*< 0.001*

APS-II acute physiology II, *AST* aspartate aminotransferase, *ASTmax* maximum AST value, *BMI* body mass index, *HH* hypoxic hepatitis, *IABP* intra-aortic balloon pump, *ICU* intensive care unit, *LOS* length of stay, *LV* left ventricle, *P* P value, *Q1* first quartile, *Q3* third quartile, *RV* right ventricle, *SAPS-II* simplified acute physiology II, *SOI* severity of illness, *T-ASTmax* time point of maximum AST value, *ULN* upper limit of normal

Italics indicate the significant *P* values

[a] % (*n*)

[b] Median (Q1–Q3)

[c] At T-ASTmax ± 12 h

Table 2 Characteristics of patients with HH classified by ASTmax subgroup

Variable	Patients				Variable	Patients			
	ASTmax subgroup			P		ASTmax subgroup			P
	5× ULN–10× ULN (n = 395)	10× ULN–20× ULN (n = 261)	> 20× ULN (n = 460)			5× ULN–10× ULN (n = 395)	10× ULN–20× ULN (n = 261)	> 20× ULN (n = 460)	
Sex[a]					SOI scores[c]				
Male	60.5% (239)	62.5% (163)	61.3% (282)	0.882	APS-II[b]	24.0 (18.0–31.0)	26.5 (20.0–32.2)	32.0 (24.0–37.9)	*< 0.001*
Age[b] (year)	63.0 (45.0–73.5)	66.0 (56.0–75.0)	67.0 (55.8–75.0)	*0.014*	SAPS-II[b]	57.0 (36.2–74.0)	60.0 (41.0–78.2)	73.0 (56.0–86.5)	*< 0.001*
BMI[b] (kg/m²)	25.5 (23.1–28.7)	25.5 (22.9–29.2)	25.1 (22.9–28.9)	0.647	Supportive therapy[c]				
Cause[a]					Ventilation[a]	71.9% (284)	72.4% (189)	78.9% (363)	*0.035*
Overall				0.135	Medication				
Cardiac failure	50.6% (200)	49.8% (130)	47.4% (218)	–	Inotropic agents[a]	38.5% (152)	37.9% (99)	50.2% (231)	*< 0.001*
Septic shock	29.4% (116)	26.1% (68)	32.4% (149)	–	Vasopressor agents[a]	50.9% (201)	59.4% (155)	70.0% (322)	*< 0.001*
Hypovolemic shock	7.6% (30)	10.3% (27)	10.4% (48)	–	Dialysis[a]	4.8% (19)	8.4% (22)	14.1% (65)	*< 0.001*
Acute respiratory failure	7.1% (28)	9.2% (24)	4.1% (19)	–	IABP[a]	13.7% (54)	20.7% (54)	18.9% (87)	*0.041*
Acute on chronic respiratory failure	3.3% (13)	1.9% (5)	4.1% (19)	–	LOS				
Pulmonary embolism	1.5% (6)	1.5% (4)	1.3% (6)	–	ICU[b] (day)	4.6 (1.6–11.2)	4.8 (1.4–11.2)	4.0 (0.7–12.4)	0.325
Hyperthermia	0.5% (2)	1.1% (3)	0.2% (1)	–	Hospital[b] (day)	12.5 (6.5–29.5)	13.1 (4.1–27.6)	10.2 (0.9–29.8)	0.250
Comorbidities					Duration				
Echocardio[a]					Episode of HH[b] (h)	23.6 (11.4–37.2)	56.8 (40.5–79.6)	104.7 (78.1–132.0)	*< 0.001*
Normal	43.8% (173)	34.5% (90)	39.8% (183)	0.234	Recovery of HH[b] (h)	12.6 (6.1–22.2)	36.2 (22.7–52.0)	77.7 (56.6–102.4)	*< 0.001*
LV dysfunction	20.5% (81)	27.6% (72)	27.1% (136)	0.136	28-day mortality				
Missing	25.3% (100)	26.8% (70)	17.0% (78)	*0.008*	ICU[a]	29.4% (116)	38.3% (100)	52.0% (239)	*< 0.001*
LV and RV dysfunction	5.8% (23)	8.4% (22)	9.6% (44)	0.452	In-hospital[a]	33.2% (131)	44.4% (116)	55.4% (255)	*< 0.001*
RV dysfunction	4.6% (18)	2.7% (7)	6.1% (28)	0.422					
DM[a]	14.9% (59)	21.1% (55)	20.7% (95)	0.055					
Chronic respiratory failure[a]	12.2% (48)	10.7% (28)	11.1% (51)	0.826					

APS-II acute physiology II, *AST* aspartate aminotransferase, *ASTmax* maximum AST value, *BMI* body mass index, *HH* hypoxic hepatitis, *IABP* intra-aortic balloon pump, *ICU* intensive care unit, *LOS* length of stay, *LV* left ventricle, *P* P value, *Q1* first quartile, *Q3* third quartile, *RV* right ventricle, *SAPS-II* simplified acute physiology II, *SOI* severity of illness, *T-ASTmax* time point of maximum AST value, *ULN* upper limit of normal

Italics indicate the significant *P* values

[a] % (*n*)

[b] Median (Q1–Q3)

[c] At T-ASTmax ± 12 h

Table 3 Characteristics of patients with HH classified by clinical cause

Variable	Cause							
	Cardiac failure (*n* = 548)	Septic shock (*n* = 333)	Hypovolemic shock (*n* = 105)	Acute respiratory failure (*n* = 71)	Acute on chronic respiratory failure (*n* = 37)	Pulmonary embolism (*n* = 16)	Hyperthermia (*n* = 6)	*P*
Sex[a]								
Male	63.1% (346)	61.6 (205)	57.1% (60)	54.9% (39)	54.1% (20)	62.5 (10)	66.7% (4)	0.721
Age[b] (year)	68.0 (58.0–76.0)	64.0 (52.0–74.0)	64.0 (56.0–73.0)	59.0 (48.5–71.5)	65.0 (61.0–72.0)	57.5 (47.5–61.5)	54.5 (35.8–64.2)	*0.003*
BMI[b] (kg/m^2)	25.5 (23.3–28.7)	25.0 (22.1–29.3)	26.2 (23.4–28.9)	24.2 (22.0–27.8)	24.6 (22.1–27.3)	27.8 (25.1–31.0)	27.6 (23.7–29.3)	0.202
Comorbidities								
Echocardio[a]								
Normal	32.7% (179)	51.1% (170)	43.8% (46)	36.6% (26)	48.6% (18)	18.8% (3)	66.7% (4)	*< 0.001*
LV dysf.	36.5% (200)	15.9% (53)	5.7% (6)	21.1% (15)	10.8% (4)	6.2% (1)	16.7% (1)	*< 0.001*
Missing	13.3% (73)	26.1% (87)	46.7% (49)	35.2% (25)	24.3% (9)	25.0% (4)	16.7% (1)	*< 0.001*
LV and RV dysf.	13.0% (71)	3.3% (11)	1.0% (1)	4.2% (3)	2.7% (1)	12.5% (2)	0.0% (0)	*< 0.001*
RV dysf.	4.6% (25)	3.6% (12)	2.9% (3)	2.8% (2)	13.5% (5)	37.5% (6)	0.0% (0	*< 0.001*
DM[a]	20.8% (114)	19.2% (64)	10.5% (11)	12.7% (9)	24.3% (9)	12.5% (2)	0.0% (0)	0.103
Chronic respiratory failure[a]	8.4% (46)	9.6% (32)	9.5% (10)	0.0% (%)	100.0% (37)	12.5% (2)	0.0% (0)	*< 0.001*
SOI scores[c]								
APS-II[b]	28.0 (23.0–35.0)	26.0 (21.0–35.0)	26.0 (18.5–32.5)	30.0 (28.0–34.0)	26.5 (24.2–30.8)	36.5 (36.2–36.8)	21.5 (19.2–25.0)	0.590
SAPS-II[b]	66.0 (44.0–79.0)	67.0 (49.0–84.0)	65.0 (48.0–82.0)	63.0 (31.0–79.0)	67.5 (55.0–73.5)	83.0 (69.2–99.2)	41.5 (34.0–48.2)	0.171
ASTmax[a]								
Overall								0.135
5–10× ULN	36.5% (200)	34.8% (116)	28.6% (30)	39.4% (28)	35.1% (13)	37.5% (6)	33.3% (2)	–
10–20× ULN	23.7% (130)	20.4% (68)	25.7% (27)	33.8% (24)	13.5% (5)	25.0% (4)	50.0% (3)	–
> 20× ULN	39.8% (218)	44.7% (149)	45.7% (48)	26.8% (19)	51.4% (19)	37.5% (6)	16.7% (1)	–
Supportive therapy[c]								
Ventilation[a]	79.2% (434)	73.0% (243)	70.5% (74)	60.6% (43)	64.9 (24)	75.0% (12)	100.0% (6)	*0.004*
Medication								
Inotropic agents[a]	63.1% (346)	26.4% (88)	21.0% (22)	12.7% (9)	21.6% (8)	43.8% (7)	33.3% (2)	*< 0.001*
Vasopressor agents[a]	58.6% (321)	69.1% (230)[d]	61.9% (65)	46.5% (33)	43.2% (16)	75.0% (12)	16.7% (1)	*< 0.001*
Dialysis[a]	10.4% (57)	11.1% (37)	2.9% (3)	9.9% (7)	2.7% (1)	0.0% (0)	16.7% (1)	0.090
IABP[a]	32.8% (180)	4.2% (14)	0.0% (0)	1.4% (1)	0.0% (0)	0.0% (0)	0.0% (0)	*< 0.001*
LOS								
ICU[b] (day)	4.6 (1.4–10.5)	4.7 (0.9–15.8)	2.6 (0.7–7.8)	6.3 (2.3–15.0)	3.2 (1.4–7.8)	2.2 (0.3–4.1)	7.7 (6.6–14.2)	0.135
Hospital[b] (day)	11.1 (4.6–25.7)	12.3 (1.1–37.9)	11.2 (0.9–28.8)	14.3 (5.2–30.2)	20.6 (7.6–27.7)	5.4 (0.3–19.4)	43.4 (10.2–97.4)	*0.037*
Duration								
Episode of HH[b] (h)	50.6 (24.9–99.3)	54.5 (25.1–87.2)	69.4 (36.8–89.5)	71.3 (39.0–90.0)	28.4 (15.1–77.2)	69.5 (28.0–139.0)	54.6 (35.4–74.0)	0.137

died within 24 h, its 28-day mortality of 41.4% ranked fourth among all subgroups. The acute respiratory failure and acute on chronic respiratory failure subgroups had similar survival curves and outcome, with 39.4 and 37.8% mortality at 28 days. The lowest mortality rate of 33.3% at 28 days was observed in the hyperthermia subgroup. The survival curves by cause of HH are presented in Fig. 2.

The 28-day mortality also increased significantly (P < 0.001) with severity of HH, ranging from 33.2% in the "5–10× ULN" subgroup to 55.4% in the "> 20× ULN"

Table 3 continued

Variable	Cause							
	Cardiac failure ($n=548$)	Septic shock ($n=333$)	Hypovolemic shock ($n=105$)	Acute respiratory failure ($n=71$)	Acute on chronic respiratory failure ($n=37$)	Pulmonary embolism ($n=16$)	Hyperthermia ($n=6$)	P
Recovery of HH[b] (h)	33.8 (3.4–67.5)	34.3 (14.3–60.9)	41.7 (21.1–65.1)	31.0 (16.2–62.1)	39.9 (11.6–89.3)	35.3 (10.5–65.4)	29.6 (21.7–43.3)	0.810
28-day mortality								
ICU[a]	37.8% (207)	48.3% (161)	40.0% (42)	33.8% (24)	27.0% (10)	56.2% (9)	33.3% (2)	*0.012*
In-hospital[a]	41.4% (227)	52.9% (176)	43.8% (46)	39.4% (28)	37.8% (14)	56.2% (9)	33.3% (2)	*0.029*

APS-II acute physiology II, *AST* aspartate aminotransferase, *ASTmax* maximum AST value, *BMI* body mass index, *HH* hypoxic hepatitis, *IABP* intra-aortic balloon pump, *ICU* intensive care unit, *LOS* length of stay, *LV* left ventricle, *P* P value, *Q1* first quartile, *Q3* third quartile, *RV* right ventricle, *SAPS-II* simplified acute physiology II, *SOI* severity of illness, *T-ASTmax* time point of maximum AST value, *ULN* upper limit of normal

[a] % (*n*)

[b] Median (Q1–Q3)

[c] At T-ASTmax ± 12 h

[d] A condition for septic shock was the need of vasopressor agents. In this table, the proportion of patients receiving vasopressor agents only at T-ASTmax is given

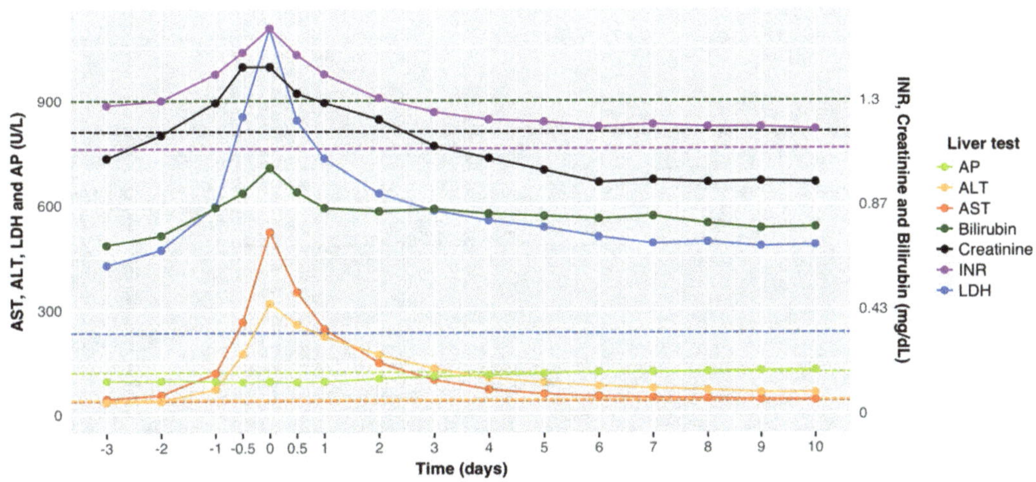

Fig. 3 Time trend of liver tests in hypoxic hepatitis. Time trend of the median AP, ALT, AST, bilirubin, creatinine, INR and LDH levels in hypoxic hepatitis. T-ASTmax is designated as time 0. AST, ALT, LDH and AP levels are measured in U/L and are plotted using the left *y*-axis. Bilirubin and creatinine levels are measured in mg/dL and plotted using the right y-axis. INR has no unit, but is also plotted using the right *y*-axis. *AP* alkaline phosphatase, *ALT* alanine aminotransferase, *AST* aspartate aminotransferase, *INR* international normalized ratio, *LDH* lactate dehydrogenase

subgroup. There was no significant difference ($P=0.363$) in 28-day mortality between men (39.8%) and women (42.4%).

Discussion

Hypoxic hepatitis is a type of acute hepatic injury in critically ill patients caused by cardiac, circulatory or respiratory failure. While commonly known and referred to as "shock liver" in daily clinical practice, little research has been done. However, early recognition of HH and management of its underlying cause and complications may improve ultimate outcome. For a long time, only studies with a relatively small number of patients have been conducted. In 2015, a meta-analysis of 24 studies that included 1782 patients summarized the available evidence, but still lacked detailed information on important patient characteristics, biochemical findings and clinical course [2]. To overcome these shortcomings, Aboelsoud et al. recently performed an extensive analysis of the Medical Information Mart for Intensive Care III

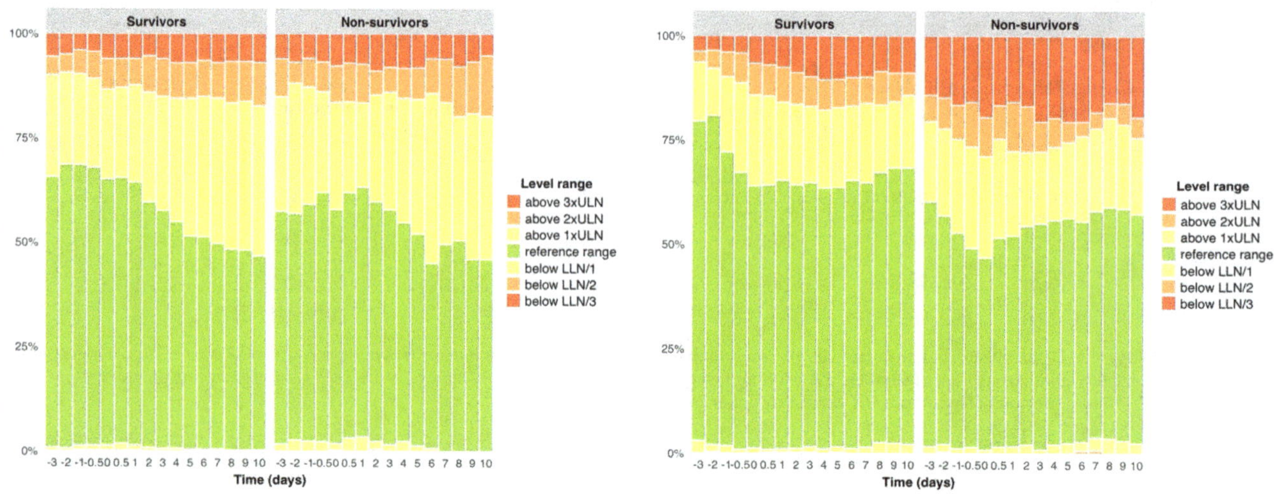

Fig. 4 a AP level range over time; **b** bilirubin level range over time. Evolution of the proportion of survivors and non-survivors with alkaline phosphatase (left) and bilirubin (right) levels within and outside the reference range. T-ASTmax is designated as time 0. *AP* alkaline phosphatase, *LLN* lower limit of normal, *ULN* upper limit of normal

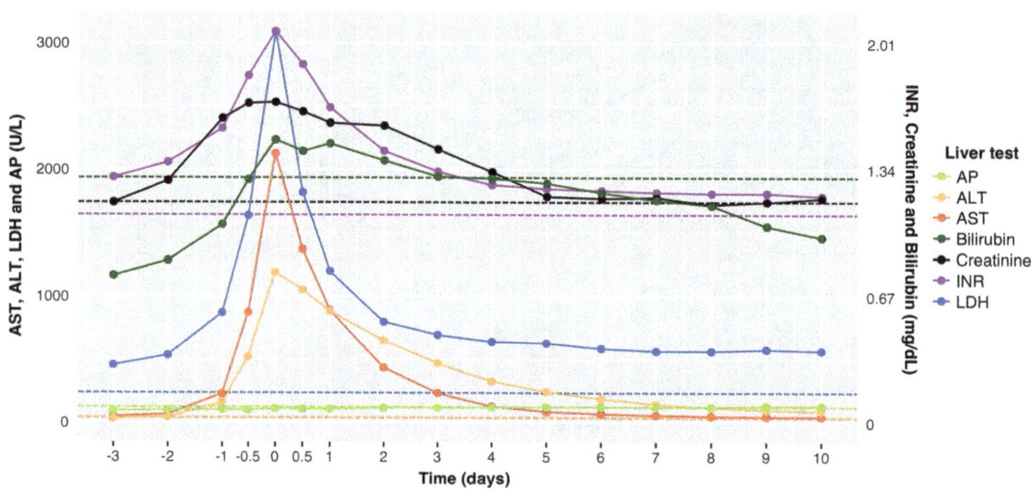

Fig. 5 Time trend of liver tests in hypoxic hepatitis of the ASTmax subgroup 5-10x ULN. Time trend of the median AP, ALT, AST, bilirubin, creatinine, INR and LDH levels in hypoxic hepatitis. T-ASTmax is designated as time 0. AST, ALT, LDH and AP levels are measured in U/L and are plotted using the left y-axis. Bilirubin and creatinine levels are measured in mg/dL and plotted using the right y-axis. INR has no unit, but is also plotted using the right y-axis. AP alkaline phosphatase, ALT alanine aminotransferase, AST aspartate aminotransferase, INR international normalized ratio, LDH lactate dehydrogenase

(MIMIC-III) research database. Their study comprised 565 patients with HH and was the largest cohort study published to date [8].

In our study of 1116 critically ill patients with HH, we investigated in detail its incidence, causes, evolution and outcome. We used an AST cutoff of at least 5 times the ULN (i.e., 155 and 185 U/L for females and males, respectively) to define HH, while other studies have used higher cutoff values ranging from 400 to 3000 U/L [2]. HH has been histologically proven to occur even in patients with moderately elevated AST levels (at AST levels of 252 and 300 IU/L in the cohort of Cohen et al. [13] and Bynum et al. [14], respectively). Additionally, by using a lower cutoff, the sensitivity to identify patients with HH could be increased. However, this approach could also result in a lower specificity, leading to an increased number of patients that are falsely diagnosed as having HH. In order to maintain a high specificity, we have thoroughly reviewed the clinical notes, the time trend of liver tests and the discharge summaries of the 4012 identified

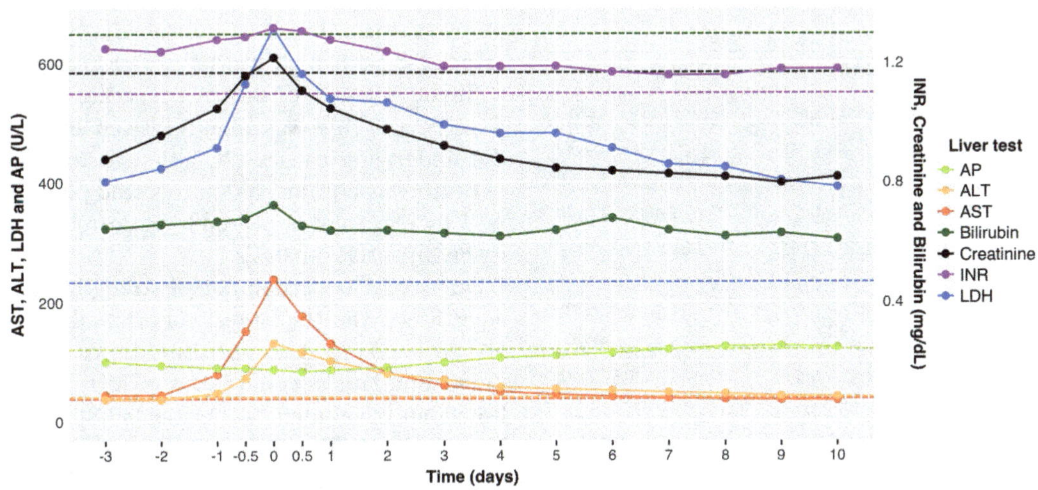

Fig. 6 Time trend of liver tests in hypoxic hepatitis of the ASTmax subgroup 10-20x ULN. Time trend of the median AP, ALT, AST, bilirubin, creatinine, INR and LDH levels in hypoxic hepatitis. T-ASTmax is designated as time 0. AST, ALT, LDH and AP levels are measured in U/L and are plotted using the left y-axis. Bilirubin and creatinine levels are measured in mg/dL and plotted using the right y-axis. INR has no unit, but is also plotted using the right y-axis. AP alkaline phosphatase, ALT alanine aminotransferase, AST aspartate aminotransferase, INR international normalized ratio, LDH lactate dehydrogenase

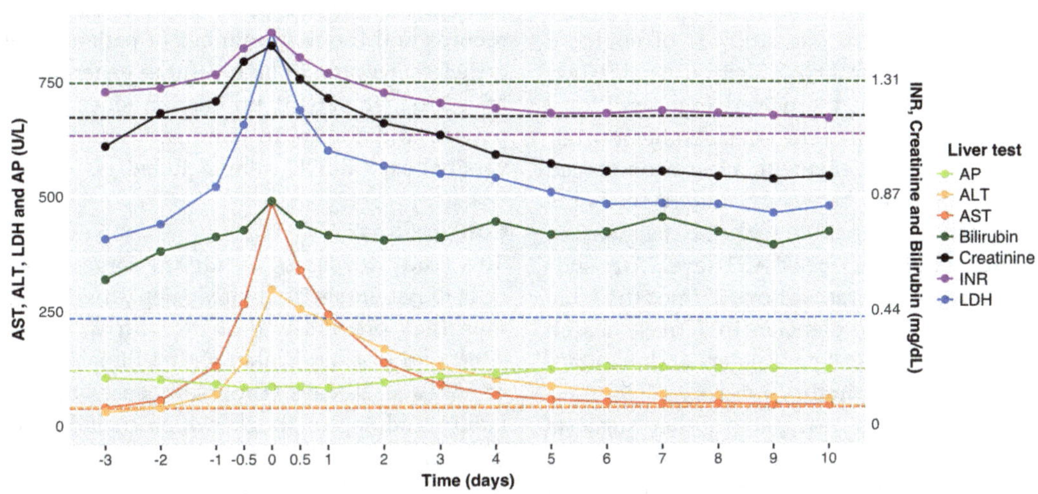

Fig. 7 Time trend of liver tests in hypoxic hepatitis of the ASTmax subgroup >20x ULN. Time trend of the median AP, ALT, AST, bilirubin, creatinine, INR and LDH levels in hypoxic hepatitis. T-ASTmax is designated as time 0. AST, ALT, LDH and AP levels are measured in U/L and are plotted using the left y-axis. Bilirubin and creatinine levels are measured in mg/dL and plotted using the right y-axis. INR has no unit, but is also plotted using the right y-axis. AP alkaline phosphatase, ALT alanine aminotransferase, AST aspartate aminotransferase, INR international normalized ratio, LDH lactate dehydrogenase

patients whose AST level exceeded our cutoff value. Our high number of excluded patients (70.0%) after applying extensive exclusion criteria may reflect a high specificity. In contrast, Aboelsoud et al. [8] used a cutoff of 800 U/L for both AST and ALT to include patients, but only excluded 24.3% of these patients based on evidence of acetaminophen poisoning, acute viral hepatitis or liver surgery.

Our study uncovered interesting results. Firstly, it indicated that HH may be more common than previously thought. In our study, an incidence of 4.0% was observed, which is higher than the pooled incidence of 2.5% from a meta-analysis of 1782 patients [2] and the incidence of 1.5% in the MIMIC-III cohort [8]. Moreover, approximately one in five critically ill patients that have died during their ICU stay had developed HH. This

Table 4 Median laboratory values (Q1–Q3) at different time stages

Variable	At start of HH	At T-ASTmax
AST (U/L)	185.0 (155.0–185.0)	521.2 (269.1–1581.6)
ALT (U/L)	120.8 (70.1–193.5)	317.0 (143.5–924.5)
LDH (U/L)	691.8 (465.8–1025.7)	1106.4 (624.8–2602.8)
Bilirubin (mg/dL)	0.8 (0.5–1.6)	1.0 (0.6–2.0)
GGT (U/L)	73.1 (36.2–160.4)	82.5 (41.7–167.0)
AP (U/L)	88.2 (61.8–150.9)	94.0 (62.9–167.0)
Lipase (U/L)	32.4 (18.9–58.9)	33.5 (18.5–66.4)
INR	1.4 (1.2–1.8)	1.6 (1.3–2.2)
PC (10^3/μL)	165.7 (103.6–241.0)	146.0 (79.5–218.0)
WBC (10^3/μL)	12.5 (8.8–17.6)	13.2 (9.0–18.5)
Hb (g/dL)	10.1 (8.8–12.0)	9.8 (8.6–11.5)
CK (U/L)	214.0 (77.2–747.2)	322.2 (105.1–1102.9)
Creatinine (mg/dL)	1.4 (0.9–2.1)	1.4 (0.9–2.2)
Urea (mg/dL)	57.1 (38.9–91.3)	61.6 (40.6–96.4)
Lactate (mg/dL)	31.3 (16.2–62.2)	27.4 (14.7–56.2)

AP alkaline phosphatase, *ALT* alanine aminotransferase, *AST* aspartate aminotransferase, *CK* creatine kinase, *GGT* gamma-glutamyl transpeptidase, *Hb* hemoglobin, *INR* international normalized ratio, *LDH* lactate dehydrogenase, *PC* platelet count, *WBC* white blood cell count

higher incidence observed in our study is of course a direct consequence of the lower AST cutoff used. However, it should be noted that the underlying conditions, the typical liver test pattern and the considerable mortality of 33.2% at 28 days in patients with a less pronounced rise of AST (peak AST level between 5 and 10 times the ULN) are just as much compatible with the diagnosis of HH as in patients with higher peak AST level. Any sudden increase in aminotransferases above 5 times the ULN should therefore prompt the clinician to actively search for any changes in physiological parameters and maintain strict hemodynamic and respiratory control.

Secondly, the typical liver test pattern that suggests diagnosis of HH was observed in all subgroups of our study cohort. HH was characterized by (1) a sudden and significant increase of aminotransferases with an AST/ALT ratio greater than 1, (2) a similar rise in LDH mostly exceeding both AST and ALT and (3) a steady decline of aminotransferases with reversal of the AST/ALT ratio approximately 1.5 days after T-ASTmax. In survivors, LDH normalized first, followed by AST and finally ALT (median of 5.1, 6.4 and 8.6 days after T-ASTmax, respectively). Bilirubin followed a similar pattern as the aminotransferases, but the magnitude of its increase was much less pronounced, with median levels never exceeding the ULN. The associated prolongation of INR and impairment of renal function as described by Raurich et al. [6] were also confirmed in this study.

Finally, we observed a 28-day mortality of 45.0%, which is in line with the reported mortality of 49% from a meta-analysis of 1782 patients [2] and the mortality of 44.1% in the MIMIC-III cohort [8]. HH was especially associated with high mortality rates early in its course, with roughly 40% of deaths occurring within 24 h after T-ASTmax. This was mainly driven by the severity of the underlying causes [2], although the ultimate cause of death was not inferred in this study. The magnitude of AST increase also appeared to be correlated with mortality on univariate analysis.

Our study has a number of strengths. To our knowledge, it is by far the largest cohort study of patients with HH ($n = 1116$). It comprises twice as many patients as the second largest cohort study, which was recently published and included 565 patients [8]. Additionally, by using a low AST cutoff of 5 times the ULN while simultaneously excluding many conditions that could mimic HH, we are confident that we could identify nearly all patients with HH at our center with a low risk of misdiagnosis. Our study may have some limitations inherent in its retrospective design. However, we believe that the retrospective design had little to no impact on our results given the entirely computerized monitoring and management at our ICU, the detailed review of patient records and the high number of patients included. Nevertheless, we should be careful to generalize these results to a broader patient population since only critically ill patients older than 18 years and only from a single university hospital ICU were included.

Conclusions

This study surpasses by far the largest cohort of critically ill patients with hypoxic hepatitis. HH is more common than previously thought with an ICU incidence of 4.0%, and it is associated with a high all-cause mortality of 45.0% at 28 days. The main causes of HH are cardiac failure and septic shock, which include more than 3/4 of all episodes. Clinicians should search actively for any underlying hemodynamic or respiratory instability even in patients with moderately increased AST levels.

Abbreviations

HH: hypoxic hepatitis; AST: aspartate aminotransferase; ICU: intensive care unit; ALT: alanine aminotransferase; LDH: lactate dehydrogenase; ULN: upper limit of normal; CK: creatine kinase; AP: alkaline phosphatase; INR: international normalized ratio; BMI: body mass index; APS-II: acute physiology II; SAPS-II: simplified acute physiology II; T-ASTmax: time point of maximum AST value; ASTmax: maximum AST value; Q1: first quartile; Q3: third quartile; MIMIC-III: Medical Information Mart for Intensive Care III.

Authors' contributions

AV and LV designed the study, collected data, performed and interpreted statistical analysis, and drafted the manuscript. Both authors contributed equally to this study and are the joint first authors. AD performed and interpreted statistical analysis, and drafted the manuscript. KC, HV and DB designed the study and revised the manuscript. JD designed the study, interpreted statistical analysis and revised the manuscript. All authors read and approved the final manuscript.

Author details

[1] Faculty of Medicine and Health Sciences, Ghent University, Ghent, Belgium. [2] Department of Internal Medicine, Ghent University Hospital, Ghent, Belgium. [3] Department of Intensive Care Medicine, Ghent University Hospital, De Pintelaan 185, 9000 Ghent, Belgium. [4] Department of Hepatology and Gastro-Enterology, Ghent University Hospital, Ghent, Belgium.

Acknowledgements

Not applicable.

Competing interests

The authors declare that they have no competing interests.

Funding

None.

References

1. Henrion J. Hypoxic hepatitis. Liver Int. 2012;32(7):1039–52.
2. Tapper EB, Sengupta N, Bonder A. The incidence and outcomes of ischemic hepatitis: a systematic review with meta-analysis. Am J Med. 2015;128(12):1314–21.
3. Henrion J, Schapira M, Luwaert R, Colin L, Delannoy A, Heller FR. Hypoxic hepatitis: clinical and hemodynamic study in 142 consecutive cases. Medicine (Baltimore). 2003;82(6):392–406.
4. Birrer R, Takuda Y, Takara T. Hypoxic hepatopathy: pathophysiology and prognosis. Intern Med. 2007;46(14):1063–70.
5. Fuhrmann V, Kneidinger N, Herkner H, Heinz G, Nikfardjam M, Bojic A, et al. Hypoxic hepatitis: underlying conditions and risk factors for mortality in critically ill patients. Intensive Care Med. 2009;35(8):1397–405.
6. Raurich JM, Llompart-Pou JA, Ferreruela M, Colomar A, Molina M, Royo C, et al. Hypoxic hepatitis in critically ill patients: incidence, etiology and risk factors for mortality. J Anesth. 2011;25(1):50–6.
7. Fuchs S, Bogomolski-Yahalom V, Paltiel O, Ackerman Z. Ischemic hepatitis: clinical and laboratory observations of 34 patients. J Clin Gastroenterol. 1998;26(3):183–6.
8. Aboelsoud MM, Javaid AI, Al-Qadi MO, Lewis JH. Hypoxic hepatitis—its biochemical profile, causes and risk factors of mortality in critically-ill patients: a cohort study of 565 patients. J Crit Care. 2017;41:9–15.
9. Dunn GD, Hayes P, Breen KJ, Schenker S. The liver in congestive heart failure: a review. Am J Med Sci. 1973;265(3):174–89.
10. Ebert EC. Hypoxic liver injury. Mayo Clin Proc. 2006;81(9):1232–6.
11. Whitehead MW, Hawkes ND, Hainsworth I, Kingham JG. A prospective study of the causes of notably raised aspartate aminotransferase of liver origin. Gut. 1999;45(1):129–33.
12. Johnson RD, O'Connor ML, Kerr RM. Extreme serum elevations of aspartate aminotransferase. Am J Gastroenterol. 1995;90(8):1244–5.
13. Bynum TE, Boitnott JK, Maddrey WC. Ischemic hepatitis. Dig Dis Sci. 1979;24(2):129–35.
14. Cohen JA, Kaplan MM. Left-sided heart failure presenting as hepatitis. Gastroenterology. 1978;74(3):583–7.
15. Core Team R. R: a language and environment for statistical computing. Vienna: R Foundation for Statistical Computing; 2016.

19

Clinical assessment and train-of-four measurements in critically ill patients treated with recommended doses of cisatracurium or atracurium for neuromuscular blockade

Pierre Bouju[1,2], Jean-Marc Tadié[1,2,4], Nicolas Barbarot[3], Julien Letheulle[1,2], Fabrice Uhel[1,2,4], Pierre Fillatre[1,2], Guillaume Grillet[1], Angélique Goepp[3], Yves Le Tulzo[1,2,4] and Arnaud Gacouin[1,2,4*]

Abstract

Background: Despite few studies, a monitoring of a neuromuscular blockade with a train of four (TOF) is recommended in intensive care unit (ICU). Our objective was to compare the results of ulnar and facial TOF measurements with an overall clinical assessment for neuromuscular blockade in ICU patients treated with recommended doses of atracurium or cisatracurium, including patients with acute respiratory disease syndrome (ARDS).

Methods: We prospectively included in two ICUs 119 patients, 94 with ARDS, who required a neuromuscular blockade for more than 24 h. Three levels of neuromuscular blockade were defined: "over-paralyzed" (TOF = 0), "well-paralyzed" (TOF = 1–2), and "under-paralyzed" (TOF = 3–4). Physicians blinded for TOF counts were asked to classify patients clinically as "over-paralyzed," "well-paralyzed," or "under-paralyzed". Patients were assessed two times daily.

Results: For the whole population 996 ulnar and facial TOF measurements and clinical assessments were obtained (846 with cisatracurium and 150 with atracurium). Proportions of patients classified as over-paralyzed, well-paralyzed, and under-paralyzed based on TOF measurements and clinical assessments differed significantly ($p < 0.0001$). The number of observed agreements between clinical assessments and facial TOF measurements was of 19.08% ($\kappa = 0.06$) and of 17.37% with ulnar TOF measurements ($\kappa = 0.04$), while it was of 62.75% between ulnar and facial TOF measurements ($\kappa = 0.45$). Results were similar for cisatracurium and atracurium. Repeated facial TOF measurements performed on the first 4 days of mechanical ventilation in ARDS patients showed that the proportion of patients TOF = 1–2 was around 8% and did not vary significantly with time ($p = 0.9$), proportion of patients TOF = 3–4 increased from 24 to 40% ($p = 0.01$), proportion of patients TOF = 0 decreased from 71 to 53% ($p = 0.005$) while objectives for protective ventilation were achieved. Proportions of facial and ulnar TOF = 0 were significantly higher among patients with ICU-acquired weakness (ICU-AW) versus those who did not develop ICU-AW (51 vs. 40%, $p = 0.03$, and 76 vs. 62%, $p = 0.006$, respectively).

Conclusions: The study provides data on clinical and TOF monitoring of neuromuscular blockade, which are widely divergent in ICU patients receiving recommended doses of benzylisoquinoliniums.

Keywords: Intensive care unit, Muscular weakness, Neuromuscular blockade, Train-of-four monitoring, Benzylisoquinoliniums

*Correspondence: arnaud.gacouin@chu-rennes.fr
[1] Service des Maladies Infectieuses et Réanimation Médicale, CHU Rennes, 2 rue Henri Le Guilloux, 35033 Rennes, France
Full list of author information is available at the end of the article

Background

Neuromuscular blocking agents (NMBAs) are often used in association with adequate analgesia and sedation for the following conditions: management and facilitation of mechanical ventilation (MV), management of elevated intracranial or intraabdominal pressure, treatment of muscle spasms, and reduction in oxygen consumption [1, 2]. Recently, NMBAs became common intravenous medications used within the intensive care unit (ICU) since Papazian et al. [3] enhanced the role of NMBAs when they found a beneficial effect of a neuromuscular blockade on the mortality in acute respiratory distress syndrome (ARDS). The previous recommendations of the American and French critical care societies for sustained neuromuscular blockade are of C grade for indications and of B grade for monitoring [2, 4]. In the clinical practice guidelines for sustained neuromuscular blockade in the adult critically ill patient published in 2016 [5], NMBAs are suggested in ARDS patients with a ratio PaO2/FiO2 less than 150 (weak recommendation) but no dosage is mentioned. All these recommendations [2, 4, 5] suggest that in ICU patients the appropriate depth of neuromuscular block may be variable and depends on the reason for neuromuscular blockade, the expected patient outcome, and the phase of the disease. Monitoring the depth of a neuromuscular blockade with peripheral nerve stimulation (PNS) is recommended only in combination with a clinical assessment by critical care societies [2, 4, 5]. The most commonly used tool is the train of four (TOF), and previous recommendations suggest dosing titration of NMBAs to one or two visualized muscle twitches [2, 4]. Of note, in the study of Papazian et al. [3], PNS was not permitted and in the 2016 practice guidelines [5] no TOF objective is recommended. North American surveys performed in the 2000s reported that 84–91% of physicians used PNS for monitoring but also that neuromuscular blockade practices varied greatly between intensive care units (ICUs) [6, 7]. Using TOF monitoring in the ICU may result in a reduction of NMBAs' dose and a subsequent decrease risk of complications related to prolonged and/or excessive blockade, such as intensive care unit-acquired weakness (ICU-AW) [8, 9]. The benefits and limitations of TOF stimulation were primarily determined from studies performed in operative room patients [10, 11], with results that may not be generalizable to ICU patients. In critically ill patients, the duration of neuromuscular blockade is longer, sepsis and/or shock is often present, and pharmacokinetic is difficult to predict [12–14]. Lastly, agreement between subjective and objective means of assessing the degree of neuromuscular blockade has been little studied in ICU [15–17]. Thus, we designed a prospective observational study in two ICUs using NMBAs with infusion rates following recommendations with the aims (1) to describe and compare TOF measurements obtained at ulnar and facial sites with clinical evaluation of depth blockade, (2) to focus on the results obtained in ARDS patients with time analysis, and (3) to evaluate when available muscle strength 7 days after awakening the patient.

Methods

Patients and setting

The study was conducted between April 1, 2014, and March 31, 2015, in two different ICUs: in a 21-bed medical ICU in Rennes University Hospital (center 1) and in a 14-bed mixed medical-surgical ICU in Saint-Brieuc General Hospital (center 2). The study was approved by the Rennes University Hospital's ethic committee (No. 14-17), and no informed consent was required because of the observational nature of the study. A non-opposition form was provided to families.

All patients aged over 18 years with a planned duration of a neuromuscular blockade for more than 24 h were screened, and those treated at least 24 h with NMBAs were finally included for analysis. Exclusion criteria were contraindications to NMBAs (malignant hyperthermia, history of anaphylaxis with NMBAs), the inability to assess muscle strength or TOF count (neuromuscular disease, admission for cardiac arrest, body core temperature below 36.5 °C), pregnancy, moribund state, decision to withhold life-sustaining treatment, refusal of the family, and continuous infusion of NMBAs for more than 12 h before screening.

Neuromuscular blockade

Before neuromuscular blockade, sedatives and opioids were titrated by nurses according to the Ramsay Sedation Scale in center 1 [18] with an objective of 6 and the Richmond Agitation Sedation Scale in center 2 [19] with an objective of −5. There was no daily sedation interruption. Sedatives used were midazolam or propofol, and opioids used were sufentanil or morphine. The NMBAs used were benzylisoquinoliniums: cisatracurium in center 1 and atracurium in center 2. Boluses and initial infusion rates followed the 2002 and 2008 recommendations using patient's body weight on admission: 0.15 ± 0.05 and 0.5 ± 0.2 mg kg^{-1} h^{-1} for cisatracurium and atracurium, respectively [2, 4]. The management of the neuromuscular blockade was left to the physician in charge, who was blinded about results of the TOF, according to its clinical evaluation. Total doses, durations of treatment, and NMBAs' infusion rates were recorded daily.

The PNS used were TOF-Watch-S® (Organon Ltd., Dublin, Ireland) in center 1, and Innervator® (Fisher-Paykel Health Care, Baxter, Maurepas, France) in center 2. The TOF delivers 4 supramaximal electrical impulses that involve four equally strong twitches of the stimulated muscle. A fade of the twitches appears when the neuromuscular blockade increases [10, 11]. To homogenize practices, both neuromuscular monitors were used in the same way, without acceleromyography: the intensity of the stimulating current was set at 50 mA, and the TOF count was visually assessed. After cleaning the skin, monitoring of the neuromuscular blockade was performed using surface electrodes (Red Dot®, 3M Health Care, Neuss, Germany) on the temporal branch of the facial nerve and on the ulnar nerve at the wrist, with assessment of twitches of the orbicularis oculi and adductor pollicis muscles, respectively [20, 21]. The presence or absence of edema was noted before each measurement. Electrodes were changed at least once per day. Monitoring was performed twice a day by one of the investigators. At each assessment, we asked the senior physician in charge, blinded about results of the TOF, to evaluate comprehensively the depth of muscle relaxation as "over-paralyzed," "well-paralyzed," or "under-paralyzed." In both ICUs, the clinical assessment was based on the attentive observation of patient's movements, ventilator asynchronies, respiratory pressures, and presence of cough or not [22]. Measurements of the TOF on the ulnar nerve were performed arbitrary 4 h after the end of the infusion of the NMBAs, that is beyond five elimination half-lives, to record residual paralysis, and patients with TOF < 4 were reassessed at 8 h.

Data collection

The following variables were recorded: age, gender, body mass index, Simplified Acute Physiologic Score II [23], and Sequential Organ Failure Assessment the day of NMBA initiation [24]. In addition, comorbidities, which could affect the pharmacokinetics of NMBAs or risk of ICU-AW, were noted: diabetes mellitus, cirrhosis, renal disease, corticosteroid treatment [1, 25]. We also noted the reasons for ICU admission and neuromuscular blockade, total doses, and duration of hypnotics and opioids.

All ARDS patients received protective ventilation and were ventilated as follows: assist-control mode, initial tidal volume targeted at 6 mL per kilogram of predicted body weight, positive end-expiratory pressure (PEEP) level was selected from the PEEP-FiO2 table proposed by the ARDS network [26], and end-inspiratory pressure was measured to be kept below 30 cm of water. Therefore, we recorded the major components of these parameters at the time of each measurement, i.e., the plateau pressure, the calculated driving pressure, and the ratio of the partial pressure of arterial oxygen (PaO2) to the fraction of inspired oxygen (FiO2). Of the treatments received, we noted the duration of catecholamines and use of renal replacement therapy. Duration of MV, duration of ICU and hospital stay, ICU and hospital mortality were finally recorded.

Muscle strength was evaluated with the use of the Medical Research Council (MRC) scale, 7 days after awakening the patient, as previously described [27]. This scale assesses six muscle groups, with a score for each group from 0 (paralysis) to 5 (normal strength). ICU-AW was defined by an overall score of less than 48/60 [27].

Definitions and endpoints

Based on 2002 and 2008 recommendations [2, 4], three levels of neuromuscular blockade were determined: "over-paralyzed" defined by a TOF = 0/4, "well-paralyzed" defined by a TOF = 1–2/4, and "under-paralyzed" defined by a TOF = 3–4/4. At each measurement, the patient was classified in one of the three categories for the facial and the ulnar sites. Regarding clinical assessment, physicians were asked to judge the adequacy of the muscle relaxation, taking into account the clinical context. Consequently in some cases depth of neuromuscular blockade could be considered as excessive by some physicians.

The primary endpoint was to compare the proportions of patients classified as "over-paralyzed," "well-paralyzed," or "under-paralyzed" between the ulnar and facial TOF and physicians' clinical assessment and to assess agreements between measurements. The secondary endpoints included an analysis of trends in the TOF values over time and comparisons of recorded plateau pressures, calculated driving pressures, and PaO2/FiO2 ratios according to the facial TOF levels in the subgroup of ARDS patients. The third endpoint was to determine whether results for TOF measurements were associated with ICU-AW.

Statistical analysis

Continuous variables were expressed as medians and interquartile ranges and were compared using a non-parametric Mann–Whitney *U* test or a Kruskal–Wallis test. Categorical variables were expressed as numbers and percentages and were compared using a Chi-square test or a Fisher exact test and a Chi-square test for trends when required. The tests were two-sided, and we considered a p value of less than 0.05 to be statistically significant. Treating the levels of neuromuscular blockade as categorical, a kappa statistic was calculated to analyze the agreement between the facial TOF measurements, the ulnar TOF measurements, and the clinical assessments. Statistical analyses were performed using MedCalc, version 11.3.3.0 (MedCalc Software, Mariakerke, Belgium).

Results

Patients' characteristics

During the study period, 254 patients who received NMBAs were screened for the study. Of these patients,

134 could not be included. One of the 120 patients included was finally excluded because of a chronic neurological disease unknown at the time of inclusion (Fig. 1). Of the 119 patients included in the study, 97 (82%) patients were hospitalized in center 1 and 22 (18%) in center 2. The main characteristics of the patients are shown and distinguished according to the inclusion center in Table 1. The main reason for the neuromuscular blockade was ARDS. Patients differed significantly between the two centers for main reason for ICU admission and neuromuscular blockade. Of note, all patients in center 1 received cisatracurium and all patients in center 2 received atracurium.

For the whole population, the duration of invasive MV was 11 days [7–24]; the length of stay in the ICU was 14 days [8–26]; and the length of stay in the hospital was 27 days [15–56]. Forty-seven (39%) patients died in the ICU, and 6 (5%) additional patients died in the hospital. ICU mortality rates did not differ between centers after comparison ($p = 0.15$).

Neuromuscular blockade

At inclusion, the NMBA infusion rates were 0.18 mg kg^{-1} h^{-1} [0.16–0.22] for cisatracurium and 0.52 mg kg^{-1} h^{-1} [0.47–0.63] for atracurium. For the whole population, the median duration of the NMBA infusion was 67 h [38–121], without differences between the two centers (64 h [38–124] for center 1 vs. 85 h [40–118] for center 2, $p = 0.37$). At the end of the NMBA infusion, the ulnar TOF was performed in all the assessable patients ($n = 98$). Six (6%) had TOF < 4 at 4 h. Of them, 4 could be reassessed at 8 h, and they all had a TOF of 4/4.

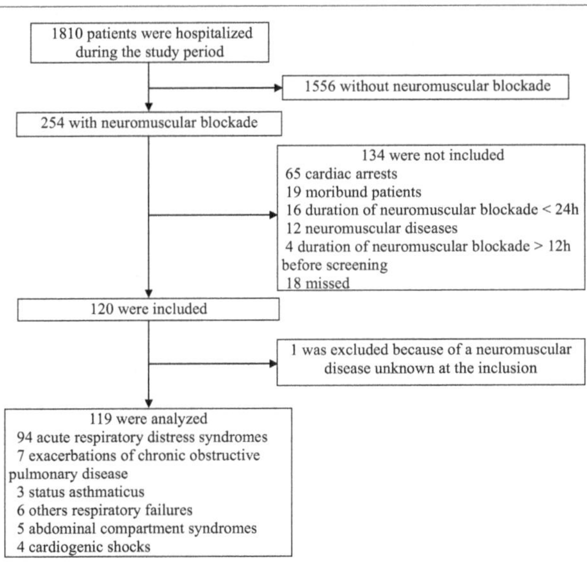

Fig. 1 Flowchart of patients

Comparisons between TOF measurements and clinical assessments

On the whole population 996 TOF facial and ulnar measurements and 996 clinical assessments were performed, 846 groups of measurements in patients receiving cisatracurium (center 1) and 150 groups of measurements in patients receiving atracurium (center 2).

On the whole population proportions of patients classified as "over-paralyzed," "well-paralyzed," or "under-paralyzed" differed significantly when results for clinical assessments were compared with results obtained with facial and ulnar TOF measurements (Fig. 2). Based on clinical assessment patients were considered to have adequate muscle relaxation nearly 9 out of 10 times while only 1 patient out of 10 was considered well-paralyzed according to TOF measurements. Statistical results were similar whether comparisons were performed on the whole population or in subgroups of patients receiving cisatracurium or atracurium (Additional file 1: Table S1).

When compared, results obtained with facial and ulnar TOF measurements differed significantly. Compared to results obtained at ulnar site, patients were classified twice as often under-paralyzed based on results obtained at facial site.

Of note, edema did not modify TOF values since there was no difference in patients with edema compared to patients without edema (data not shown).

Agreement between TOF measurements and clinical assessments

Based on kappa statistic, we found similar levels of agreement for comparisons between TOF measurements and clinical assessments in center 1 and center 2 (Additional file 2: Tables S2a–S2i). When the whole population was considered, the number of observed agreements was 190 (19.08%) ($\kappa = 0.06$) between clinical assessments and facial TOF measurements and of 173 (17.37%) ($\kappa = 0.04$) between clinical assessments and ulnar TOF measurements. The level of agreement was slightly higher for comparison between facial und ulnar measurements since the number of observed agreements was of 625 (62.75%) ($\kappa = 0.45$).

Subgroup analysis on ARDS patients

We analyzed data recorded on the first 4 days of MV for time analysis. Results for clinical assessments did not vary significantly with time. Based on ulnar and facial TOF measurements, from day 0 to day 3 of MV the proportion of patients considered "well-paralyzed" did not vary significantly while the proportion of

Table 1 Patients' characteristics at the inclusion

Characteristics	All patients $N = 119$	Center 1 (cisatracurium use) $N = 97$	Center 2 (atracurium use) $N = 22$
Age (years)	62 (52–73)	62 (51–72)	63 (52–73)
Male [*n* (%)]	78 (66)	61 (63)	17 (77)
Body mass index (kg/m^2)	25.5 (23.4–29.6)	25.3 (23.1–29.6)	26.6 (23.7–32.2)
SAPS II (points)	51 (40–62)	50 (40–62)	51 (44–60)
SOFA (points)	9 (6–12)	9 (7–12)	9 (6–12)
Length of stay before ICU (days)	1 (0–4)	1 (0–4)	1 (0–3)
Main reason for ICU admission [*n* (%)]			
Medical	111 (93)	93 (96)	18 (82)*
Surgical	8 (7)	4 (4)	4 (18)
Main reason for neuromuscular blockade [*n* (%)]			
ARDS	94 (79)	78 (80)	16 (73)*
Exacerbations of COPD	7 (6)	5 (5)	2 (9)
Status asthmaticus	3 (3)	3 (3)	0
Other respiratory failures	6 (5)	5 (5)	1 (4.5)
Abdominal compartment syndromes	5 (4)	2 (2)	3 (13.5)
Miscellaneous	4 (3)	4 (4)	0
Main comorbidities [*n* (%)]			
Diabetes	16 (13)	14 (14)	2 (9)
Renal disease	8 (7)	7 (7)	1 (5)
Cirrhosis	16 (13)	14 (14)	2 (9)
Corticosteroid treatment	12 (10)	11 (11)	1 (5)
Sepsis [*n* (%)]	85 (71)	68 (70)	17 (77)
Catecholamines [*n* (%)]	78 (66)	62 (64)	16 (73)
Renal replacement therapy [*n* (%)]	9 (8)	6 (6)	3 (14)

Continuous variables are reported as medians and interquartile ranges (25th–75th percentiles), and categorical variables as numbers and percentages

SAPS II Simplified Acute Physiologic Score II, *SOFA* Sequential Organ Failure Assessment, *ICU* intensive care unit, *ARDS* acute respiratory distress syndrome, *COPD* chronic obstructive pulmonary disease

* $p < 0.05$ center 1 versus center 2

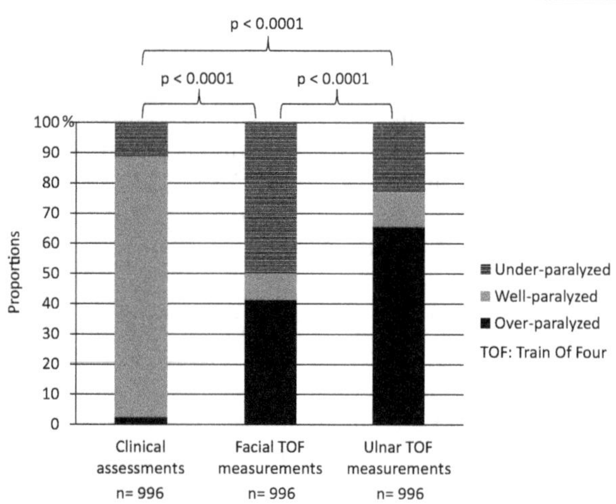

Fig. 2 Comparison of results obtained by the train of four and the clinical assessment of neuromuscular blockade recorded over the entire study period

patients "under-paralyzed" increased significantly. The proportion of patients "over-paralyzed" decreased significantly with time according to facial TOF measurements and tended to decrease significantly according to ulnar measurements (Fig. 3). Similar results were found whether patients received cisatracurium or atracurium (Additional file 3: Table S3). When PaO2/FiO2 ratios, plateau pressures, and calculated driving pressures were compared daily between the three different levels of neuromuscular blockade defined by the facial measurements of the TOF on the first 4 days of MV, no significant difference was found (Table 2). The daily dose of cisatracurium used in center 1 increased from 150 mg (90–240, day 0) to 300 mg (166–330, day 3) ($p < 0.01$ after comparison), and the daily dose of atracurium used in center 2 increased from 219 mg (153–235, day 0) to 362 mg (217–454, day 3) ($p = 0.03$ after comparison).

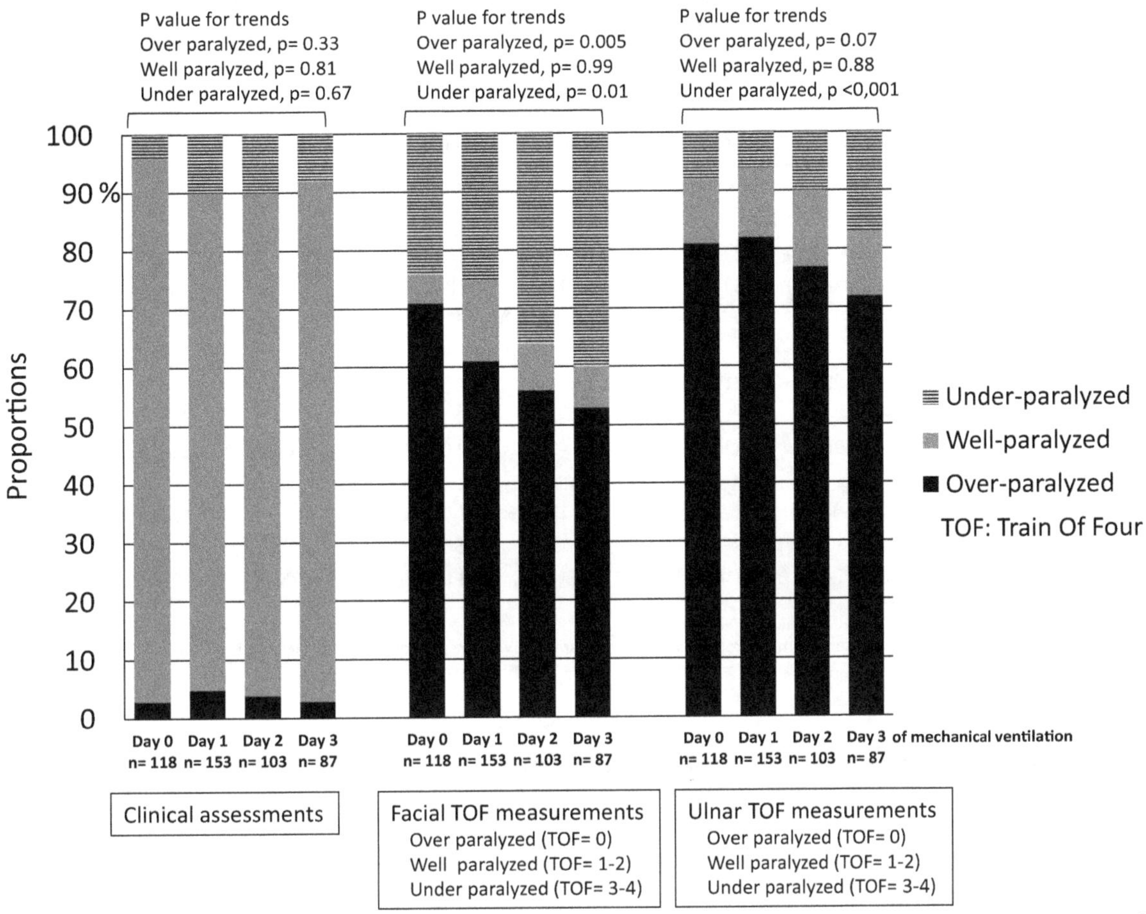

Fig. 3 Clinical, facial, and ulnar train-of-four (TOF) measurements recorded on the first 4 days of mechanical ventilation from the diagnosis of ARDS

ICU-acquired weakness 7 days after awakening the patient

The MRC score could be assessed in 47 patients who were able to follow commands 7 days after awakening. ICU-AW was diagnosed in 14 patients (30%). After comparisons between patients with and without ICU-AW, proportions of patients with liver cirrhosis [0 (0%) vs. 5 (15%), respectively, $p = 0.32$], diabetes mellitus [1 (14%) vs. 2 (6%), respectively, $p = 0.45$], renal disease [0 (0%) vs. 3 (9%), respectively, $p = 0.42$] and who received concomitant administration of steroids during the ICU stay [9(64%) vs. 15 (33%), respectively, $p = 0.23$] did not differ significantly. The other risk factors for ICU-AW assessed in the study did not differ significantly between patients with and without ICU-AW (Additional file 4: Table S4). Proportion of ulnar and facial TOF = 0 during treatment with NMBAs was significantly higher in patients with ICU-AW than in patient without ICU-AW, although it was not significant for total doses and duration of cisatracurium and atracurium (Table 3).

Discussion

To our knowledge, here we report the largest prospective cohort of critically ill patients paralyzed with the recommended doses of benzylisoquinoliniums and assessed for neuromuscular blockade by both a clinical evaluation and ulnar and facial TOF measurements. As expected we found that the evaluation of neuromuscular blockade differed vastly between the TOF and clinical assessment but also that TOF counts differed significantly between evaluation of facial and hand muscles. Furthermore, we found that the proportion of TOF = 0 measurements was significantly higher in patients with ICU-AW than in patients with no ICU-AW. An important result is that findings did not differ whether patients received cisatracurium or atracurium.

As it is already known in the operating room setting [10, 11], our study shows that an overall clinical assessment of the depth of a neuromuscular blockade is not correlated with the TOF count in critically ill patients. This finding has already been described in three previous

Table 2 PaO2/FiO2 ratios, plateau pressure, and calculated driving pressure recorded on the first 4 days of mechanical ventilation (MV) from the diagnosis of ARDS, distinguished according to results for facial train of four (TOF), and compared day by day

Day of MV	Day 0		Day 1		Day 2		Day 3	
	First	Second	First	Second	First	Second	First	Second
Measurements (*n*)	80	38	88	65	66	37	51	36
PaO2/FiO2 (mmHg), median (IQR)*								
Facial TOF = 0	115 (82–154)	170 (100–209)	148 (116–231)	171 (143–192)	178 (128–212)	151 (105–196)	160 (118–201)	136 (114–183)
Facial TOF = 1–2	111 (93–206)	160 (107–220)	203 (121–269)	142 (121–178)	198 (154–228)	–	183 (146–213)	121 (113–130)
Facial TOF = 3–4	98 (77–148)	168 (137–246)	159 (128–198)	195 (162–239)	185 (140–232)	220 (210–240)	187 (130–211)	154 (140–184)
Plateau pressure, cmH2O, median (IQR)*								
Facial TOF = 0	24 (19–26)	22 (20–25)	23 (19–25)	22 (20–24)	22 (20–24)	24 (20–25)	23 (20–25)	23 (22–26)
Facial TOF = 1–2	27 (23–27)	23 (23–24)	21 (17–23)	21 (19–27)	20 (18–20)	–	24 (21–26)	21 (17–25)
Facial TOF = 3–4	22 (20–27)	21 (20–22)	22 (20–24)	22 (21–24)	22 (20–24)	22 (20–24)	22 (19–24)	23 (20–25)
Driving pressure, cmH2O, median (IQR)*								
Facial TOF = 0	11 (9.5–18)	11 (8.5–14)	11 (9–13)	10 (9–12)	11 (9–13)	12 (10–14)	12 (11–17)	13 (11–17)
Facial TOF = 1–2	12 (12–14)	11 (10–12)	9 (9–11.5)	10 (8–15)	9.5 (8–11.5)	–	11.5 (10–14)	10 (9–11)
Facial TOF = 3–4	12 (10–16)	10.5 (8.5–12)	11 (10–14)	11 (9.5–13)	11 (9–13)	11 (8.5–12.5)	10 (9.5–13.5)	12 (9.5–15)

IQR interquartile ranges

* No significant difference for the daily first and second measurements when compared between results obtained for facial TOF = 0, facial TOF = 1–2, and facial TOF = 3–4

Table 3 Neuromuscular blockade, train-of-four (TOF) measurements, and intensive care unit-acquired weakness (ICU-AW) 7 days after awaking

	ICU-AW = Yes	ICU-AW = No	*p* value
Whole population	*N* = 14	*N* = 33	
Measures of facial TOF = 0/all measures of facial TOF	75/147 (51%)	97/243 (40%)	0.03
Measures of ulnar TOF = 0/all measures of ulnar TOF	111/147 (76%)	151/243 (62%)	0.006
Center 1	*N* = 12	*N* = 29	
Cisatracurium total dose (mg)	1482 (635–3257)	998 (591–1470)	0.25
Cisatracurium duration (h)	89 (42–210)	65 (35–110)	0.28
Center 2	*N* = 2	*N* = 4	
Atracurium total dose (mg)	1056 (1092–1320)	472 (418–749)	0.06
Atracurium duration (h)	190 (186–195)	93 (76–105)	0.07

Continuous variables are reported as medians and interquartile ranges (25th–75th percentiles)

ICU-AW intensive care unit-acquired weakness, *NMBAs* neuromuscular blocking agents, *TOF* train of four

studies, where the clinical assessment was performed by nurses and not by physicians, and two of these studies took place in pediatric ICUs [15–17]. Our results highlight the major discrepancy between clinical assessment and measures obtained after PNS but also between ulnar and facial TOF measurements.

A major finding of this study was that the objective of TOF count of 1 or 2 was obtained in only less than 10% of the measurements when patients are monitored only according to clinical assessment, even though the NMBA infusion rates were in accordance with the recommendations [2, 4]. Few studies supported the recommendations of monitoring the TOF in the ICU. Rudis et al. [8] compared in one group of patients paralyzed with an aminosteroid managed with a clinical assessment and one group managed with a TOF for an objective of 1/4. These authors observed a decreased amount of infused NMBAs and a faster recovery of muscle paralysis and spontaneous ventilation in the TOF group. However, in studies using benzylisoquinoliniums, there was no advantage for amount of infused NMBAs or residual weakness with a TOF compared to a clinical assessment [22, 28]. It is noteworthy that in the 2016 American recommendations, the only indication for NMBAs is ARDS with a ratio PaO2/FiO2 less than 150, and that no dosage and no objective of TOF are advocated [5].

A favorable impact of a neuromuscular blockade on the 90-day survival for severe ARDS patients was demonstrated in a well-designed study [3] with higher doses than recommended (i.e., 37.5 mg/h of cisatracurium), without monitoring the TOF. These doses were based on two previous studies from the same group with a goal of zero twitch for everyone during 48 h [29, 30]. This favorable effect of the NMBAs on ARDS may be due to an improvement in adjustment of tidal volume and plateau pressure with a reduction of asynchronies and ventilator-induced lung injuries, to an improvement of oxygenation, and finally to an anti-inflammatory effect [3, 29–31]. In one study, an objective of a TOF at 0/4 was compared to an objective at 2/4 [32]. As in our study, the plateau pressure and ratio PaO2/FiO2 did not differ between the TOF values. However, we did not assess asynchronies and we did not measure levels of cytokines, and thus, we cannot exclude that a deeper level of neuromuscular blockade is required to prevent lesions induced by bio-traumatism. Repeated measurements suggest also that higher than recommended and increasing doses of NMBAs during the first days of MV are required to obtain no facial TOF response and consequently total paralysis of the diaphragmatic and accessory muscles [3, 29, 30].

The proportion of TOF 3 or 4 increased significantly with time while patients receive the recommended doses of NMBAs. This has already been attributed to an up-regulation of acetylcholine receptors, although some authors did not find the same results [13, 22]. The pharmacokinetics of NMBAs in critically ill patients can be affected by many conditions, such as sepsis and/or shock [12]. In addition, it has been shown that ICU patients are less sensitive to neuromuscular blockade than patients in the operating room [14].

The link between NMBAs and ICU-AW, especially with benzylisoquinoliniums, is debated [1, 25, 27, 33, 34]. We diagnosed ICU-AW in 30% of our patients able to perform the MRC score on day 7 after their awakening, which is in accordance with the literature [25, 27]. The percentages of the ulnar and facial TOF = 0 measurements were higher in the cases of ICU-AW, while total doses and duration of NMBAs were not associated with a higher risk of ICU-AW. Further studies are required to determine whether that aiming for an objective of TOF count of 1 or 2 rather than zero could reduce amounts of infused NMBAs, thus lowering the risk of ICU-AW. In addition, there are many risk factors for ICU-AW which could be confounders [25, 27] and the present study was underpowered to assess most of them.

The results showing that TOF = 0 is more frequent at the ulnar site is not surprising since the orbicularis oculi muscle is known to be less sensitive to NMBAs than the adductor pollicis muscle. We monitored the TOF on the facial and the ulnar nerves because the facial site is advised in the French recommendations, but not in the recommendations from the Society of Critical Care Medicine [2, 4]. The orbicularis oculi muscle better assesses the depth of relaxation of the diaphragm, which is often the goal of a neuromuscular blockade in the ICU, especially in cases of ARDS [29, 30]. Although our study was not designed to, it seems more appropriate to monitor the facial TOF in ARDS patients to provide the adequate dose of NMBAs, at least during the first 48 h of MV in order to totally paralyze the diaphragmatic muscle as suggested by Papazian et al. [3]. Nevertheless, it is currently impossible to determine the aim of TOF to achieve in ARDS patients because in the only study [3] that shown a benefit in the use of NMBAs, no monitoring of TOF was done. Of note, the two centers did not use the same peripheral nerve stimulator and we believe that differences in NMBAs and TOF monitors between centers increase the external validity of the study.

Our study has some limitations. We included mainly medical patients so our results may not be generalized to all ICUs. We did not use an automated TOF measurement. More measurements would have provided a more accurate assessment, although the best frequency for measurement is not specified in the literature [1, 2, 4]. Ideally, the intensity of the stimulating current has to be tested for each patient before an NMBA infusion, which is difficult in real practice. Thus, we chose an intensity of the stimulating current of 50 mA for all patients, which was in agreement with some authors [20, 21]. Although we restrained ourselves to follow the advice published in the literature, the measurement of the TOF can be impaired by technical pitfalls such as incorrect positioning of electrodes [20, 21, 35]. The clinical evaluation of a neuromuscular blockade by physicians was not recorded in a standardized form, and we did not find models in the literature. The depth of sedation may have influenced the clinical evaluation of the neuromuscular blockade. Asynchronies and spontaneous breathing efforts were not precisely and extensively recorded in ARDS patients. Finally, we did not assess results of TOF on extubation times mainly because weaning process differed slightly between the two centers.

In conclusion, our study shows that there is a huge discrepancy between the clinical assessment and the TOF measurements in critically ill patients, that TOF count of 1 or 2 is a goal rarely achieved at usual doses of NMBAs, but also that respiratory objectives for plateau pressure and oxygenation can be obtained in ARDS patients without TOF monitoring. Our results do not suggest that the need for monitoring NMBAs could itself be questioned but rather that site for nerve stimulation and objective for TOF count could differ according to critically ill patients, reasons for neuromuscular blockade, and courses of the diseases. Nevertheless, more studies are needed to establish the best target of the TOF count to provide necessary and sufficient muscle relaxation and avoid residual muscular weakness.

Additional files

Additional file 1. Comparisons of results obtained by the train of four and the clinical assessment of neuromuscular blockade recorded over the entire study period.

Additional file 2. Results for agreements between clinical assessment of neuromuscular blockade with the train of four on the facial and ulnar nerves on whole population, in center 1 and in center 2.

Additional file 3. Clinical, facial and ulnar train of four measurements recorded on the first 4 days on mechanical ventilation from the diagnosis of acute respiratory distress syndrome.

Additional file 4. Factors associated with the diagnosis of intensive care unit-acquired weakness seven days after awaking the patient.

Abbreviations

ARDS: acute respiratory distress syndrome; ICU-AW: intensive care unit-acquired weakness; MRC: Muscular Research Council; MV: mechanical ventilation; NMBAs: neuromuscular blocking agents; PaO2/FiO2: ratio of the partial pressure of arterial oxygen (PaO2) to the fraction of inspired oxygen (FiO2); PEEP: positive end-expiratory pressure; PNS: peripheral nerve stimulation; TOF: train of four.

Authors' contributions

PB, AGa, JL, JMT, and YLT designed the study; PB, NB, AGa, FU, JL, PF, GG, AGo, and JMT participated in patient recruitment and data collection; PB and AGa analyzed data; PB, NB, AGa, JMT, and YLT involved in writing the manuscript. All authors read and approved the final manuscript.

Author details

[1] Service des Maladies Infectieuses et Réanimation Médicale, CHU Rennes, 2 rue Henri Le Guilloux, 35033 Rennes, France. [2] Faculté de Médecine, Biosit, Université Rennes 1, 35043 Rennes, France. [3] Réanimation polyvalente, CH Saint-Brieuc, 22000 Saint-Brieuc, France. [4] Inserm-CIC-1414, Université Rennes I, IFRI 40, 35033 Rennes, France.

Competing interests

The authors declare that they have no competing interests.

References

1. Greenberg SB, Vender J. The use of neuromuscular blocking agents in the ICU: where are we now? Crit Care Med. 2013;41:1332–44.
2. Murray MJ, Cowen J, DeBlock H, Erstad B, Gray AW, Tescher AN, et al. Clinical practice guidelines for sustained neuromuscular blockade in the adult critically ill patient. Crit Care Med. 2002;30:142–56.
3. Papazian L, Forel J-M, Gacouin A, Penot-Ragon C, Perrin G, Loundou A, et al. Neuromuscular blockers in early acute respiratory distress syndrome. N Engl J Med. 2010;363:1107–16.
4. Sauder P, Andreoletti M, Cambonie G, Capellier G, Feissel M, Gall O, et al. Sedation and analgesia in intensive care (with the exception of new-born babies). Ann Fr Anesth Réanim. 2008;27:541–51.
5. Murray MJ, DeBlock H, Erstad B, Gray A, Jacobi J, Jordan C, et al. Clinical practice guidelines for sustained neuromuscular blockade in the adult critically ill patient. Crit Care Med. 2016;44:2079–103.
6. Mehta S, Burry L, Fischer S, Martinez-Motta JC, Hallett D, Bowman D, et al. Canadian survey of the use of sedatives, analgesics, and neuromuscular blocking agents in critically ill patients. Crit Care Med. 2006;34:374–80.
7. Rhoney DH, Murry KR. National survey of the use of sedating drugs, neuromuscular blocking agents, and reversal agents in the intensive care unit. J Intensive Care Med. 2003;18:139–45.
8. Rudis MI, Sikora CA, Angus E, Peterson E, Popovich J, Hyzy R, et al. A prospective, randomized, controlled evaluation of peripheral nerve stimulation versus standard clinical dosing of neuromuscular blocking agents in critically ill patients. Crit Care Med. 1997;25:575–83.
9. Frankel H, Jeng J, Tilly E, St Andre A, Champion H. The impact of implementation of neuromuscular blockade monitoring standards in a surgical intensive care unit. Am Surg. 1996;62:503–6.
10. Thilen SR, Bhananker SM. Qualitative neuromuscular monitoring: how to optimize the use of a peripheral nerve stimulator to reduce the risk of residual neuromuscular blockade. Curr Anesthesiol Rep. 2016;6:164–9.
11. Brull SJ, Murphy GS. Residual neuromuscular block: lessons unlearned. Part II: M ethods to reduce the risk of residual weakness. Anesth Analg. 2010;111:129–40.
12. Boyd AH, Eastwood NB, Parker CJ, Hunter JM. Comparison of the pharmacodynamics and pharmacokinetics of an infusion of cis-atracurium (51W89) or atracurium in critically ill patients undergoing mechanical ventilation in an intensive therapy unit. Br J Anaesth. 1996;76:382–8.
13. Newman PJ, Quinn AC, Grounds RM, Hunter JM, Boyd AH, Eastwood NB, et al. A comparison of cisatracurium (51W89) and atracurium by infusion in critically ill patients. Crit Care Med. 1997;25:1139–42.
14. Dieye E, Minville V, Asehnoune K, Conil C, Georges B, Cougot P, et al. Pharmacodynamics of cisatracurium in the intensive care unit: an observational study. Ann Intensive Care. 2014;4:3.
15. Corso L. Train-of-four results and observed muscle movement in children during continuous neuromuscular blockade. Crit Care Nurse. 2008;28:30–8.
16. Greer R, Harper NJ, Pearson AJ. Neuromuscular monitoring by intensive care nurses: comparison of acceleromyography and tactile assessment. Br J Anaesth. 1998;80:384–5.
17. Peña O, Prestjohn S, Guzzetta CE. Agreement between muscle movement and peripheral nerve stimulation in critically ill pediatric patients receiving neuromuscular blocking agents. Heart Lung J Crit Care. 2000;29:309–18.
18. Ramsay MA, Savege TM, Simpson BR, Goodwin R. Controlled sedation with alphaxalone–alphadolone. Br Med J. 1974;2:656–9.
19. Ely EW, Truman B, Shintani A, Thomason JWW, Wheeler AP, Gordon S, et al. Monitoring sedation status over time in ICU patients: reliability and validity of the Richmond Agitation-Sedation Scale (RASS). JAMA. 2003;289:2983–91.
20. Helbo-Hansen HS, Bang U, Nielsen HK, Skovgaard LT. The accuracy of train-of-four monitoring at varying stimulating currents. Anesthesiology. 1992;76:199–203.
21. Rudis MI, Guslits BG, Zarowitz BJ. Technical and interpretive problems of peripheral nerve stimulation in monitoring neuromuscular blockade in the intensive care unit. Ann Pharmacother. 1996;30:165–72.
22. Strange C, Vaughan L, Franklin C, Johnson J. Comparison of train-of-four and best clinical assessment during continuous paralysis. Am J Respir Crit Care Med. 1997;156:1556–61.
23. Le Gall JR, Lemeshow S, Saulnier F. A new Simplified Acute Physiology Score (SAPS II) based on a European/North American multicenter study. JAMA. 1993;270:2957–63.
24. Vincent JL, Moreno R, Takala J, Willatts S, De Mendonça A, Bruining H, et al. The SOFA (Sepsis-related Organ Failure Assessment) score to describe organ dysfunction/failure. On behalf of the Working Group on Sepsis-Related Problems of the European Society of Intensive Care Medicine. Intensive Care Med. 1996;22:707–10.
25. Kress JP, Hall JB. ICU-acquired weakness and recovery from critical illness. N Engl J Med. 2014;371:287–8.
26. Ventilation with lower tidal volumes as compared with traditional tidal volumes for acute lung injury and the acute respiratory distress syndrome. The Acute Respiratory Distress Syndrome Network. N Engl J Med 2000;342:1301–1308.

27. De Jonghe B, Sharshar T, Lefaucheur J-P, Authier F-J, Durand-Zaleski I, Boussarsar M, et al. Paresis acquired in the intensive care unit: a prospective multicenter study. JAMA. 2002;288:2859–67.
28. Baumann MH, McAlpin BW, Brown K, Patel P, Ahmad I, Stewart R, et al. A prospective randomized comparison of train-of-four monitoring and clinical assessment during continuous ICU cisatracurium paralysis. Chest. 2004;126:1267–73.
29. Forel J-M, Roch A, Marin V, Michelet P, Demory D, Blache J-L, et al. Neuromuscular blocking agents decrease inflammatory response in patients presenting with acute respiratory distress syndrome. Crit Care Med. 2006;34:2749–57.
30. Gainnier M, Roch A, Forel J-M, Thirion X, Arnal J-M, Donati S, et al. Effect of neuromuscular blocking agents on gas exchange in patients presenting with acute respiratory distress syndrome. Crit Care Med. 2004;32:113–9.
31. Slutsky AS. Neuromuscular blocking agents in ARDS. N Engl J Med. 2010;363:1176–80.
32. Lagneau F, D'honneur G, Plaud B, Mantz J, Gillart T, Duvaldestin P, et al. A comparison of two depths of prolonged neuromuscular blockade induced by cisatracurium in mechanically ventilated critically ill patients. Intensive Care Med. 2002;28:1735–41.
33. Alhazzani W, Alshahrani M, Jaeschke R, Forel JM, Papazian L, Sevransky J, et al. Neuromuscular blocking agents in acute respiratory distress syndrome: a systematic review and meta-analysis of randomized controlled trials. Crit Care. 2013;17:R43.
34. Fan E, Dowdy DW, Colantuoni E, Mendez-Tellez PA, Sevransky JE, Shanholtz C, et al. Physical complications in acute lung injury survivors: a two-year longitudinal prospective study. Crit Care Med. 2014;42:849–59.
35. Lagneau F, Benayoun L, Plaud B, Bonnet F, Favier J, Marty J. The interpretation of train-of-four monitoring in intensive care: what about the muscle site and the current intensity? Intensive Care Med. 2001;27:1058–63.

20

The pain, agitation, and delirium practice guidelines for adult critically ill patients: a post-publication perspective

Yoanna Skrobik[1*] and Gerald Chanques[2]

Abstract

The recently published Clinical Practice Guidelines for the Management of Pain, Agitation, and Delirium in Adult Patients in the Intensive Care Unit differ from earlier guidelines in the following ways: literature searches were performed in eight databases by a professional librarian; psychometric validation of assessment scales was considered in their recommendation; discrepancies in recommendation votes by guideline panel members are available in online supplements; and all recommendations were made exclusively on the basis of evidence available until December of 2010. Pain recognition and management remains challenging in the critically ill. Patient outcomes improve with routine pain assessment, use of co-analgesics and administration as well as dose adjustment of opiates to patient needs. Thoracic epidurals help ease patients undergoing abdominal aortic surgery. Little data exists to guide clinicians as to the type or dose of co-analgesics; no opiate choice is associated with better patient outcomes. Lighter or no sedation is beneficial, and interruption is desirable in patients who require deep sedation for specific pathologic states. Delirium screening is probably useful; no treatment modality can be unequivocally recommended, and the benefit of prophylaxis is established only for early mobilization. The details of these recommendations, as well as more recent publications that complement the guidelines, are provided in this commentary.

Review

Introduction

The Clinical Practice Guidelines for the Management of Pain, Agitation, and Delirium in Adult Patients in the Intensive Care Unit was recently published [1]. This commentary summarizes the guidelines process, its efforts to ensure transparency and scientific rigor as well as describing some areas that remain controversial. How these guidelines differ from earlier versions, knowledge gaps, and which questions they do and do not answer are described below.

How these guidelines differ from others

Four methodological characteristics differentiate these guidelines from earlier versions. First, technical support was provided by a research librarian, Charlie Kishman, from the University of Cincinnati, who provided ongoing searches from eight distinct databases. Expertise in compiling data from a maximum of high-yield sources, and the thoroughness and methodology required to collate search terms and compile the results, impacts the quality guidelines or systematic reviews [2]. The convenience of having all relevant triaged articles land in an e-mail inbox (to be screened by team members from the pain and analgesia, agitation and sedation, delirium, and related clinical outcomes teams) cannot be overstated. The relevant articles were triaged in an online reference RefWorks site accessible to all members, for more manageable ongoing discussions and subsequent referencing. Second, all team members committed to focusing on published evidence in critically ill adults. No clinical experience-based opinion was incorporated in these guidelines, nor was any recommendation made where no evidence existed. Third, team member votes on the various recommendations were made public for readers to have access to the vote distribution. The intent, in addition to transparency and rigor, was to

* Correspondence: skrobik@sympatico.ca
[1]Soins Intensifs, Hôpital Maisonneuve Rosemont, Montréal, QC H1T 2M4, Canada
Full list of author information is available at the end of the article

underscore that even in the context of rigorous evidence judgment plays a role in final attribution of scientific value and of importance. The GRADE method of assessment was chosen for ranking the evidence [3]. GRADE's value as a barometer of evidence has not been demonstrated, nor has its reliability and agreement among experts [4]. Publishing the votes allows the guidelines reader to independently view the extent of concordance among voters grading the evidence contained within these guidelines. Fourth, the guidelines incorporate a variety of bedside behavioral assessment tools used to detect and evaluate pain, assess depth of sedation and degree of agitation, and detect delirium. No comparative assessments of the psychometric properties (i.e., scale reliability and validity) and feasibility of these tools for use in intensive care unit (ICU) patients are published. The assessment of the psychometric properties of applying pain, sedation and delirium scales to ICU patients [5] was undertaken, another first for this type of guideline.

Behavioral pain scales used in adult ICU patients were analyzed and compared adapting a previously published process [6]. Psychometric scoring systems were not available to evaluate and compare the psychometric properties of sedation and delirium scales, which have different validation strategies from those used for pain scales. The task force members undertook the development of similar psychometric scoring systems to assess and compare sedation and delirium scales, calling upon the expertise of psychometric experts and using accepted theoretical principles of health scale development and psychometric testing [5].

Conflict of interest declarations were left up to the individual authors; each author chose whether associations with different pharmaceutical industry partners constituted conflict. Experts with no conflicts are hard to find; some argued that being conflicted does not affect your judgment as to the quality of evidence [7]. Consensus among experts is subject to halo effects because of the group discussion process, where influence is challenging to differentiate from learning from each other and exchanging information. The strength of recommendations were ranked as strong (1) or weak (2), and either in favor of an intervention (+) or against (–) an intervention. For all strong recommendations, the phrase "*We recommend...*" was used. A weak recommendation indicated a less clear trade-off or weaker evidence; the phrase "*We suggest...*" was then used. In the absence of sufficient evidence, or when group consensus could not be achieved, no recommendation (0) was made.

Pain assessment and analgesia

The current guidelines address several new dimensions of pain assessment and management described below. Several other areas remain unexplored, largely because of a dearth in publications; these also are summarized below.

Pain in ICU patients

Incidence, consequences and outcomes

The current guidelines emphasize that pain is frequent in ICU patients [8], with an incidence of up to 50% in medical and surgical patients at rest [9], and increasing up to 80% during common care procedures. Since tracheal suctioning and drain removal as well as turning the patients for nursing-care procedures is reported as the most painful routine care procedures [10], routine preemptive analgesics in these circumstances are recommended. Pain in medical patients, which often is attributable to immobilization, can be addressed with early physiotherapy [11] and lighter sedation regimens as the current sedation and delirium portions of the guidelines suggest [1] ("*We recommend performing early mobilization of adult ICU patients whenever feasible to reduce the incidence and duration of delirium (+1B); and We recommend either daily sedation interruption or a light target level of sedation be routinely used in mechanically ventilated adult ICU patients (+1B)*").

Long-term outcomes associated with pain or its management

The association between pain in ICU patients and the development of chronic pain syndrome in ICU survivors is not addressed [12] as studies published after December 2010 were not included in the evidence review and voting process. Posttraumatic stress disorder (PTSD) is attributed to pain memories in some studies [13-15]. Although one pediatric and one war-trauma study suggest more frequent use of morphine might reduce the risk of subsequent development of PTSD-related symptoms after injury [16,17], these findings have not been documented in an adult critical care population.

As these guidelines point out, improved pain management is clearly associated with better patient outcome in the ICU [8,18,19]. At least three studies performed in surgical, trauma, and medical ICUs report that a protocolized approach to assess and manage pain, agitation, and delirium [20] is associated with a reduced duration of mechanical ventilation, ICU acquired infections, length of stay and costs in ICU, and hospital as well as 30-day mortality [8,18-21]; accordingly, the guidelines recommend protocolized pain screening and assessing analgesic needs first to palliate the current under-recognition and treatment of pain [22].

Pain assessment

In patients able to communicate, self-report is without a doubt the most reliable method to assess pain [23]. The most commonly used are the Visual Analogue Scale

(VAS), the Verbal Descriptor Scale (VDS) and the 0–10 Numeric Rating Scale (NRS). A prospective comparison of five popular self-report pain scales in terms of their feasibility, validity, and performance suggests that NRS-V is the most feasible and the pain scale preferred by patients [24]. Self-report pain tools were not rated by, but the NRS-V was considered preferable for pain detection in ICU patients. The thresholds for pain that usually trigger therapeutic interventions are defined by a V-NRS score greater than 3 points (scale range 0–10).

Since the review of pain measurement instruments available for ICU patients by Hamill-Ruth and Marohn [23] more than a decade ago highlighting the absence of validated instruments for critically ill patients, several new behavioral pain instruments have been described in the literature and were reviewed for guideline purposes [19,25-29]. Recent reviews [6,30] of these instruments concluded that only the Behavioral Pain Scale (BPS) [19] and the Critical Care Pain Observation Tool (CPOT) [27] provide acceptable levels of validity and reliability; these two behavioral scales now constitute the two recommended nonverbal pain screening techniques. The BPS was initially elaborated to assess pain in nonverbal, mechanically ventilated patients without severe head injury [19,31,32] with three behavioral domains: facial expression, upper limb movements, and compliance with ventilation. The CPOT has a fourth domain (muscle tension), which may be the most psychometrically valid of all in selected patients [27], such as the neurologically critically ill [33]. The BPS requires that ventilator asynchrony be observed while the patient undergoes a painful stimulus before attributing the asynchrony to pain, whereas the CPOT does not stipulate this requirement; this limitation is not addressed in the current guidelines. In addition, the CPOT has a vocalization domain to allow pain assessment in nonintubated patients, but this dimension's psychometric properties have yet to be validated. More recently, a vocalization domain was added to the BPS, demonstrating good psychometric properties in ICU nonintubated patients [34]. Vital signs, such as heart rate and blood pressure, are unreliable as pain assessment surrogates in ICU patients compared with behavioral parameters [33-35]; the guidelines make this point and emphasize the need for systematic and rigorous pain assessment, particularly because ICU patients' pain is consistently underrated by ICU caregivers [36-38]. Behavioral pain tools should not be used in communicative patients, because correlation coefficients between BPS and self-reported pain scales are low [24].

Treatment

No analgesic medication is associated with improved patient outcome. Opioids were used in up to 90% of mechanically ventilated patients in a multicenter patient-based study [39]. Accordingly, the guidelines "*...recommend that IV opioids should be considered as the first-line drug class of choice to treat nonneuropathic pain in critically ill patients (+1C).*" How these opioids should be administered is not addressed. The continuous use of opioids may lead to drug and metabolite accumulation [40,41]. Intravenous perfusions are not mandatory; indeed, escalation of bolus opioids with or without continuous opiate infusion in ICU patients is feasible patients and associated with improved outcome [8,18,20].

A study performed in ICU patients (70% of whom were surgical) used a gradual escalation of analgesics from nonopioid drugs to incrementally powerful opioids [8]. In that study, tramadol use increased significantly, whereas incidence of pain and duration of mechanical ventilation decreased. Co-analgesia with nonopioids was introduced two decades ago [42] and is widely practiced for treating postoperative pain. In keeping with this rationale and despite the dearth of studies addressing co-analgesia effectiveness in critically ill patients, the guidelines suggest "*...that nonopioid analgesics be considered to decrease the quantity of opioids administered (or to eliminate the need for IV opioids altogether) and to decrease opioid-related side effects (+2C).*" In patients with end-stage liver disease, reduced dosing acetaminophen appears to be safe [43]. Nefopam, a centrally acting nonopioid agent proposed as an adjuvant to opioid analgesics, relieves moderate to severe pain in ICU patients without respiratory or neurological effects [44]. This description was published in 2011, after the final ratings and votes had been established for the publications being reviewed. Finally, gabapentin is effective for pain treatment opioid consumption reduction in ICU patients with Guillain-Barré syndrome [45]. This, and a similar study by the same group [46], led to the recommendation "*...that either enterally administered gabapentin or carbamazepine, in addition to intravenous IV opioids, should be considered for treatment of neuropathic pain (+1A).*"

Regional analgesia (continuous epidural or peripheral nerve blocks) is known to improve the efficacy of traditional analgesic interventions and to decrease pulmonary complications in many postoperative patients [47]. Its integration into practice is variable over time and by European geographic region [48-50]. A multicenter study that included 1,416 continuous peripheral nerve blocks identified ICU stay as an independent factor associated with complications, such as hypoesthesia/paresthesia, local inflammation, and infection [50]. Use of regional analgesia in ICU patients deserves further evaluation in regards of its benefits, feasibility, side effects, and contraindications. Accordingly, the guidelines recommendations are cautious and limit their recommendation for regional anesthesia in the only population where it has been unequivocally demonstrated to be beneficial [51,52]. "*We recommend that thoracic epidural anesthesia/analgesia should be considered for postoperative analgesia in patients undergoing abdominal aortic surgery (+1B). We provide no recommendation for the use of a lumbar epidural over parenteral opioids for postoperative analgesia in patients undergoing abdominal aortic aneurysm surgery, due to a lack of benefit when these routes of administration are compared in this patient population (0,A). We provide no recommendation for the use of thoracic epidural analgesia in patients undergoing either intrathoracic or nonvascular abdominal surgical procedures, because of insufficient and conflicting evidence for this mode of analgesic delivery in these patients (0, B). We suggest that thoracic epidural analgesia may be considered for patients with traumatic rib fractures (+2B). We provide no recommendation for neuraxial/regional analgesia over systemic analgesia in medical ICU patients, due to lack of evidence in this patient population (0, No Evidence)*".

Critical care analgesia research perspectives: beyond the guidelines

The biology underpinning pain syndromes remains underexplored, particularly in medical ICU patients. Hyperalgesia associated with sepsis could contribute to a possible "diffuse ICU pain syndrome." Indeed, myalgia and arthralgia are common clinical features associated with sepsis and fever [53], partly because of inflammation and muscle hypercatabolism induced by thermogenesis [54]. Inflammatory cytokines and sympathetic amines are associated with a nociceptive state associated with inflammation and sepsis [55,56].

Barriers associated with pain not being evaluated by health caregivers should be better elucidated [55,56]. In patients unable to communicate, electrophysiological measurements could allow for objective measurement of pain. The measurement of pupil size (pupillometry) appears to be more sensitive than behavioral parameters in a population of ICU patients undergoing nociceptive procedures [57]; whether pupillometry is useful compared with behavioral parameters during suctioning is less clear [58]. Which pain threshold should trigger analgesic administration is not well established. Randomized, controlled studies are still needed to demonstrate the association between pain assessment, analgesia, and short- and long-term outcomes (PTSD, chronic pain syndromes, and quality of life). Which pharmacologic interventions are useful, particularly with regards to co-analgesia, is uncertain. Surprisingly, there is a dearth of information on the use of acetaminophen/paracetamol or of anti-inflammatory agents in the ICU population [59,60].

Nonpharmacological adjuncts or substitutes to pharmacological intervention also are of interest. Music therapy and music are beneficial for critically ill patients. This unaddressed area in the literature is acknowledged in the current guidelines, which state: "*Complimentary, nonpharmacologic interventions for pain management, such as music therapy and relaxation techniques, can be considered as complementary therapies in pain management; they may be opioid-sparing and analgesia-enhancing choices, and they are low cost, easy to provide, and safe.*" Although a multimodal approach to pain management in ICU patients has been recommended, few studies have demonstrated the effectiveness of nonpharmacologic interventions [20,61,62].

Sedation assessment and management

The current guidelines support the minimization of sedation so that patients are responsive and able to communicate. In clinical contexts where this is not possible or not desirable, daily interruption of sedation is encouraged. The recommendations take into account subsequently published data suggesting that interruption confers no additional advantage to sedation minimization [63]; although these publications were not available to the guidelines committee, the preliminary data were known and thought to be harmonious with the statements put forward earlier. These suggestions are novel compared with earlier guidelines, where the emphasis was on patient comfort but not necessarily of the harm inherent to sedatives. At the heart of earlier deliberations stood the conviction on the part of many caregivers that sedation mitigates how traumatic the patient perceives the ICU experience to be. This notion is slowly being contradicted by data from follow-up studies [64]. There is emerging understanding that excessive sedation, even when limited to 48 hours [65], is common and is associated with increased morbidity, mortality, and expenditure [65,66]. Daily interruption of sedative infusions, titration of sedative dose and opiates to symptoms [8,20,67], and minimization of drug administration is associated with patient benefit, reduced costs [21], and does not lead to accidental device removal or psychological stress [68]. The contrast to earlier guidelines is the explicit statement that harm is likely with iatrogenic coma; this point is made both in the sedation and delirium sections.

Despite review of the literature for the 10 years preceding the inception of the guidelines and during the 7 years spent in its creation, no clear recommendation could be put forward with regard to preferred sedation agent. Few topics generated as much controversy and discussion as the use or avoidance of benzodiazepines, leading to heated debates during panel discussions and to perspective-defining publications [69,70]. The answer to the question: *Should nonbenzodiazepine-based sedation, instead of sedation with benzodiazepines, be used in mechanically ventilated adult ICU patients?* (actionable) was reworded numerous times.

In parallel with the literature on continuously administered analgesic agents, few data report the pharmacokinetic properties of continuously administered benzodiazepines, propofol, and dexmedetomidine [71]. Any comparison of these agents should take into account the variability in half-life, terminal half-life, and changes associated with co-administration of competitive metabolic pathway agents, inflammatory status, and renal and hepatic dysfunction [70]. Dexmedetomidine was not labeled as preferable sedative agent except in delirious patients' continuous sedation, where it is preferable to benzodiazepines. Cost also is a concern; benzodiazepines remain the least expensive molecule, albeit one subject to pharmacokinetic properties specific to the critically ill; the benefits of choosing any agent have to be considered in the light of the current context of health care cost containment policies in America and Europe [72,73].

Delirium

Routine delirium assessment in all critically ill patients is recommended, in keeping with ICU guidelines published by others [74]. This shift in attributing importance to ICU delirium screening is integrated into regional or national accreditation requirements; for instance, ICU delirium screening is now mandated across Canada. Psychometric properties were assessed based on scale reliability and validity, and feasibility in critically ill adults. Scales were then rated on 1) item selection and content validation, 2) reliability, 3) validity, 4) feasibility, and 5) relevance or impact of implementation on patient outcomes, with regard to the scoring of delirium. The Intensive Care Delirium Screening Checklist (ICDSC) and the Confusion Assessment Method-ICU (CAM-ICU) were considered best. The presence of the original creators of these scales on the guidelines panel was not considered a conflict of interest; the psychometric validation was performed independently from their input. Two caveats should be considered: 1) the psychometric validation process, although performed by experts, was not peer-reviewed (by its publication or in any other form), in contrast to all other material considered for these guidelines; 2) despite application of rigorous psychometric validation principles, the fact that these two psychometrically valid scores detect ranges of delirium from 10% to >80% in similar populations was not accounted for.

The importance of delirium screening is emphasized to reassure patients and provide prognostic indicators. The recommendation that screening be performed with a tool rather than with clinical assessments by intensive care physicians was based on studies where delirium screening was introduced de novo [18] and by the strong opinions held by guidelines writers. A recent (unpublished until March 2013) study suggests, however, that clinical assessments by critical care physicians may identify delirium more rapidly and more accurately than screening tool assessments [75], a perhaps unsurprising finding. Delirium prevention is highlighted for the first time, with emphasis on early mobility as a safe and effective way of not only preventing delirium but providing patients with a more functional outcome at hospital discharge. Risk factors for ICU delirium are inconsistent across studies; those retained had to have been identified in at least two studies: these were preexisting dementia; history of hypertension; history of alcoholism; and admission a high severity of illness on admission. Some publications associate continuously administered benzodiazepine and delirium in critically ill patients [76,77].

Because continuously sedating patients with midazolam appears to be associated with a higher incidence of delirium than sedating patients with dexmedetomidine [78], and because this difference is not seen when morphine is compared to dexmedetomidine [79], midazolam has been presumed to be linked to delirium occurrence. A more recently published study suggests midazolam levels are in fact lower in patients who develop delirium [80]. The Confusion Assessment Method (CAM-ICU) screening tool was used to detect ICU delirium in studies that described less delirium with dexmedetomidine, a molecule that is associated with greater wakefulness than midazolam. Some authors have suggested that the CAM-ICU scoring may be affected by sedation [81]; the potential that the greater sedation seen and expected with midazolam was a confounder for delirium remains to be clarified before convincing conclusions can be drawn. With regard to more recently established risk factors for ICU delirium, the pre-deliric score [82] had not been published at the time of guideline writing; its risk stratification was not included in the guidelines document, and the risk prediction is currently being validated in an international multicenter study.

Delirium prophylaxis was addressed for the first time in these guidelines. To the question: "*Should a nonpharmacological delirium protocol in the ICU be used in the ICU to reduce the incidence or duration of delirium? (actionable)*," the guidelines provide the following answer: "*We recommend that performing early mobilization of adult ICU patients be performed whenever feasible to reduce the incidence and duration of delirium (+1B).*" This recommendation is based on the first multicenter, randomized, controlled trial of early mobility [11] and a subsequent implementation study, where investigators noted striking reductions in the incidence of delirium in mobilized patients. These studies also indicate that early and aggressive mobilization is unlikely to harm

ICU patients, while reducing ICU and hospital LOS. Ongoing studies aiming to prove the benefit of multicomponent prevention [83] are currently under way.

No recommendations were made with regard to pharmacological delirium prevention. Six randomized studies evaluating a pharmacologic intervention for ICU patients had been published at the time of review. Although a reduction in delirium was observed in five of the studies, important methodological differences and limitations may have influenced some of the results [84,85], whereas other studies were limited to very narrow patient population [86,87]. Although use of dexmedetomidine as a sedative during elective cardiac surgery was associated with less delirium than propofol or midazolam [85], a subsequent study that was nearly four times larger found that use of dexmedetomidine resulted in a similar incidence of delirium compared with morphine-only sedation regimen [79]. In both of these sedation studies, delirium incidence was measured using the CAM–ICU; it remained unclear whether some of the patients deemed to have delirium actually had delirium or were simply sedated [88].

Given these data, no pharmacologic prophylaxis recommendation for delirium was made; a recent systematic review of delirium prophylaxis in the critically ill concurs with the lack of evidence to support this practice [89]. However, the reduction in subsyndromal delirium shown in one study was acknowledged as follows: *"One before/after study evaluated the impact of a multidisciplinary protocol for managing pain, agitation, and delirium in ICU patients."* This study demonstrated a reduction in the incidence of *subsyndromal* delirium (but not delirium), with improved pain control, and without compromising sedation or anxiolysis, and a 15% reduction in their total ICU costs [20,21]. Subsyndromal delirium in ICU patients is defined as patients who have <4 points on the ICDSC; patients with subsyndromal delirium have worse clinical outcomes than those without delirium [90].

After the guidelines had been written, the largest ICU delirium prophylaxis study published to date described that a low-dose, 12-hour infusion of haloperidol reduces the incidence of delirium in surgical patients from 23% to 15% ($p = 0.03$) [91]. As the average APACHE scores were 9, the generalizability of these findings to the broad ICU population is not clear. However, encouraging preliminary single-center pre-post European pilot studies [92] have shown reductions in delirium incidence and duration in patients considered at high risk after prophylactic low doses of haloperidol, and support moving forward with multicenter prophylaxis trials in high-risk ICU populations. All successful prophylaxis studies to date have included surgical patients exclusively. In a well-conducted, but underpowered, multicenter, randomized, controlled pilot of delirium prophylaxis in medical ICU patients with antipsychotics (either haloperidol or ziprasidone vs. placebo) did not show any benefit with either haloperidol or ziprasidone compared with placebo [93].

The guidelines are clear as to the paucity of evidence supporting any pharmacologic treatment for delirium. With the possible exception of a benefit shown in a small (n = 36) study randomizing patients on as-needed haloperidol to quetiapine [94], where patients with quetiapine had shorter delirium duration, no drug has been shown to improve delirium outcome once it as occurred. Accordingly, the treatment section of the guidelines is clear: "Question: *Does treatment with haloperidol reduce the duration of delirium in adult ICU patients? (descriptive)* Answer: *There is no published evidence that treatment with haloperidol reduces the duration of delirium in adult ICU patients (No Evidence),* and Question: *Does treatment with atypical antipsychotics reduce the duration of delirium in adult ICU patients? (descriptive)* Answer: *Atypical antipsychotics may reduce the duration of delirium in adult ICU patients (C).*" A recent review of delirium treatment in ICU patients [95] concedes that there is limited evidence on the safety and effectiveness of antipsychotics in ICU delirium.

Rivastigmine use in the critically ill is specifically discouraged in the guidelines: "*We do not recommend administering rivastigmine to reduce the duration of delirium in ICU patients (-1B).*" Although tested in only one study, when rivastigmine was compared with placebo in critically ill patients the investigation was halted because of perceived futility and potential harm by the DSMB (Data Safety Monitoring Board) [96]; rivastigmine-treated patients were found to have more severe and longer delirium, with a trend toward a higher mortality rate. Delirium in association to alcohol withdrawal was not covered in these guidelines because of space considerations; this topic is reviewed in a separate publication [95].

Conclusions

The current guidelines update the critical care clinician on the importance of pain and delirium assessments and the need to minimize or interrupt sedation. The methodological rigor with which the evidence was triaged improves the clarity and scientific basis of the recommendations; the guidelines also better identify gaps in current evidence. We hope that the current update on guideline content and process will incite critical care investigators to build on established work to address pain, sedation, and delirium issues in order to improve care and outcomes for the critically ill and to reduce the significant burden of critical illness on patients, their families, and society.

Competing interests
The authors declare that they have no competing interests.

Authors' contributions
YS was part of the Society of Critical Care Medicine's guidelines committee. Both authors wrote sections of the manuscript, and extensively reviewed its entire content. Both authors read and approved the final manuscript.

Author details
[1]Soins Intensifs, Hôpital Maisonneuve Rosemont, Montréal, QC H1T 2M4, Canada. [2]Intensive Care and Anaesthesiology Department (DAR), Saint Eloi Hospital, Montpellier University Hospital, 80, Avenue Augustin Fliche, Montpellier cedex 5 34295, France.

References
1. Barr J, *et al*: **Clinical practice guidelines for the management of pain, agitation, and delirium in adult patients in the intensive care unit.** *Crit Care Med* 2013, **41**(1):263–306.
2. McGowan J, Sampson M: **Systematic reviews need systematic searchers.** *J Med Libr Assoc* 2005, **93**(1):74–80.
3. Guyatt GH, *et al*: **GRADE: an emerging consensus on rating quality of evidence and strength of recommendations.** *BMJ* 2008, **336**(7650):924–926.
4. Kavanagh BP: **The GRADE system for rating clinical guidelines.** *PLoS Med* 2009, **6**(9):e1000094.
5. Kottner J, *et al*: **Guidelines for Reporting Reliability and Agreement Studies (GRRAS) were proposed.** *J Clin Epidemiol* 2011, **64**(1):96–106.
6. Pudas-Tahka SM, *et al*: **Pain assessment tools for unconscious or sedated intensive care patients: a systematic review.** *J Adv Nurs* 2009, **65**(5):946–956.
7. Jones DJ, Barkun A, Lu Y, Enns R, Sinclair P, Martel M, Gralnek I, Bardou M, Kuipers EJ, Sung J: **Conflicts of interest ethics: silencing expertise in the development of international clinical practice guidelines.** *Ann Intern Med* 2012, **156**:809–816.
8. Chanques G, *et al*: **Impact of systematic evaluation of pain and agitation in an intensive care unit.** *Crit Care Med* 2006, **34**(6):1691–1699.
9. Chanques G, *et al*: **A prospective study of pain at rest: incidence and characteristics of an unrecognized symptom in surgical and trauma versus medical intensive care unit patients.** *Anesthesiology* 2007, **107**(5):858–860.
10. Puntillo KA, *et al*: **Pain behaviors observed during six common procedures: results from Thunder Project II.** *Crit Care Med* 2004, **32**(2):421–427.
11. Schweickert WD, *et al*: **Early physical and occupational therapy in mechanically ventilated, critically ill patients: a randomised controlled trial.** *Lancet* 2009, **373**(9678):1874–1882.
12. Kyranou M, Puntillo K: **The transition from acute to chronic pain: might intensive care unit patients be at risk?** *Ann Intensive Care* 2012, **2**(1):36.
13. Myhren H, *et al*: **Posttraumatic stress, anxiety and depression symptoms in patients during the first year post intensive care unit discharge.** *Crit Care* 2010, **14**(1):R14.
14. Myhren H, *et al*: **Patients' memory and psychological distress after ICU stay compared with expectations of the relatives.** *Intensive Care Med* 2009, **35**(12):2078–2086.
15. Schelling G, *et al*: **Health-related quality of life and posttraumatic stress disorder in survivors of the acute respiratory distress syndrome.** *Crit Care Med* 1998, **26**(4):651–659.
16. Holbrook TL, *et al*: **Morphine use after combat injury in Iraq and post-traumatic stress disorder.** *N Engl J Med* 2010, **362**(2):110–117.
17. Nixon RD, *et al*: **Predictors of posttraumatic stress in children following injury: The influence of appraisals, heart rate, and morphine use.** *Behav Res Ther* 2010, **48**(8):810–815.
18. Robinson BR, *et al*: **An analgesia-delirium-sedation protocol for critically ill trauma patients reduces ventilator days and hospital length of stay.** *J Trauma* 2008, **65**(3):517–526.
19. Payen JF, *et al*: **Assessing pain in critically ill sedated patients by using a behavioral pain scale.** *Crit Care Med* 2001, **29**(12):2258–2263.
20. Skrobik Y, *et al*: **Protocolized intensive care unit management of analgesia, sedation, and delirium improves analgesia and subsyndromal delirium rates.** *Anesth Analg* 2010, **111**(2):451–463.
21. Awissi DK, *et al*: **I-SAVE study: impact of sedation, analgesia, and delirium protocols evaluated in the intensive care unit: an economic evaluation.** *Ann Pharmacother* 2012, **46**(1):21–28.
22. Puntillo KA, *et al*: **Practices and predictors of analgesic interventions for adults undergoing painful procedures.** *Am J Crit Care* 2002, **11**(5):415–429. quiz 430-1.
23. Hamill-Ruth RJ, Marohn ML: **Evaluation of pain in the critically ill patient.** *Crit Care Clin* 1999, **15**(1):35–54. v-vi.
24. Chanques G, *et al*: **The measurement of pain in intensive care unit: comparison of 5 self-report intensity scales.** *Pain* 2010, **151**(3):711–721.
25. Puntillo KA, Miaskowski C, Kehrle K, Stannard D, Gleeson S, Nye P: **Relationship between behavioral and physiological indicators of pain, critical care patients' self-reports of pain, and opioid administration.** *Crit Care Med* 1997, **25**:1159–1166.
26. Mateo OM, Krenzischek D: **A pilot study to assess the relationship between behavioral manifestations and self-report of pain in postanesthesia care unit patients.** *J Post Anesth Nurs* 1992, **7**:15–21.
27. Gelinas C, Fillion L, Puntillo KA, Viens C, Fortier M: **Validation of the critical-care pain observation tool in adult patients.** *Am J Crit Care* 2006, **15**:420–427.
28. Odhner M, Wegman D, Freeland N, Steinmetz A, Ingersoll GL: **Assessing pain control in nonverbal critically ill adults.** *Dimens Crit Care Nurs* 2003, **22**:260–267.
29. Puntillo KA, Stannard D, Miaskowski C, Kehrle K, Gleeson S: **Use of a pain assessment and intervention notation (P.A.I.N.) tool in critical care nursing practice: nurses' evaluations.** *Heart Lung* 2002, **31**:303–314.
30. Li D, Puntillo K, Miaskowski C: **A review of objective pain measures for use with critical care adult patients unable to self-report.** *J Pain* 2008, **9**(1):2–10.
31. Aissaoui Y, *et al*: **Validation of a behavioral pain scale in critically ill, sedated, and mechanically ventilated patients.** *Anesth Analg* 2005, **101**(5):1470–1476.
32. Young J, *et al*: **Use of a Behavioural Pain Scale to assess pain in ventilated, unconscious and/or sedated patients.** *Intensive Crit Care Nurs* 2006, **22**(1):32–39.
33. Gelinas C, *et al*: **Exploring the validity of the bispectral index, the Critical-Care Pain Observation Tool and vital signs for the detection of pain in sedated and mechanically ventilated critically ill adults: a pilot study.** *Intensive Crit Care Nurs* 2011, **27**(1):46–52.
34. Chanques G, Payen J, Mercier G, de Lattre S, Viel E, Jung B, Cisse M, Lefrant JY, Jaber S: **Assessing pain in non-intubated critically ill patients unable to self report: an adaptation of the Behavioral Pain Scale.** *Intensive Care Med* 2009, **35**:2060–2067.
35. Gelinas CAC: **Behavioral and physiologic indicators during a nociceptive procedure in conscious and unconscious mechanically ventilated adults: similar or different?** *J Crit Care* 2009, **24**(17):628.
36. Desbiens NA, Mueller-Rizner N: **How well do surrogates assess the pain of seriously ill patients?** *Crit Care Medicine* 2000, **28**:1347–1352.
37. Hall-Lord ML, Larsson G, Steen B: **Pain and distress among elderly intensive care unit patients: comparison of patients' experiences and nurses' assessments.** *Heart Lung* 1998, **27**:123–132.
38. Whipple JK, Lewis K, Quebbeman EJ, Wolff M, Gottlieb MS, Medicus-Bringa M, Hartnett KR, Graf M, Ausman RK: **Analysis of pain management in critically ill patients.** *Pharmacotherapy* 1995, **15**:592–599.
39. Payen JF, *et al*: **Current practices in sedation and analgesia for mechanically ventilated critically ill patients: a prospective multicenter patient-based study.** *Anesthesiology* 2007, **106**(4):687–695. quiz 891-2.
40. Kapila A, *et al*: **Measured context-sensitive half-times of remifentanil and alfentanil.** *Anesthesiology* 1995, **83**(5):968–975.
41. Ethuin F, *et al*: **Pharmacokinetics of long-term sufentanil infusion for sedation in ICU patients.** *Intensive Care Med* 2003, **29**(11):1916–1920.
42. Kehlet H, Dahl JB: **The value of "multimodal" or "balanced analgesia" in postoperative pain treatment.** *Anesth Analg* 1993, **77**(5):1048–1056.
43. Chandok N, Watt KD: **Pain management in the cirrhotic patient: the clinical challenge.** *Mayo Clin Proc* 2010, **85**(5):451–458.
44. Chanques G, *et al*: **Analgesic efficacy and haemodynamic effects of nefopam in critically ill patients.** *Br J Anaesth* 2011, **106**(3):336–343.

45. Pandey CK, *et al*: **The comparative evaluation of gabapentin and carbamazepine for pain management in Guillain-Barre syndrome patients in the intensive care unit.** *Anesth Analg* 2005, **101**(1):220–225. table of contents.
46. Pandey CK, Bose N, Garg G, *et al*: **Gabapentin for the treatment of pain in guillain-barre syndrome: A double-blinded, placebo-controlled, crossover study.** *Anesth Analg* 2002, **95**:1719–1723.
47. Popping DM, *et al*: **Protective effects of epidural analgesia on pulmonary complications after abdominal and thoracic surgery: a meta-analysis.** *Arch Surg* 2008, **143**(10):990–999. discussion 1000.
48. Martin J, *et al*: **Changes in sedation management in German intensive care units between 2002 and 2006: a national follow-up survey.** *Crit Care* 2007, **11**(6):R124.
49. Low JH: **Survey of epidural analgesia management in general intensive care units in England.** *Acta Anaesthesiol Scand* 2002, **46**(7):799–805.
50. Constantin JM, *et al*: **Current use of sedation and analgesia: 218 resuscitations in France services practices survey.** *Ann Fr Anesth Reanim* 2010, **29**(5):339–346.
51. Park WY, Thompson JS, Lee KK: **Effect of epidural anesthesia and analgesia on perioperative outcome: a randomized, controlled Veterans Affairs cooperative study.** *Ann Surg* 2001, **234**(4):560–569. discussion 569-71.
52. Nishimori M, *et al*: **Epidural pain relief versus systemic opioid-based pain relief for abdominal aortic surgery.** *Cochrane Database Syst Rev* 2012, **7**:CD005059.
53. Atkins E, Bodel P: **Fever.** *N Engl J Med* 1972, **286**(1):27–34.
54. Rabuel C, *et al*: **Human septic myopathy: induction of cyclooxygenase, heme oxygenase and activation of the ubiquitin proteolytic pathway.** *Anesthesiology* 2004, **101**(3):583–590.
55. Broyles LM, *et al*: **Clinicians' evaluation and management of mental health, substance abuse, and chronic pain conditions in the intensive care unit.** *Crit Care Med* 2008, **36**(1):87–93.
56. Pasero C, *et al*: **Structured approaches to pain management in the ICU.** *Chest* 2009, **135**(6):1665–1672.
57. Li D, *et al*: **Evaluations of physiologic reactivity and reflexive behaviors during noxious procedures in sedated critically ill patients.** *J Crit Care* 2009, **24**(3):472. e9-13.
58. Jeitziner MM, *et al*: **Assessment of pain in sedated and mechanically ventilated patients: an observational study.** *Acta Anaesthesiol Scand* 2012, **56**(5):645–654.
59. Rapanos T, *et al*: **Rectal indomethacin reduces postoperative pain and morphine use after cardiac surgery.** *Can J Anaesth* 1999, **46**(8):725–730.
60. Hynninen MS, *et al*: **Non-steroidal anti-inflammatory drugs in treatment of postoperative pain after cardiac surgery.** *Can J Anaesth* 2000, **47**(12):1182–1187.
61. Erstad BL, Chopda S, Esser MJ: **Prescribing of analgesics in trauma patients.** *Am J Ther* 1997, **4**(1):27–30.
62. Puntillo K, Ley SJ: **Appropriately timed analgesics control pain due to chest tube removal.** *Am J Crit Care* 2004, **13**(4):292–301. discussion 302; quiz 303-4.
63. Mehta S, *et al*: **Daily sedation interruption in mechanically ventilated critically ill patients cared for with a sedation protocol: a randomized controlled trial.** *JAMA* 2012, **308**(19):1985–1992.
64. Shehabi Y, *et al*: **Early intensive care sedation predicts long-term mortality in ventilated critically ill patients.** *Am J Respir Crit Care Med* 2012, **186**(8):724–731.
65. Shehabi Y, *et al*: **Sedation depth and long-term mortality in mechanically ventilated critically ill adults: a prospective longitudinal multicentre cohort study.** *Intensive Care Med* 2013. in press.
66. Herridge MS, *et al*: **Functional disability 5 years after acute respiratory distress syndrome.** *N Engl J Med* 2011, **364**(14):1293–1304.
67. Kress JP, Herridge MS: **Medical and economic implications of physical disability of survivorship.** *Semin Respir Crit Care Med* 2012, **33**(4):339–347.
68. Treggiari MM, *et al*: **Randomized trial of light versus deep sedation on mental health after critical illness.** *Crit Care Med* 2009, **37**(9):2527–2534.
69. Ely EW, Dittus RS, Girard TD: **Point: should benzodiazepines be avoided in mechanically ventilated patients? Yes.** *Chest* 2012, **142**(2):281–284. discussion 289-90.
70. Skrobik Y: **Counterpoint: should benzodiazepines be avoided in mechanically ventilated patients? No.** *Chest* 2012, **142**(2):284–287. discussion 287-9.
71. Barletta JF, Devlin JW: **Sedation with dexmedetomidine vs lorazepam in mechanically ventilated patients.** *JAMA* 2008, **299**(13):1541–1542. author reply 1542.
72. Jakob SM, *et al*: **Dexmedetomidine vs midazolam or propofol for sedation during prolonged mechanical ventilation: two randomized controlled trials.** *JAMA* 2012, **307**(11):1151–1160.
73. Wunsch H: **Weighing the costs and benefits of a sedative.** *JAMA* 2012, **307**(11):1195–1197.
74. Martin J, *et al*: **Evidence and consensus-based German guidelines for the management of analgesia, sedation and delirium in intensive care–short version.** *Ger Med Sci* 2010, **8**:Doc02.
75. Bigatello LM, *et al*: **Effects of routine monitoring of delirium in a surgical/trauma intensive care unit.** *J Trauma Acute Care Surg* 2013, **74**(3):876–883.
76. Pisani MA, *et al*: **Benzodiazepine and opioid use and the duration of intensive care unit delirium in an older population.** *Crit Care Med* 2009, **37**(1):177–183.
77. Pandharipande P, *et al*: **Lorazepam is an independent risk factor for transitioning to delirium in intensive care unit patients.** *Anesthesiology* 2006, **104**(1):21–26.
78. Riker RR, *et al*: **Dexmedetomidine vs midazolam for sedation of critically ill patients: a randomized trial.** *JAMA* 2009, **301**(5):489–499.
79. Shehabi Y, *et al*: **Prevalence of delirium with dexmedetomidine compared with morphine based therapy after cardiac surgery: a randomized controlled trial (DEXmedetomidine COmpared to Morphine-DEXCOM Study).** *Anesthesiology* 2009, **111**(5):1075–1084.
80. Skrobik Y, *et al*: **Factors Predisposing to Coma and Delirium: Fentanyl and Midazolam Exposure; CYP3A5, ABCB1, and ABCG2 Genetic Polymorphisms; and Inflammatory Factors.** *Crit Care Med* 2013, **41**(4):999–1008.
81. Kress JP: **The complex interplay between delirium, sepsis and sedation.** *Crit Care* 2010, **14**(3):164.
82. van den Boogaard M, *et al*: **Development and validation of PRE-DELIRIC (PREdiction of DELIRium in ICu patients) delirium prediction model for intensive care patients: observational multicentre study.** *BMJ* 2012, **344**:e420.
83. Campbell NL, *et al*: **Improving delirium care in the intensive care unit: the design of a pragmatic study.** *Trials* 2011, **12**:139.
84. Aizawa K, *et al*: **A novel approach to the prevention of postoperative delirium in the elderly after gastrointestinal surgery.** *Surg Today* 2002, **32**(4):310–314.
85. Maldonado JR, *et al*: **Dexmedetomidine and the reduction of postoperative delirium after cardiac surgery.** *Psychosomatics* 2009, **50**(3):206–217.
86. Hudetz JA, *et al*: **Ketamine attenuates delirium after cardiac surgery with cardiopulmonary bypass.** *J Cardiothorac Vasc Anesth* 2009, **23**(5):651–657.
87. Prakanrattana U, Prapaitrakool S: **Efficacy of risperidone for prevention of postoperative delirium in cardiac surgery.** *Anaesth Intensive Care* 2007, **35**(5):714–719.
88. van Eijk MM, *et al*: **Routine use of the confusion assessment method for the intensive care unit: a multicenter study.** *Am J Respir Crit Care Med* 2011, **184**(3):340–344.
89. Bledowski J, Trutia A: **A review of pharmacologic management and prevention strategies for delirium in the intensive care unit.** *Psychosomatics* 2012, **53**(3):203–211.
90. Ouimet S, *et al*: **Subsyndromal delirium in the ICU: evidence for a disease spectrum.** *Intensive Care Med* 2007, **33**(6):1007–1013.
91. Wang W, *et al*: **Haloperidol prophylaxis decreases delirium incidence in elderly patients after noncardiac surgery: a randomized controlled trial*.** *Crit Care Med* 2012, **40**(3):731–739.
92. van den Boogaard M, *et al*: **Haloperidol prophylaxis in critically ill patients with a high risk for delirium.** *Crit Care* 2013, **17**(1):R9.
93. Girard TD, *et al*: **Feasibility, efficacy, and safety of antipsychotics for intensive care unit delirium: the MIND randomized, placebo-controlled trial.** *Crit Care Med* 2010, **38**(2):428–437.
94. Devlin JW, *et al*: **Efficacy and safety of quetiapine in critically ill patients with delirium: a prospective, multicenter, randomized, double-blind, placebo-controlled pilot study.** *Crit Care Med* 2010, **38**(2):419–427.

95. Awissi DK, *et al*: **Alcohol withdrawal and delirium tremens in the critically ill: a systematic review and commentary.** *Intensive Care Med* 2013, **39**(1):16–30.
96. van Eijk MM, *et al*: **Effect of rivastigmine as an adjunct to usual care with haloperidol on duration of delirium and mortality in critically ill patients: a multicentre, double-blind, placebo-controlled randomised trial.** *Lancet* 2010, **376**(9755):1829–1837.

21

Predictors of posttraumatic stress and quality of life in family members of chronically critically ill patients after intensive care

Gloria-Beatrice Wintermann[1,2,3], Kerstin Weidner[1], Bernhard Strauß[3], Jenny Rosendahl[3*†] and Katja Petrowski[4*†]

Abstract

Background: Prolonged mechanical ventilation for acute medical conditions increases the risk of chronic critical illness (CCI). Close family members are confronted with the life-threatening condition of the CCI patients and are prone to develop posttraumatic stress disorder affecting their health-related quality of life (HRQL). Main aim of the present study was to investigate patient- and family-related risk factors for posttraumatic stress and decreased HRQL in family members of CCI patients.

Methods: In a cross-sectional design nested within a prospective longitudinal cohort study, posttraumatic stress symptoms and quality of life were assessed in family members of CCI patients ($n = 83$, aged between 18 and 72 years) up to 6 months after transfer from ICU at acute care hospital to post-acute rehabilitation. Patients admitted a large rehabilitation hospital for ventilator weaning. The Posttraumatic Stress Scale-10 and the Euro-Quality of life-5D-3L were applied in both patients and their family members via telephone interview.

Results: A significant proportion of CCI patients and their family members (14.5 and 15.7 %, respectively) showed clinically relevant scores of posttraumatic stress. Both CCI patients and family members reported poorer HRQL than a normative sample. Factors independently associated with posttraumatic stress in family members were the time following ICU discharge ($\beta = .256$, 95 % confidence interval .053–.470) and the patients' diagnosis of PTSD ($\beta = .264$, 95 % confidence interval .045–.453). Perceived satisfaction with the relationship turned out to be a protective factor for posttraumatic stress in family members of CCI patients ($\beta = -.231$, 95 % confidence interval −.423 to −.015). Regarding HRQL in family members, patients' acute posttraumatic stress at ICU ($\beta = -.290$, 95 % confidence interval −.360 to −.088) and their own posttraumatic stress 3 to 6 months post-transfer ($\beta = -.622$, 95 % confidence interval −.640 to −.358) turned out to be significant predictors.

Conclusions: Posttraumatic stress and HRQL should be routinely assessed in family members of CCI patients at regular intervals starting early at ICU. Preventive family-centered interventions are needed to improve posttraumatic stress and HRQL in both patients and their family members.

Keywords: Chronic critical illness (CCI), Intensive care, Posttraumatic stress symptoms, Health-related quality of life (HRQL), Family members, Post-intensive care syndrome (PICS) family, Sepsis

*Correspondence: jenny.rosendahl@med.uni-jena.de; k.petrowskin@dshs-koeln.de
†Jenny Rosendahl and Katja Petrowski contributed equally to this work
[3] Institute of Psychosocial Medicine and Psychotherapy, Jena University Hospital, Friedrich-Schiller University, Stoystr. 3, 07743 Jena, Germany
[4] Department of Workplace Health Promotion, German Sport University Cologne, Cologne, Germany
Full list of author information is available at the end of the article

Background

Treatment on intensive care unit (ICU) for acute medical, surgical, neurologic or cardiac critical illness can go along with secondary medical complications such as severe sepsis with multiorgan failure. Elective placement of tracheotomy and prolonged mechanical ventilation for at least 21 consecutive days put these patients at risk for the development of chronic critical illness (CCI). About 5–10 % of patients requiring prolonged ventilator weaning show an unspecific clinical syndrome of additional key characteristics, e.g., neuromuscular weakness, myopathy, neuropathy, protracted coma, delirium, malnutrition, anasarca, endocrinopathy, inflammatory impairment and intense psychophysiological distress [1, 2]. After discharge from ICU or specialized weaning units, patients still show functional impairments or even ongoing need for ventilator support with an increased risk of death.

The traumatic event of acute critical illness leading to ICU treatment, the heightened 1-year mortality and associated severe physical complications lead to increased caregiving demands and psychological stress in the whole family system of CCI patients [2]. Family members of CCI patients experience a cluster of mental complications [e.g., major depression, complicated grief, acute and posttraumatic stress disorder (ASD/PTSD)] which have been referred to as post-intensive care syndrome family (PICS-F) [3]. Prevalence estimates for clinically relevant posttraumatic stress symptoms in family members of the general ICU population widely range (13–57 %) with a median point prevalence of 21 % [4–7, see systematic reviews: 3, 8, 9]. Highest prevalence rates for posttraumatic stress symptoms in family members of adult general ICU patients have been shown 3 (56 %) [10] and 6 (49 %) [6] months following ICU stay. However, few studies exist assessing the occurrence and severity of posttraumatic stress in family members of CCI patients.

A recent study has shown clinically relevant symptoms of posttraumatic stress in two-third of spouses of CCI patients even an average of 55 months after ICU discharge. Above, higher own or patients' posttraumatic stress was associated with lower mental and general health-related quality of life (HRQL) in both spouses of CCI patients [11] and in family members of general ICU patients [5]. Furthermore, spouses reported a significantly worse mental HRQL than German normative samples [11].

There is large evidence regarding predictors of posttraumatic stress and impaired HRQL in family members of ICU patients. Characteristics increasing the risk of clinically relevant posttraumatic stress in family members of critically ill patients include female gender, younger age, lower educational level, being an adult child, lifetime mental disorder, higher state or trait anxiety, involvement in decision-making process, bereavement, severity of acute illness and dissatisfaction with information [for an overview see 12]. Family members of younger-aged or critically ill patients were at increased risk of PTSD [13, 14]. Furthermore, the patients' and their family members' psychological distress was positively associated up to 6 months following the ICU discharge [e.g., 6]. Regarding the impact of time following ICU discharge on posttraumatic stress in family members, some studies show a decrease in posttraumatic stress, no impact or even an increase with time following ICU discharge [4–6, 11].

Taken together, studies concerning the occurrence of posttraumatic stress in close family members of CCI patients are rare, show heterogeneous results [12], apply various symptom cutoff scores, use either heterogeneous or selective samples of only spouses [11] and consider follow-up periods that are rather short [e.g., 5, 7: 3 months] or quite long [e.g., 11: 55 months]. However, whether results can be replicated in a large, homogeneous and representative sample of both spousal and nonspousal dyads consisting of the CCI patient and their close family members remains to be further elucidated.

Hence, the aims of the present prospective, longitudinal cohort study were the following: first, to investigate whether there were differences in the level of posttraumatic stress and HRQL between CCI patients and their close (spousal or nonspousal) family members. Second aim was to clarify the impact of distinct patient and familymember characteristics as risk factors for the prediction of posttraumatic stress and HRQL in spousal and nonspousal family members of CCI patients following up to 6 months after transfer from ICU at acute care hospital to post-acute rehabilitation.

Methods

Setting and procedure

The study was registered at the German Clinical Trials Register (No. DRKS00003386) and approved by the Local Ethics Committee of the Friedrich-Schiller University, Jena, Germany (No 3278-10/11). All patients have signed written informed consent. Family members gave informed consent orally on the telephone.

Participants and sample size

Criteria for inclusion were a principal diagnosis of critical illness polyneuropathy (CIP; ICD: G62.80) or critical illness myopathy (CIM; ICD: G72.80) with or without sepsis, age between 18 and 72 years, a minimum length of ICU stay of 6 days, sufficient German language skills, informed consent, a negative evaluation of the cognitive test Confusion Assessment Method for the Intensive Care Unit (CAM-ICU) [15, 16] and the presence of a close family member willing to participate in the present study. Patients were excluded from the present study if they were not alert, they were cognitively impaired or they had sensory deficits limiting their ability to communicate. Family members were included if they were at least 18 years of age, gave oral informed consent, showed sufficient German language skills and could be regarded as being closely interrelated with the CCI patient. A close family member was defined as a person most involved in the CCI patient's treatment and care decisions [7]. Participants were consecutively enrolled. The study was observational with longitudinal and cross-sectional data assessment. Further details describing the study design are reported in [17].

CCI patients were interviewed orally and vis à vis within 4 weeks after transfer from intensive care at acute care hospitals to the ICU in post-acute rehabilitation (t1). Patients were again interviewed via telephone contact 3 (t2) or 6 months (t3) post-transfer. In the following, we refer to the follow-up of t2/t3 as up to 6 months. At t2 or t3, patients were asked whether they had a close family member who would agree to be interviewed. Patients and the patients' family members were enrolled and interviewed (up to 6 months following transfer to post-acute rehabilitation) if both gave oral informed consent on the telephone. For the present study, a subsample of the already published sample of chronically critically ill patients with data available of their close family members was used [17].

Measures

Posttraumatic stress was assessed with the German version of the Posttraumatic Symptom Scale (PTSS-10) [18, 19]. The PTSS-10 was applied within a time frame of up to 6 months after transfer from acute care hospital to post-acute rehabilitation in both CCI patients and their close family members. The questionnaire consists of ten items assessing the symptom categories increased arousal, re-experiencing and avoidance according to DSM-III-R criteria [20]. Items are rated on a seven-point Likert scale (1 = never, 7 = always). The total score is received by summing up the scores of all items (range 10–70). A score of more than 35 points is considered as adequate cutoff for clinically relevant PTSD symptomatology [19]. The internal consistency of the PTSS-10 can be regarded as high in the present study (Cronbach's α .87 for patients and .82 for family members). Additionally, the diagnosis of PTSD was ascertained with the Structured Clinical Interview for DSM-IV (SCID) [21] in CCI patients.

Quality of life was assessed with the questionnaire Euro-Quality of Life (EQ-5D-3L) [22] up to 6 months after transfer from acute care hospital to post-acute rehabilitation in CCI patients and their close family members. The EQ-5D-3L measures the HRQL on five dimensions (mobility, self-care, usual activities, pain/discomfort and anxiety/depression) which are evaluated within three severity levels (no problems, some or moderate problems, and extreme problems or unable). Additional, the EQ-5D-3L assesses the current subjective health state via a visual analog scale ranging from 0 (worst health state) to 100 (best health state). A single one-dimensional index value is generated based on a simple sum score according to Hinz et al. [23]. In the present study, Cronbach's α for EQ-5D-3L was .74 for patients and .70 for their family members.

Medical history of the patients was assessed via patient records. Furthermore, the Barthel index was judged by an independent evaluator. Performance in 11 domains comprising activities of daily living (e.g., fecal incontinence, urinary incontinence, help with grooming/toilet use/feeding) is evaluated. Values of Barthel index range between 0 and 100. A higher value is associated with a better mobility and degree of independence from caregivers. Additionally, the early rehabilitation Barthel index was assessed with the seven domains including intensive care supervision, tracheostomy tube management and supervision, intermittent or continuous mechanical ventilation, confusion, behavioral disturbances, severe impairment of communication, and dysphagia, with a minimum value of −325 and a maximum value of 0 [24]. Both Barthel scales were summed up, yielding scores between −325 and 100. Inter-rater reliability is very high ($r = .95$). Test–retest reliability is good as well ($r = .89$) [25].

Acute posttraumatic stress in patients with CCI was measured with the German version of the Acute Stress Disorder Scale (ASDS) [26] within 4 weeks after transfer to post-acute rehabilitation. It consists of 19 items representing symptoms of re-experiencing, avoidance, arousal and dissociation. Patients rated the extent of symptoms on a five-point Likert scale (1 = not at all, 5 = very much). The items are summed up to a total score (range 19–95). In the present study, Cronbach's α was .96. Additionally, the diagnosis of ASD was ascertained with the SCID [21].

Statistical methods

Normal distribution was tested using the Kolmogorov–Smirnov test. In case of nonnormal distribution, data medians and interquartile ranges are reported. For continuous and normally distributed data, the means and standard deviations were calculated. Categorical variables are reported as absolute and relative frequencies. Bivariate correlational analyses were calculated using point-biserial correlation for a dichotomous and a continuous variable. Wilcoxon's signed-rank test was used to compare means of outcome variables (HRQL/posttraumatic stress) between patients and family members. McNemar test was conducted in case of dyadic nominal outcome data.

We compared EQ-5D-3L scores of age- and gender-stratified subgroups of our sample with the respective subgroups of a normative German sample [23]. Standardized mean differences (Cohen's *d*) with 95 % confidence interval (CI) were calculated for these comparisons. Likewise, the patients' and family members' PTSS scores were compared to a healthy control group as published by Schüffel et al. [27].

In order to identify risk factors associated with posttraumatic stress (PTSS-10 score) and HRQL (EQ-5D-3L score) in close family members of CCI patients, we first evaluated bivariate correlations (Kendall's tau, point-biserial correlation). We considered patient-related risk factors (patients' clinical, acute/chronic psychological and socioeconomic characteristics), family-related risk factors (family members' socioeconomic, chronic psychological characteristics) and partnership-related risk factors (perceived satisfaction/closeness) (see Additional file 1: Table S1, Additional file 2: Table S2, for a description of univariate correlations see Additional file 3). Second, variables that were correlated (p values <.2) with the dependent factor (ASD/PTSD symptomatology) were included in multivariable stepwise regression analyses. PTSS-10 and EQ-5D-3L up to 6 months following transfer to post-acute rehabilitation were considered as outcome variables. Standardized regression coefficients with 95 % CIs were used to quantify the strength of the association.

In the present study, normal distribution of outcome data could not be approved. Analyses were realized using original data. Since multivariate regression analysis is regarded as robust against violations against normal distribution, it was performed nevertheless [28]. Transformation of raw values (empirical T values, normal rank-transformed values) only partially revealed normal distribution. A sensitivity analysis without outliers (data>/<2 SD of mean) did not change the main results of our regression model.

We applied a significance level $\alpha = .05$ (two sided). All analyses were performed using SPSS 23 (SPSS Inc., Chicago, IL, USA).

Results

Of the $N = 352$ potential chronically critically ill patients, $n = 195$ could be successfully enrolled. Of these, $n = 60$ dyadic interviews could be conducted at follow-up about 3 months and further $n = 23$ dyadic interviews about 6 months after transfer from ICU at acute care hospital to post-acute rehabilitation hospital. Finally, data of $n = 83$ patient–family member dyads could be successfully gained up to 6 months following transfer to post-acute rehabilitation hospital (see Fig. 1). In the present study, patients who dropped out of the study revealed significantly more often the respiratory system as site of infection (59.8 %) than patients being followed up (44.6 %). Dropped-out patients showed a significantly lower Barthel index both at discharge from post-acute rehabilitation and at discharge from rehab hospital than patients being followed up (see Additional file 4: Table S3).

Most of the family members were partners ($n = 59$, 71.1 %) comprising husband/wives ($n = 54$, 65.1 %) and cohabitation ($n = 5$, 6.0 %). Other kinds of family members were mother ($n = 5$, 6.0 %), son ($n = 10$, 12.0 %), daughter ($n = 5$, 6.0 %) and sister ($n = 4$, 4.8 %). Family members were significantly younger (median age 59.9) than patients (median age 61.7). Significantly less family members (27.7 %) than patients (73.5 %) were male. Posttraumatic stress was assessed at a median time of 4.8 months following ICU discharge. Patients with CCI stayed at ICU a median time of 66.0 days. Median duration of mechanical ventilation was 50.0 days. An overview of the descriptive characteristics is given in Table 1.

Posttraumatic stress and impaired HRQL in patients and their close family members

Patients and their family members did not significantly differ with respect to median posttraumatic stress score as assessed with the PTSS-10 (median, patients: 20.0, family members: 18.0). 14.5 % of patients and 15.7 % of family members showed clinically significant posttraumatic stress symptoms without significant difference between both groups. CCI patients significantly differed regarding PTSS-10 score compared with a healthy control group ($d = .359$, 95 % CI .067–.65). Family members did not significantly differ with respect to posttraumatic stress symptoms compared with a healthy control group ($d = .245$, 95 % CI −.045 to .535). Patients with CCI showed a significantly lower HRQL than their family members. Compared with a healthy German normative sample, HRQL was significantly lower in patients with CCI ($d = -2.063$, 95 % CI −2.291 to −1.834) as well as in their close family members ($d = -.394$, 95 % CI −.614 to −.174) (see Table 2).

There was a significant association between patients' and family members' posttraumatic stress (PTSS-10, $\tau = .167$, $p = .030$). Concerning HRQL, no dyadic association could be found (EQ-5D-3L, $\tau = .108$, $p = .216$). Both groups, family members and CCI patients, showed a significant negative association between their PTSS-10 scores and their EQ-5D-3L scores (actor effect) (PTSS-10 × EQ-5D-3L, family members: $\tau = -.367$, $p < .001$;

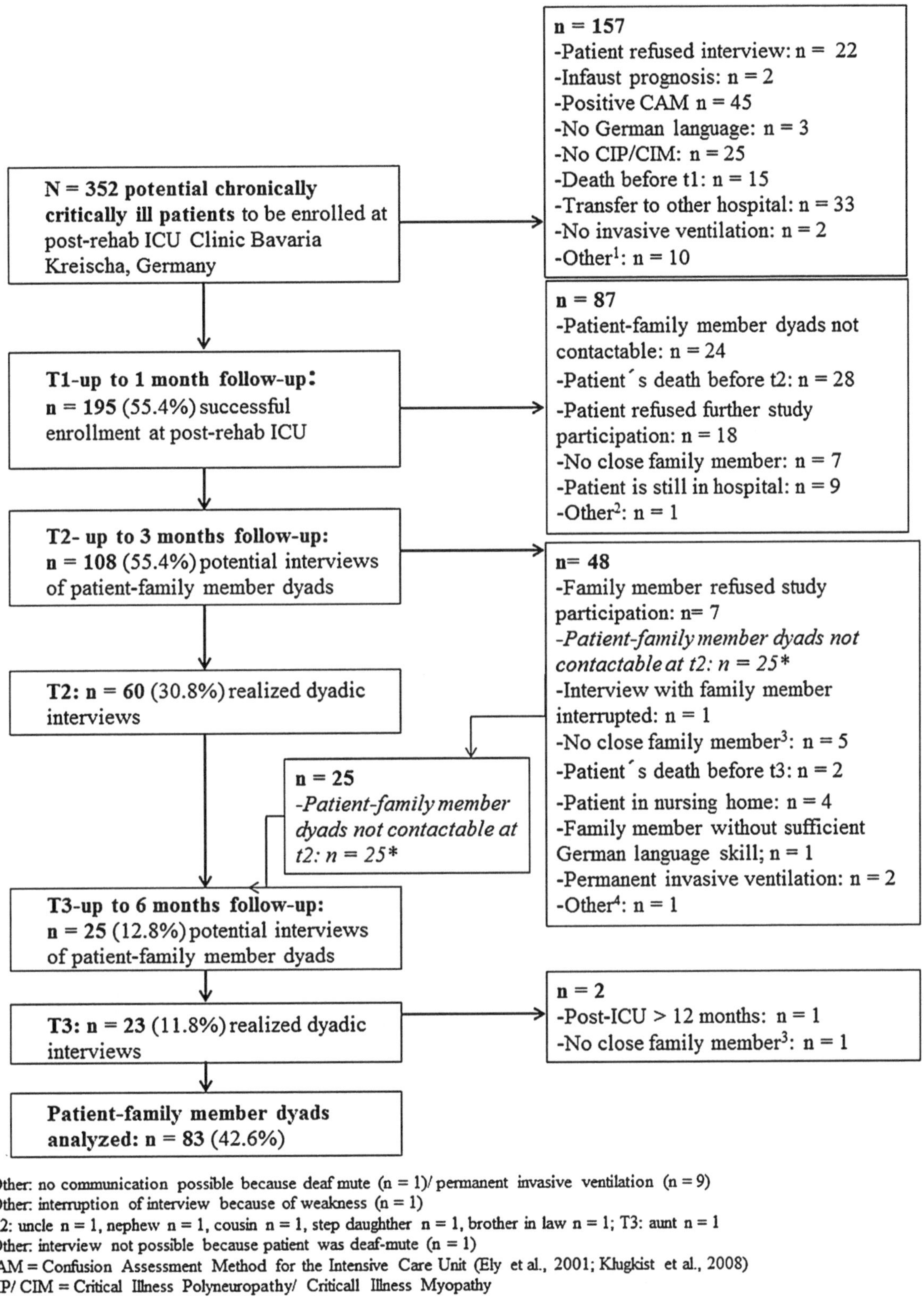

Fig. 1 Study flow diagram. $N = 83$ dyads comprising a CCI patients and their close family member were finally analyzed. [1]Other: no communication possible because deaf-mute ($n = 1$)/permanent invasive ventilation ($n = 9$). [2]Other: interruption of interview because of weakness ($n = 1$). [3]T2: uncle $n = 1$, nephew $n = 1$, cousin $n = 1$, step daughter $n = 1$, brother in law $n = 1$; T3: aunt $n = 1$. [4]Other: interview not possible because patient was deaf-mute ($n = 1$). *CAM* Confusion Assessment Method for the Intensive Care Unit [15, 16]. *CIP/CIM* critical illness polyneuropathy/critical illness myopathy

Table 1 Descriptive characteristics of the dyads of patients with chronic critical illness and their family members ($n = 83$)

Characteristic	Patients	Family members	χ^2/Z	*p*
Age [years median (IQR)]	61.7 (56.0 to 65.7)	59.9 (48.6 to 64.4)	−2.853	*.004**** (*Z*)[a]
Gender [*n* (%)]				
Male	61 (73.5)	23 (27.7)		
Female	22 (26.5)	60 (72.3)	19.014	*<.001**** (χ^2)[b]
Family status [*n* (%)]				
Single	6 (7.2)			
Married/cohabited	63 (75.9)			
Divorced/living apart	8 (9.6)			
Widowed	6 (7.2)			
Characteristics of relationship [median (IQR)]				
Length of partnership[c]		37.0 (25.8 to 43.0)		
Satisfaction with relationship		10.0 (8.0 to 10.0)		
Closeness of relationship		10.0 (9.0 to 10.0)		
Living together in mutual household, yes/no [*n* (%)]		62 (74.7)/21 (25.3)		
Caring for ill patient at the moment, yes/no [*n* (%)]		45 (54.2)/38 (45.8)		
Education [*n* (%)][d]				
<10 years	26 (31.3)			
≥10 years	54 (65.1)			
ICU stay [days median (IQR)]	66.0 (49.0 to 97.0)			
Mechanical ventilation [days median (IQR)]	50.0 (33.0 to 76.0)			
Sepsis [*n* (%)]				
No sepsis	29 (34.9)			
Sepsis	28 (33.7)			
Severe sepsis or septic shock	26 (31.3)			
Site of infection [*n* (%)]				
Respiratory	37 (44.6)			
Urinary/genitals	8 (9.6)			
Abdominal	8 (9.6)			
Bones/soft tissue	5 (6.0)			
Wound infection	2 (2.4)			
Heart	1 (1.2)			
Multiple	9 (10.8)			
Others[e]	4 (4.8)			
Unknown	4 (4.8)			
Barthel index, median (IQR)				
At admission at post-acute ICU	−200.0 (−225.0 to 140.0)			
At discharge from post-acute rehabilitation	−25.0 (−80.0 to 10.0)			
At discharge from rehab hospital	70.0 (45.0 to 85.0)			
Time following ICU discharge [months median (IQR)]	4.7 (3.8 to 6.4) Min 3.1, Max 9.2	4.8 (3.9–6.5) Min 3.1, Max 9.2	−4.096	*<.001**** (*Z*)[a]
Time following mechanical ventilation [months median (IQR)]	3.9 (3.2 to 5.9) Min 1.3, Max 8.5	4.2 (3.3–6.1) Min 1.3, Max 9.4	−4.089	*<.001**** (*Z*)[a]

*p ≤ .05

***p ≤ .001

[a] *Z* value and *p* value from Wilcoxon's signed-rank test

[b] χ^2 (chi-square) value and *p* value from McNemar test

[c] $n = 25$ missing values

[d] $n = 3$ missing values

[e] $n = 1$ brain, $n = 3$ central venous catheter

Table 2 Psychological characteristics of the dyads of patients with CCI and their close family member ($n = 83$)

Characteristic	Patients	Family members	Z/χ^2	p
Posttraumatic Stress Scale				
Median (IQR)[a]	20.0 (14.0–29.0)	18.0 (14.0–28.0)	−1.029	.303 (Z)[b]
Posttraumatic Stress Scale[a] ≥ 35 (%)	12 (14.5)	13 (15.7)	.000	1.000 (χ^2)[c]
Quality of life[d]				
Median (IQR)	70.0 (50.0–80.0)	90.0 (80.0–100.0)	−6.529	*<.001**** (Z)[b]
History of traumatic life experiences				
Yes [n (%)][e]	24 (28.9)[e]	46 (55.4)	5.281	*.022** (χ^2)[c]

*p ≤ .05

***p ≤ .001

[a] PTSS-10 [19]; [b] Z value and p value from Wilcoxon's signed-rank test; [c] χ^2 (chi-square) value and p value from McNemar test; [d] EQ-5D-3L formula according to Hinz et al. [23]; [e] $n = 14$ (16.9 %) missing values

patients: $\tau = -.384$, $p < .001$). Patients and family members with higher posttraumatic stress reported lower HRQL. Regarding the effect of posttraumatic stress on their respective partners' HRQL (partner effect), there was no significant impact in neither of the two groups (PTSS-10 × EQ-5L, family members: $\tau = -.135$, $p = .095$; patients: $\tau = -.068$, $p = .413$).

Predictors of posttraumatic stress in family members of CCI patients

Up to 6 months following discharge from ICU of CCI patients, the time following ICU discharge ($\beta = .262$, 95 % CI .061–.476) and a diagnosis of PTSD up to 6 months following ICU discharge in CCI patients ($\beta = .254$, 95 % CI .089–1.102) could be identified as significant patient-related characteristics predictive of posttraumatic stress in family members. With respect to family-related characteristics, the perceived satisfaction with the relationship could be identified ($\beta = -.229$, 95 % CI −.425 to −.013). The model explained an adjusted total variance of 17.9 % [$R^2 = .18$, $F(3, 77) = 6.828$, $p < .001$] (Table 3).

Predictors of HRQL in family members of CCI patients

Within 3 to 6 months following discharge from ICU of the CCI patient, their own PTSS-10 score ($\beta = -.622$, 95 % CI −.640 to −.358) and the acute posttraumatic stress at ICU as assessed with the ASDS in CCI patients ($\beta = -.290$, 95 % CI −.360 to −.088) could be identified as significant predictors of HRQL in close family members. The model explained an adjusted total variance of 47.4 % [$R^2 = .47$, $F(2, 66) = 31.583$, $p < .001$] (see Additional file 5: Table S4).

Discussion

The primary aim of the present study was the investigation of the level of posttraumatic stress and HRQL in close family members of CCI patients with or without sepsis following 3 to 6 months after ICU discharge. The secondary aim was on the examination of dyadic associations between posttraumatic stress and HRQL between patients and their family members. Third, we intended to specify patient- and family-related predictors of posttraumatic stress and HRQL in close family members of CCI patients.

Clinically relevant symptomatology of PTSD was a problem for both patients and their close family members. Nearly every sixth close family member and every seventh patient surviving CCI displays symptoms of clinically significant posttraumatic stress up to 6 months following ICU. Both groups showed a significantly reduced HRQL compared with a German normative sample [23]. CCI patients displayed an EQ-5D-3L score approximately

Table 3 Multiple stepwise regression analysis with patient and family member characteristics as regressors and posttraumatic stress in family member of CCI patients as dependent variable $N = (83)$

Predictors of posttraumatic stress in family members of CCI patients	β	95 % CI	T	p
Characteristics of patients with CCI				
Diagnosis of PTSD, 3–6 months following ICU	.254	.089 to 1.102	2.342	*.022**
Time following ICU	.262	.061 to .476	2.571	*.012**
Characteristics of close family members				
Satisfaction with relationship	−.229	−.425 to −.013	−2.122	*.037**

*p ≤ .05

two standard deviations below the mean of a representative healthy German sample. Regarding the effect of posttraumatic stress on HRQL, actor effects but no partner effects could be elucidated. Significant patient-related predictors for posttraumatic stress in family members of CCI patients 3 to 6 months following ICU discharge were the time following ICU and a diagnosis of post-ICU PTSD. The perceived satisfaction with the relationship was associated with a decreased PTSS-10 score. Regarding HRQL in close family members of patients with CCI, a higher posttraumatic stress at post-rehab ICU in patients and their own posttraumatic stress were significant predictors.

Clinically significant posttraumatic stress symptoms are among the most common psychological long-term sequelae in intensive care unit survivors with a median point prevalence of 19 % [e.g., 29, 30]. Also family members of critically ill patients are at risk of posttraumatic stress disorder both during and after the ICU stay as second-order patients. The critical illness and admission to the ICU are life-threatening events putting the whole family on a severe emotional crisis with profound changes in family roles and responsibilities [31]. Moreover, caregiver of CCI patients experiences distress which presumably arises from patients' problem behaviors such as negative emotions or pain. Above, family members perceive restrictions in social life and personal recreation [32]. The rate of clinically relevant posttraumatic stress symptoms in our study was 15.7 % for close family members and 14.5 % for CCI patients. This frequency is a bit higher than the rate found in a sample of older adults seeking medical services in primary health clinics (11.1 %) [33] but in line with a former study showing a prevalence rate of 14.0 % for family members of patients dying at the ICU [13]. Jubran et al. [34] also found a lower prevalence rate of 12.0 % for diagnosed PTSD in patients surviving weaning from prolonged mechanical ventilation. Lower prevalence rates in the present study contradict higher prevalence rates in former studies [e.g., 4–6, 11]. This might be justified by differences in the applied methods and cutoffs to assess posttraumatic stress. For instance, the lowest prevalence rates of PTSD have been found in studies using self-report symptom checklists as item mapping approach based on DSM-IV criteria for PTSD [13, 35]. Moreover, higher prevalence rates were more common in homogeneous sample of spouses than other kinship relations [e.g., 11, 14]. In contrast, other studies also comprising nonspousal family members, patient's next of kins or designated power of attorney for healthcare even found higher rates of posttraumatic stress [4–6, 36]. Thus, the specific characteristics of the respective study samples might have played a major role. Former studies could show highest prevalence rates in family members whose relative died in the ICU and who shared in end-of-life decisions [5, 12, 37]. In the present study, only CCI patients who survived the follow-up period were included. Moreover, former studies could approve younger age as significant predictor of post-ICU posttraumatic stress. Following, lower prevalence rates in the present study might be ascribed to older age since nearly 50 % of the family members were aged 60 years or older [37, 38].

The present study could confirm a negative association between posttraumatic stress and HRQL in both CCI patients and their close family member after intensive care [11]. Our results are also in line with the study by Chung et al. [39] showing a significant actor effect for depressive and anxiety symptoms on quality of life in both patients with heart failure and their spouses. The increased and ongoing need for care during the post-acute recovery phase demands close interactions between patients and their family members. This launches a contagious process of emotional transmission leading to the induction of feelings of empathy in the members of the dyad. Consequently, a patient's HRQL can be affected not only by his/her own mental health status (actor effect) but also by their respective family member's one (partner effect) [11]. In the present study, no partner effects could be shown. Also former studies could not consistently reveal partner effects. Chung et al. [39] could only show partner effects for spouses of patients with heart failure. Those spouses with high depressive/anxiety symptoms negatively impacted the quality of life in the respective patients. Rosendahl et al. [11] could only show partner effects for posttraumatic stress symptoms of patients surviving severe sepsis on their spouses' mental HRQL. Another study in cancer patients showed a transmission of emotional stress only from male patients to their female partners [40]. A possible explanation of the missing partner effects for the present study might be the inclusion of a heterogeneous sample of both spouses and other family members (sister, daughter, son, etc.). Moreover, the EQ-5D-3L is not sufficiently sensitive for the assessment of the mental component of HRQL or a differential representation of social and emotional role functioning which might be disturbed in family members of CCI patients.

Another influential factor displays the time frame for the assessment of posttraumatic stress symptoms in CCI patients and their close family members. Former studies have shown the highest prevalence rates for posttraumatic stress symptoms associated with a moderate to major risk of PTSD 3 months [e.g., 5, 7, 10] and 6 months [e.g., 6] following ICU discharge. Findings even suggest that intensity of PTSD symptoms declines in the follow-up of the ICU experience [7] and there is a considerable rate showing recovery with decreasing PTSD symptoms post-ICU [41]. However, in the present study family members' posttraumatic stress could be significantly predicted by the time following ICU discharge. Since illness-associated morbidity in this particular sample of CCI patients persists for years, it is well known that several months after ICU discharge the physical and emotional burden of disease endures in these patients and their family [2]. CCI patients exhibit an increased hospital lethality of about 50 % and a 1-year survival rate of only 25 % [42, 43]. Following, the patient's hospital discharge does not resolve psychological stress for the family system. Hospital readmissions and the development of new or worsening impairments in physical, cognitive or mental health status [30] expose the family members to a chronic state of psychological arousal. Thus, vulnerability for clinically relevant symptoms of posttraumatic stress is increased even in the follow-up after ICU discharge. This finding is further corroborated by a considerable rate of delayed onset or chronic/persistent course of PTSD during longer follow-up periods in the aftermath of ICU stay [41, 44].

Another major finding of the present study is the prediction of HRQL in family members of CCI patients by the patients' acute posttraumatic stress at ICU. To the best of our knowledge, this is the first study prospectively assessing patient-related characteristics and associating them with HRQL in close family members of CCI patients. The intensity of acute posttraumatic stress experienced by CCI patients within 1 month following transfer from acute care hospital mirrors the severity of the traumatic event the patients were exposed to and the acute psychological reactions in the ICU (e.g., agitation, extreme fear, early intrusive memories, delirious symptoms, mood disturbance) putting those patients at increased risk of persistent or delayed PTSD in the follow-up [45]. Following, the more distressed and emotionally aroused patients are during ICU stay the more they impact their close family members' emotional as well as physical well-being. This could be shown in the present study by a, although small, but significantly positive correlation between posttraumatic stress in CCI patients and their close family member [see also 46]. Furthermore and up to a certain extent, the present finding could be corroborated by a study showing an association between psychological distress in patients 2 weeks after ICU discharge and PTSD scores in their close family members at 6-month follow-up [6]. Another predictor of family members' posttraumatic stress was the satisfaction with the relationship. This family-related factor turned out to be protective and might moderate the relationship between emotional distress and quality of life [39].

We could not find a significant effect of the severity of illness, the length of ICU stay, family member's age and gender. This is in line with existing findings [e.g., 11, 47] but on the other hand contradicts results showing a significant impact of caregivers' sex and length of ICU stay [48]. Jones et al. [6] did not find any association between the family members' posttraumatic stress and demographic characteristics related to the patient's ICU stay which confirms our findings. Above, sepsis has not been consistently elucidated as significant risk factor for post-ICU psychological morbidity in patients and their family members [17, 49–51]. The present findings confirm lower HRQL in women and participants of older age. This has been already shown in former studies [e.g., 23].

For the present study, some methodological shortcomings should be addressed. First, for the assessment of posttraumatic stress disorder a self-report measure (PTSS-10) instead of a clinician administered structured diagnostic interview was applied. The PTSS-10 is based on subjectively reported symptom intensities. Thus, a potential overestimation of the frequency of posttraumatic stress might have occurred. Above, the PTSS-10 has some limitations since it is based on DSM-III criteria, items on numbing or flashbacks are missing and only one item assesses avoidance. Future study should rather use the PTSS-14 [52] as extended version for a more accurate assessment of posttraumatic symptomatology. Second, the recruitment of family members by phone contact might have been prone to socially desirable answers and bias. Third, since the nature of the present study design is, although nested within a prospective study, rather observational and cross-sectional, no causal interference is possible. There is no information about posttraumatic stress in close family members of CCI patients at different time points following ICU discharge. Also, there is no information concerning the number of family members demanding psychological support or having been treated for their PTSD. Fourth, longitudinal and multicenter trials are needed and should focus on the long-term course of physical and mental health in patient–family member dyads after critical illness taking into account salutogenetic aspects of dyadic dynamics. Above, future studies should address the effectiveness of interventions (e.g., realization of the recommendations suggested in the pain, agitation and delirium clinical practice guidelines, establishment of Critical Care Recovery Centers (CCRC) [53]; family-centered interventions improve dyadic coping strategies [8]) in preventing post-intensive care syndrome, enhancing post-critical illness rehabilitation and improving quality of life in patients and their families after the ICU experience [3]. Additionally, future research should address the impact the family members' PTSD might have on the dyadic relationship and the CCI patients' recovery process. Moreover, the patients' family history of PTSD should be more closely focused on in order to identify genetic or sociological risk factors allowing targeted interventions in a risk population. With the aim to launch preventive interventions for effective care of clinically relevant PTSD in close family members of CCI patients, the early ascertainment of patient- as well as family-related risk factors and diagnostic markers for post-traumatic stress in close family members of CCI patients is highly warranted.

Conclusions

There is a considerable rate of clinically relevant post-traumatic stress symptoms and significantly diminished HRQL in close family members of CCI patients following ICU stay. Close family members of CCI patients display second-order patients which also suffer from impaired mental and physical long-term sequelae following CCI and intensive care. We suggest a routine assessment of patient- and family-related risk factors while the chronically critically ill patient is in the ICU and up to 6 months following discharge from ICU at acute care hospital. Posttraumatic stress and quality of life should be ascertained at regular intervals starting at ICU admission and being followed up at least 6 months post-ICU.

Additional files

Additional file 1: Table S1. Unadjusted univariate analyses to determine the association between risk factors (patient-related clinical, socioeconomic, acute psychological and chronic psychological factors; family-related socioeconomic, chronic psychological factors, characteristics of the partnership) and post-ICU posttraumatic stress as assessed with the PTSS-10 (Posttraumatic Stress Scale, Raphael et al., 1989) in close family members of patients with chronically critical illness up to six months after discharge from ICU at acute care hospital (sample: n = 83).

Additional file 2: **Table S2.** Unadjusted univariate analyses to determine the association between risk factors (patient-related clinical, socioeconomic, acute psychological and chronic psychological factors; family -related socioeconomic, acute psychological and chronic psychological factors, characteristics of the partnership) and post-ICU health-related quality of life as assessed with the EQ-5D-3L (Rabin & de Charro, 2001) in close relatives of patients with chronically critical illness up to six months after discharge from ICU (sample: n = 83).

Additional file 3: Description of univariate correlations.

Additional file 4: Table S3. Socio-demographic and clinical characteristics of the patients being followed up (n = 83) and drop outs (n = 112).

Additional file 5:Table S4. Multiple stepwise regression analysis with patient and family member characteristics as regressors and health-related quality of life in family member of CCI patients as dependent variable N = (83).

Abbreviations

ASDS: Acute Stress Disorder Scale; ASD: acute stress disorder; CCI: chronic critical illness; CAM-ICU: Confusion Assessment Method for the Intensive Care Unit; CI: confidence interval; EQ-5D-3L: Euro-Quality of Life; ICU: intensive care unit; PICS-F: post-intensive care syndrome family; PTSS-10: Posttraumatic Symptom Scale; PTSD: posttraumatic stress disorder; SCID: Structured Clinical Interview for DSM-IV.

Authors' contributions

GBW wrote the manuscript and was responsible for study coordination and final data assessment. JR developed the study design, mainly supported data assessment, the statistical analyses and profoundly improved the final version of the manuscript. KP proofread the manuscript and systematically contributed to the development of the main concept of the present manuscript. BS and KW supported the realization of the present study and contributed to manuscript improvement. All authors read and approved the final manuscript.

Author details

[1] Department of Psychotherapy and Psychosomatic Medicine, Medizinische Fakultät Carl Gustav Carus, Technische Universität Dresden, Dresden, Germany. [2] Center for Sepsis Control and Care, Jena University Hospital, Friedrich-Schiller University, Jena, Germany. [3] Institute of Psychosocial Medicine and Psychotherapy, Jena University Hospital, Friedrich-Schiller University, Stoystr. 3, 07743 Jena, Germany. [4] Department of Workplace Health Promotion, German Sport University Cologne, Cologne, Germany.

Acknowledgements

This study was supported by the German Federal Ministry of Education and Research grant 01EO1002. We would like to kindly thank Stefan Rueckriem, Sara Wüstemann, Clara Luise Buck, Christine Schlitter and Corinna Illgen for their support in data assessment and patient recruitment. Moreover, we would like to thank André Scherag for his statistical advice. We acknowledge support by the German Research Foundation and the Open Access Publication Funds of the TU Dresden.

Competing interests

The authors declare that they have no competing interests.

References

1. Marchioni A, Fantini R, Antenora F, Clini E, Fabbri L. Chronic critical illness: the price of survival. Eur J Clin Invest. 2015;45:1341–9.
2. Nelson JE, Cox CE, Hope AA, Carson SS. Chronic critical illness. Am J Respir Crit Care Med. 2010;182:446–54.
3. Davidson JE, Jones C, Bienvenu OJ. Family response to critical illness: postintensive care syndrome-family. Crit Care Med. 2012;40:618–24.
4. Anderson WG, Arnold RM, Angus DC, Bryce CL. Posttraumatic stress and complicated grief in family members of patients in the intensive care unit. J Gen Intern Med. 2008;23:1871–6.
5. Azoulay E, Pochard F, Kentish-Barnes N, Chevret S, Aboab J, Adrie C, et al. Risk of post-traumatic stress symptoms in family members of intensive care unit patients. Am J Respir Crit Care Med. 2005;171:987–94.
6. Jones C, Skirrow P, Griffiths RD, Humphris G, Ingleby S, Eddleston J, et al. Post-traumatic stress disorder-related symptoms in relatives of patients following intensive care. Intensive Care Med. 2004;30:456–60.
7. McAdam JL, Fontaine DK, White DB, Dracup KA, Puntillo KA. Psychological symptoms of family members of high-risk intensive care unit patients. Am J Crit Care. 2012;21:386–93 **(quiz 394)**.
8. Petrinec AB, Mazanec PM, Burant CJ, Hoffer A, Daly B. Coping strategies and posttraumatic stress symptoms in post-ICU family decision makers. Crit Care Med. 2015;43:1205–12.
9. van Beusekom I, Bakhshi-Raiez F, de Keizer NF, Dongelmans DA, van der Schaaf M. Reported burden on informal caregivers of ICU survivors: a literature review. Crit Care. 2016;20:16.
10. Lautrette A, Darmon M, Megarbane B, Joly LM, Chevret S, Adrie C, et al. A communication strategy and brochure for relatives of patients dying in the ICU. N Engl J Med. 2007;356:469–78.
11. Rosendahl J, Brunkhorst FM, Jaenichen D, Strauss B. Physical and mental health in patients and spouses after intensive care of severe sepsis: a

dyadic perspective on long-term sequelae testing the Actor–Partner Interdependence Model. Crit Care Med. 2013;41:69–75.
12. Hickman RL Jr, Douglas SL. Impact of chronic critical illness on the psychological outcomes of family members. AACN Adv Crit Care. 2010;21:80–91.
13. Gries CJ, Engelberg RA, Kross EK, Zatzick D, Nielsen EL, Downey L, et al. Predictors of symptoms of posttraumatic stress and depression in family members after patient death in the ICU. Chest. 2010;137:280–7.
14. Siegel MD, Hayes E, Vanderwerker LC, Loseth DB, Prigerson HG. Psychiatric illness in the next of kin of patients who die in the intensive care unit. Crit Care Med. 2008;36:1722–8.
15. Ely EW, Inouye SK, Bernard GR, Gordon S, Francis J, May L, et al. Delirium in mechanically ventilated patients: validity and reliability of the Confusion Assessment Method for the Intensive Care Unit (CAM-ICU). JAMA. 2001;286:2703–10.
16. Klugkist M, Sedemund-Adib B, Schmidtke C, Schmucker P, Sievers HH, Hüppe M. Confusion Assessment Method for the Intensive Care Unit (CAM-ICU): diagnosis of postoperative delirium in cardiac surgery. Anaesthesist. 2008;57:464–74.
17. Wintermann GB, Brunkhorst FM, Petrowski K, Strauss B, Oehmichen F, Pohl M, et al. Stress disorders following prolonged critical illness in survivors of severe sepsis. Crit Care Med. 2015;43:1213–22.
18. Raphael B, Lundin T, Weisaeth L. A research method for the study of psychological and psychiatric aspects of disaster. Acta Psychiatr Scand Suppl. 1989;353:1–75.
19. Stoll C, Kapfhammer HP, Rothenhausler HB, Haller M, Briegel J, Schmidt M, et al. Sensitivity and specificity of a screening test to document traumatic experiences and to diagnose post-traumatic stress disorder in ARDS patients after intensive care treatment. Intensive Care Med. 1999;25:697–704.
20. American Psychiatric Association. Diagnostic and statistical manual of mental disorders. 3rd ed. Washington: American Psychological Association; 1980.
21. Wittchen HU, Wunderlich U, Gruschwitz S, Zaudig M. Structured Clinical Interview for DSM disorders (SCID). Göttingen: Hogrefe; 1997.
22. Rabin R, de Charro F. EQ-5D: a measure of health status from the EuroQol Group. Ann Med. 2001;33:337–43.
23. Hinz A, Brahler E, Schwarz R, Schumacher J, Stirn A. How useful is the calculation of total scores for questionnaires concerning health related quality of life? Psychother Psychosom Med Psychol. 2005;55:221–8.
24. Rollnik JD. The Early Rehabilitation Barthel Index (ERBI). Rehabilitation (Stuttg). 2011;50:408–11.
25. O'Sullivan SB, Schmitz TJ. Physical rehabilitation, vol. 5. Philadelphia: FA Davis Company; 2006.
26. Helfricht S, Landolt MA, Moergeli H, Hepp U, Wegener D, Schnyder U. Psychometric evaluation and validation of the German version of the Acute Stress Disorder Scale across two distinct trauma populations. J Trauma Stress. 2009;22:476–80.
27. Schüffel W, Schade B, Schunk T. A brief inventory to investigate stress reactions: Posttraumatic Symptom Scale, 10 Items (PTSS-10) by Raphael, Lundin & Weisaeth. Marburg, Paper. http://psydok.sulb.uni-saarland.de/volltexte/2004/437/pdf/artikel.pdf. Accessed 17 Mar 2016.
28. van Belle G. Statistical rules of thumb. New York: Wiley; 2002.
29. Davydow DS, Gifford JM, Desai SV, Needham DM, Bienvenu OJ. Posttraumatic stress disorder in general intensive care unit survivors: a systematic review. Gen Hosp Psychiatry. 2008;30:421–34.
30. Needham DM, Davidson J, Cohen H, Hopkins RO, Weinert C, Wunsch H, et al. Improving long-term outcomes after discharge from intensive care unit: report from a stakeholders' conference. Crit Care Med. 2012;40:502–9.
31. Johnson SK, Craft M, Titler M, Halm M, Kleiber C, Montgomery LA, et al. Perceived changes in adult family members' roles and responsibilities during critical illness. Image J Nurs Sch. 1995;27:238–43.
32. Choi J, Donahoe MP, Zullo TG, Hoffman LA. Caregivers of the chronically critically ill after discharge from the intensive care unit: six months' experience. Am J Crit Care. 2011;20:12–22 **(quiz 23)**.
33. Preville M, Lamoureux-Lamarche C, Vasiliadis HM, Grenier S, Potvin O, Quesnel L, et al. The 6-month prevalence of posttraumatic stress syndrome (PTSS) among older adults: validity and reliability of the PTSS scale. Can J Psychiatry. 2014;59:548–55.
34. Jubran A, Lawm G, Duffner LA, Collins EG, Lanuza DM, Hoffman LA, et al. Post-traumatic stress disorder after weaning from prolonged mechanical ventilation. Intensive Care Med. 2010;36:2030–7.
35. Jackson JC, Pandharipande PP, Girard TD, Brummel NE, Thompson JL, Hughes CG, et al. Depression, post-traumatic stress disorder, and functional disability in survivors of critical illness in the BRAIN-ICU study: a longitudinal cohort study. Lancet Respir Med. 2014;2:369–79.
36. Sundararajan K, Martin M, Rajagopala S, Chapman MJ. Posttraumatic stress disorder in close Relatives of Intensive Care unit patients' Evaluation (PRICE) study. Aust Crit Care. 2014;27:183–7.
37. Fumis RR, Ranzani OT, Martins PS, Schettino G. Emotional disorders in pairs of patients and their family members during and after ICU stay. PLoS ONE. 2015;10:e0115332.
38. Girard TD, Shintani AK, Jackson JC, Gordon SM, Pun BT, Henderson MS, et al. Risk factors for post-traumatic stress disorder symptoms following critical illness requiring mechanical ventilation: a prospective cohort study. Crit Care. 2007;11:R28.
39. Chung ML, Moser DK, Lennie TA, Rayens MK. The effects of depressive symptoms and anxiety on quality of life in patients with heart failure and their spouses: testing dyadic dynamics using Actor–Partner Interdependence Model. J Psychosom Res. 2009;67:29–35.
40. Moser MT, Kunzler A, Nussbeck F, Bargetzi M, Znoj HJ. Higher emotional distress in female partners of cancer patients: prevalence and patient-partner interdependencies in a 3-year cohort. Psychooncology. 2013;22:2693–701.
41. Myhren H, Ekeberg O, Toien K, Karlsson S, Stokland O. Posttraumatic stress, anxiety and depression symptoms in patients during the first year post intensive care unit discharge. Crit Care. 2010;14:R14.
42. Angus DC, Carlet J. Surviving intensive care: a report from the 2002 Brussels Roundtable. Intensive Care Med. 2003;29:368–77.
43. Marik PE. Handbook of evidence-based critical care. New York: Springer; 2010.
44. Schelling G, Briegel J, Roozendaal B, Stoll C, Rothenhäusler HB, Kapfhammer HP. The effect of stress doses of hydrocortisone during septic shock on posttraumatic stress disorder in survivors. Biol Psychiatry. 2001;50:978–85.
45. Wade DM, Howell DC, Weinman JA, Hardy RJ, Mythen MG, Brewin CR, et al. Investigating risk factors for psychological morbidity three months after intensive care: a prospective cohort study. Crit Care. 2012;16:R192.
46. Hagedoorn M, Sanderman R, Bolks HN, Tuinstra J, Coyne JC, et al. Distress in couples coping with cancer: a meta-analysis and critical review of role and gender effects. Psychol Bull. 2008;134:1–30.
47. Paparrigopoulos T, Melissaki A, Efthymiou A, Tsekou H, Vadala C, Kribeni G, et al. Short-term psychological impact on family members of intensive care unit patients. J Psychosom Res. 2006;61:719–22.
48. Andresen M, Guic E, Orellana A, Diaz MJ, Castro R. Posttraumatic stress disorder symptoms in close relatives of intensive care unit patients: prevalence data resemble that of earthquake survivors in Chile. J Crit Care. 2015;30:1152.e7–11.
49. Bienvenu OJ, Gellar J, Althouse BM, Colantuoni E, Sricharoenchai T, Mendez-Tellez PA, et al. Post-traumatic stress disorder symptoms after acute lung injury: a 2-year prospective longitudinal study. Psychol Med. 2013;43:2657–71.
50. Boer KR, Mahler CW, Unlu C, Lamme B, Vroom MB, Sprangers MA, et al. Long-term prevalence of post-traumatic stress disorder symptoms in patients after secondary peritonitis. Crit Care. 2007;11:R30.
51. Davydow DS, Hough CL, Langa KM, Iwashyna TJ. Depressive symptoms in spouses of older patients with severe sepsis. Crit Care Med. 2012;40:2335–41.
52. Twigg E, Humphris G, Jones C, Bramwell R, Griffiths RD. Use of a screening questionnaire for post-traumatic stress disorder (PTSD) on a sample of UK ICU patients. Acta Anaesthesiol Scand. 2008;52:202–8.
53. Khan BA, Lasiter S, Boustani MA. CE: critical care recovery center: an innovative collaborative care model for ICU survivors. Am J Nurs. 2015;115:24–31 **(quiz 34, 46)**.

22

Cytomegalovirus infection in immunocompetent critically ill adults

Awad Al-Omari[1,2*], Fadi Aljamaan[3], Waleed Alhazzani[4], Samer Salih[5] and Yaseen Arabi[6]

Abstract

Cytomegalovirus (CMV) infection is increasingly recognized in critically ill immunocompetent patients. Some studies have demonstrated an association between CMV disease and increased mortality rates, prolonged intensive care unit and hospital length of stay, prolonged mechanical ventilation, and nosocomial infections. However, there is a considerable controversy whether such association represents a causal relationship between CMV disease and unfavorable outcomes or just a marker of the severity of the critical illness. Detection of CMV using polymerase chain reaction and CMV antigenemia is the standard diagnostic approach. CMV may have variety of clinical manifestations reflecting the involvement of different organ systems. Treatment of CMV in critical care is challenging due to diagnostic challenge and drug toxicity, and building predictive model for CMV disease in critical care setting would be promising to identify patients at risk and starting prophylactic therapy. Our objective was to broadly review the current literature on the prevalence and incidence, clinical manifestations, potential limitations of different diagnostic modalities, prognosis, and therapeutic options of CMV disease in critically ill patients.

Keywords: Cytomegalovirus, Infection, Immunocompetent, Critical illness

Background

CMV disease is usually a disease acquired by adolescence and follows a benign course, while it might reactivate in patients with immune suppression and associated with high mortality and morbidity.

There is growing evidence that critically ill immunocompetent patients can develop CMV disease. Studies have described CMV infection in immunocompetent surgical, septic, burn, or trauma critically ill patients [1, 2]. Some studies have demonstrated an association between CMV disease and increased mortality rates, prolonged (ICU) and hospital length of stay, prolonged mechanical ventilation, and increased rate of nosocomial infections [2, 3]. However, there is a considerable controversy whether such association represents a causal relationship between CMV disease and unfavorable outcomes, or whether CMV disease only represents a marker for severe illness that carries poor clinical outcomes.

The objective of this review is to examine the up-to-date literature regarding CMV disease in critically ill patients. We will review the studies that assessed prevalence and incidence of CMV disease refuting the differences among them leading to different results, clinical manifestations, pathogenesis, potential limitations of different diagnostic modalities, association with outcomes, and treatment options of CMV disease in critically ill patients.

Definitions

Primary CMV infection usually occurs during childhood and early adolescence and is usually asymptomatic or mild and self-limiting disease in immunocompetent patients. After the resolution of acute infection, CMV establishes latent phase mainly within leukocytes, namely mononuclear cells, and this stage is diagnosed with a positive anti-CMV IgG serology (seropositivity) and is characterized by maintenance of the viral genome in the

*Correspondence: dr_awad_ksa@yahoo.com
[1] Critical Care and Infection Control Department, Dr. Sulaiman Al Habib Medical Group, Riyadh, Saudi Arabia
Full list of author information is available at the end of the article

absence of production of lytic infectious virions but with the ability of the viral genome to reactivate under certain conditions [3].

CMV literature focused on immunocompromized population like transplant and AIDS populations; therefore, CMV disease statuses and definitions were based on that literature which defined CMV infection as detection of CMV genetic or molecular material in the patients' serum or body fluids, indicating active replication of the virus. CMV infection according to that literature can occur as a result of reactivation of latent CMV or reinfection with an exogenous strain. Recurrent infection in immunocompromized patients is the detection of CMV genetic or molecular material in a patient who had previous documented infection and who has not had virus detected for an interval of at least 4 weeks during active surveillance [4]. Recurrent infection could be due to reactivation (if the detected strain is the same as the primary infecting strain) which is the most common mechanism of acquiring the disease in adulthood, especially in immunocompromized population (seropositivity of the donor or recipient has been recognized as the most likely mechanism of acquiring the disease after organ transplant; therefore, it is the recommended strategy for starting CMV prophylactic treatment across most guidelines) [5–7], or new infection (different strains) [4]. Additionally, de novo primary infection may occur in adults but is rare. However, the distinction between the three scenarios, reactivation, new strain infection, and de novo primary infection, is difficult in practice, unless the patient is followed for a long time or the infecting source CMV genetic strains have been characterized.

CMV disease in critically ill adults will probably fall under one of these three mechanisms. Meta-analysis done by Osawa and Singh [8] has shown that CMV-seronegative critically ill patients rarely developed CMV infection across most studies, suggesting that reactivation is the most likely mechanism of CMV disease in this population. However, the other two mechanisms may be responsible for the infection in some cases.

CMV end-organ disease has been defined as evidence of virus replication associated with clinical manifestations due to viremia or the invasion of organs such as the lungs, bone marrow, and colon [4].

The scope of this article is to examine CMV disease literature in critically ill overtly immunocompetent patients.

In summary, CMV is usually acquired in childhood, and the most common mechanism of the disease in adulthood is reactivation of latent virus whether in immunocompromized or critically ill population, followed by rare incidence of recurrent new or de novo new infection.

Virus genome, pathogenesis, and virulence

CMV is the most common member of the herpes viruses to infect humans. Its double-stranded linear DNA duplex contains 165 genes that encode viral proteins that mimic and interact with human cellular proteins and are related to its virulence and latency.

CMV is maintained in a latent or low production state within monocytes mainly and dendritic cells (DC). They do not usually express viral genes in significant number due to the robust CD8+ cytotoxic T lymphocyte response and T memory cells. In immunocompetent individuals, asymptomatic viral shedding may be detectable in the saliva or urine; however, cell-mediated host immune responses prevent the development of overt CMV disease [3].

CMV genome is detected within early progenitor myeloid CD34+ cells, and monocytes and (DC) differentiation will be the only lineage that will pass the CMV genome. Viral expression is closely related to expression of immediate early (IE) genes within monocytes and (DC), but expression of infectious (lytic) virions only happens within (DC), a process regulated by major IE enhancer promoter (MIEP) which is normally under repressors closely related to other factors and cytokines within the cells [3].

CMV disease occurs as a result of immunosuppression associated with critical illness. A landmark study by Clari showed that CMV infection in critically ill patients was consistently associated with undetectable IFN-γ T cell responses within the first 2 days of admission to the ICU, and that viral load was inversely related to IFN-γ T cell responses [9]. A study by Venet showed that septic patients display immune system paralysis, manifesting as reduced Th1 B cell function, increased IL-10 production (anti-inflammatory), and global lymphopenia affecting natural killer cells (NK) specifically quantitatively and most importantly qualitatively related to their interferon production, which is pivotal in attacking CMV-infected cells [10, 11]. CMV disease has also been linked to the cytokine storm associated with critical illness, specifically tumor necrosis factor alpha that activates nuclear factor κB, which enhances the replication of the dormant CMV DNA inside leukocytes, while enhancing the production of cytokines and other proteins [12]. In animal models with bacterial sepsis, Toll-like receptor 4 signaling and secreted inflammatory cytokines all have been found to be potential triggers for reactivation of latent CMV in immunocompetent mice lungs [13].

Under such critical conditions observed during sepsis, burns, trauma, or major surgery, the CMV genes are expressed and viral replication is initiated [14, 15], invading cells in the lung, kidney, liver, bone marrow, and intestine [3], and exerts direct cytotoxic effects.

In addition, when CMV starts to replicate within leukocytes, it has inherent escape mechanisms from the host immune system, and the CMV unique short (US 2, 3, 6, 10, and 11) proteins down-regulate the surface expression levels of HLA-1 and HLA-2 on leukocytes that mark these cells to be attacked by CD8+ T lymphocytes [16].

Other CMV genes encode structural proteins, such as the matrix protein pp65, that is involved in down-regulation of HLA-1 leukocytes surface markers and used as a target of antigen detection immune assays [17].

In addition, virulence is also related to boosting immune response causing more tissue damage, and this is due to homology of some of CMV proteins to inflammatory cytokines as human tumor necrosis factor alpha receptor and CXC chemokine such as interleukin-8 [18].

Animal model studies suggested that the outcome after reactivation might be determined by the viral load of the original infection, which correlates with the number of CMV-specific T memory cells, i.e., immunological responses (higher IgG levels), CD-8 cytotoxic cells, and hence inflated immune response during reactivation, and this might be a promising marker to predict the outcome in patients with reactivation [13, 19].

In addition, the virus has an immunosuppressive effect via its modulatory effect on cytokine production, which may enhance the susceptibility to secondary bacterial and fungal infections. CMV also has a direct suppressive effect on the bone marrow.

Some CMV proteins are also related to antiviral mechanisms, including the viral DNA polymerase UL54 and UL97, which encodes a protein phosphotransferase enzyme that phosphorylates the antiviral drug ganciclovir, an essential activation step required for its inhibitory effect on CMV DNA replication [20–22].

In summary, CMV has a complicated genome that allows the virus to go into latent state and facilitate its evasion from immune response and homology to human chemokines, all of which is involved in its pathogenesis.

Risk factors

Several factors have been identified to be associated with CMV disease in critically ill patients (Table 1), including requirement of mechanical ventilation on admission [8], an inflammatory status like sepsis [23–25]. Other reports have linked CMV disease to steroid use, but this finding has not yet been confirmed [26–28]. In addition, catecholamines surge associated with critical illness has been linked to CMV disease in myocardial infarction patients [25]. Several studies failed to show a correlation between age and CMV infection [1, 24, 27, 29, 30], while the reported association with gender is inconsistent across the literature [1, 2, 24, 27–29, 31]. Interestingly, higher disease severity scores such as the acute physiology and chronic health evaluation (APACHE) II [1, 27, 29] and sepsis-related organ failure assessment (SOFA) [30] scores have not been found to be associated with increased risk of CMV disease. Active malignancy has not been shown to be a risk factor for CMV disease in critically ill patients [2, 24, 28].

Table 1 Risk factors for CMV disease in critical care setting and their strength of association

Risk factor	Strength of association
Immune compromised	Strong association [49]
Age	No evidence [8]
Gender	Inconsistent data [8]
Mechanical ventilation	Strong association [1, 8]
Sepsis	Strong association [8, 47]
Corticosteroids use	Weak evidence [27]
Blood transfusion	Weak association [1, 27, 28]
Disease severity scores	No association [1, 24, 27–31]
Active malignancy	No association [2, 24, 28]
Stress (catecholamines surge)	Weak association [25]

Blood transfusion, especially in the first 24 h of critical illness, has been shown to be an important risk factor for CMV disease [1], which has been linked to the timing and the amount of blood transfused, although the mechanisms involved are unclear. Contamination of transfused blood with CMV-infected leukocytes may be responsible for some cases, especially in cases where the blood bank does not perform leukocyte depletion pre-transfusion [32, 33], even though leukocyte-depleted blood is not completely clear of leukocytes; hence, its use does not completely eliminate the risk of CMV infection. In addition, the immunomodulatory effect of transfusion may also predispose patients to CMV reactivation.

In summary, mechanical ventilation and blood transfusion in the ICU have been associated with the development of CMV disease, but no association with severity scores was found.

Epidemiology

Several epidemiologic studies assessed the incidence of CMV disease in critically ill patients (Table 2), and these studies used different methodologies that lead to variation in the observed incidence of infection ranging from 0% to as high as 98%. This inconsistency in the results could be explained by many factors as variation in the definition of CMV disease (old studies considered seropositivity as evidence of CMV disease, while others used newer technologies as PCR and antigen detection), variation in inclusion criteria as some studies included only seropositive patients and hence assessed only reactivation rate of CMV rather than CMV infection rate which might be slightly higher than reactivation by including seronegative patients developing new infection in addition to reactivation, all that in addition to variation in studied populations that ranged from all ICU patients to specific population such as septic, surgical, burn, or post-cardiac surgery patients that might have different risks of CMV disease.

Variation in diagnostic methods used including selecting different specimens, some used serum, while others used urine, saliva, or bronchoalveolar lavage samples, tests were performed at different points in the ICU stay and testing time and frequency was not standardized in all studies as some left it up to the judgment of the treating team. Recent studies showed that CMV disease typically occurs within the first 2 weeks of critical illness. A study performed by Kalil and Florescu [34] showed that the diagnosis rate of CMV infection increased significantly (from 1 to 21%) when patients who spent five or more days in the ICU were screened, pointing to a threshold in timing for the window to develop CMV in critical care setting. In a recent systematic review that included 13 studies (nine prospective and four retrospective), the incidence of CMV disease in critically ill patients, defined as the detection of antigenemia, DNAemia, or positive viral culture from blood samples with or without other clinical specimens, ranged from 0 to 36%. Notably, the reported incidence of the disease was much higher in studies that screened the patients weekly than those that screened only once within the first 4 days of admission to the ICU (6–33 vs. 0.8–1.2%), indicating that the disease happens frequently beyond the first 4 days post-admission. Among the studies using PCR detection (which is the most sensitive diagnostic test for CMV), the mean and median times of detection ranged from 4 to 12 days after ICU admission [8].

In summary, the incidence and demographics of CMV disease in the ICU were highly variable across studies, as a result of variation in study design and definition of the disease.

Clinical manifestations

Identification of CMV disease in immunocompetent patients is complicated by its non-specific symptoms, multiorgan involvement, and the fact that its clinical manifestations converge with those of the critical illness. Heininger et al. [24] reported that serious organ involvement with CMV disease could occur in up to 10% of cases. A systematic review of studies reporting the clinical manifestations of severe CMV disease in immunocompetent ICU patients found that the gastrointestinal tract (hepatitis, gastroenteritis, duodenitis, enteritis, colitis, proctitis) is to be the most common, followed by central nervous system (encephalitis, myelitis, encephalomyelitis, meningitis, and meningioradiculopathy), and hematological system (hemolytic anemia, thrombocytopenia, disseminated intravascular coagulation, and pancytopenia) [35]. Other organs, such as the lungs and eyes, were rarely involved. CMV myocarditis, a recognized entity in immunocompromized patients, was not documented.

Vascular manifestations have been reported such as portal or femoropopliteal vascular thrombosis and pulmonary embolism that is thought to be related to vascular endothelial cells damage [35].

The immunomodulatory effects of CMV may be responsible for increased risk of secondary bacterial and fungal infections in critical care setting [3, 4].

CMV pneumonia is a well-known clinical manifestation of CMV disease in immunocompromized patients. However, lung involvement may be less recognizable in immunocompetent critically ill patients especially if they were intubated for other reasons, but few studies demonstrated that the prevalence of this disease in immunocompetent critically ill patients may be as high as 50% in patients with ventilator-associated pneumonia or ICU-acquired acute respiratory distress syndrome [36]. However, CMV disease is not necessarily the pathologic cause of ICU-acquired pneumonia and discrimination between a causal or associative relationship is challenging because the diagnosis depends on quality of the respiratory sample, pathologist skills, and variation of the diagnostic test. As an example of this variation, Coisel et al. [37] studied patients mechanically ventilated who are seropositive for CMV and found significant increased mortality in CMV-positive group; in addition, the diagnostic yield of BAL CMV PCR was 73% in comparison with the detection of CMV antigenemia which was 46%. Heininger et al. [38] studied patients admitted with severe sepsis of whom 31% developed ICU-acquired pneumonia and have shown slightly different diagnostic yield of tracheal aspirate CMV PCR of 70 versus 62% using blood CMV PCR. In a previous study, the same authors included only CMV surgical seropositive patients and found equal diagnostic yield between BAL PCR and blood PCR. Chiche showed different results, as the diagnostic yield of BAL was 26% (using CMV shell vial culture) compared to 85% using CMV antigenemia [26]. Papazian et al. [39] studied patients with ventilator-associated pneumonia and made histologic diagnosis of CMV pneumonia in 29% of the patients. The study found that BAL shell vial culture had a sensitivity/specificity of 53, 92% in comparison with histologic diagnosis. Ong et al. [40] studied immunocompetent patients with ARDS and found a CMV reactivation incidence of 27%, which was associated with significant increase in ICU mortality.

Table 2 Summary of studies assessing CMV disease in ICU patients

Year of publication	Study	Study design	Patient population	Patients no.	Method and specimen	Frequency of monitoring	Incidence (%)	Mortality (%)	
								CMV positive[a]	CMV negative[b]
1990	Domart et al. [31]	Prospective, single center	Mediastinitis, post-cardiac surgery Patients in whom viral cultures could be done within 10 days of surgical debridement	115	Serology for CMV IgG Viral culture blood and urine. Positive cases: positive CMV culture	Within first 10 days of debridement then every 3 weeks	25	55*	37*
1994	Docke et al. [50]	Unidentified	Septic patients	60	1—CMV culture in blood. 2—Immuno-cytological detection of CMV antigens in blood. 3—PCR amplification in blood. 4—TNF and interleukin six assays. Positive cases: any positive PCR or culture or antigen detection	Once	97.7	NA	
1996	Stephan et al. [51]	Prospective, single center	Mechanically ventilated	23	Culture, PCR Blood and BAL	Unclear	0	0	
1996	Papazian et al. [39]	Retrospective Single center	Patients with ventilator-associated pneumonia	86	Histopathology Autopsies and open lung biopsy	Once 22.4 ± 8.8 days after admission to the intensive care unit	29	NA	NA
1998	Kutza et al. [29]	Prospective, single center	SICU Septic patients with positive CMV IgG serology	34	CMV IgG serology CMV antigenemia CMV DNA PCR in blood Serum cytokines: TNF alpha, IL-1b, and IL-6 measured by ELISAs. Positive cases: positive CMV antigenemia and/or CMV DNA PCR in blood	1—Blood samples were collected on day 1 of sepsis, then twice weekly during ICU stay, then once weekly after release from the ICU, until recovery or death	32	73.9*	63.6*
1998	Cook et al. [27]	Prospective, case–control single center	Postoperative general SICU. Septic patients with no identifiable bacterial or fungal source. Positive BAL or blood or sputum CMV culture	12	CMV and HSV viral culture from BAL, blood or sputum. All cases included had positive CMV culture	CMV was cultured in diploid human foreskin fibroblast culture for 6 weeks Plasma was evaluated by shell vial technique to IE antigen at 24 h. HSV cultures	100	65[a]	35[a]

Table 2 continued

Year of publication	Study	Study design	Patient population	Patients no.	Method and specimen	Frequency of monitoring	Incidence (%)	Mortality (%)	
								CMV positive[a]	CMV negative[b]
2001	Heininger et al. [24]	Prospective, single center	SICU Patients with SAPS II >40 and positive serology	56	CMV DNA PCR and/or viral culture Leukocytes, plasma, and lower respiratory tract secretions Positive cases: positive PCR	Once weekly	35.6	55*	36.2*
2002	Razonable et al. [52]	Prospective Case–control Single center	Mixed ICU	120	CMV and HHV-6 and HHV-7 DNA by PCR in blood Positive cases: positive PCR	4th days after ICU admission	<1	NA	
2003	Cook et al. [23]	Prospective Single center	SICU Patients staying for 5 days or more in SICU	104	Serology in blood CMV and HSV cultures in blood and sputum Positive cases: positive CMV culture	Once weekly until discharge from SICU	9.6	50*	26.5*
2005	Jaber et al. [28]	Retrospective, matched case–control, single center	Medical, surgical, and transplant unit Non-immune-compromised patients	237	PP65 antigen Blood Positive cases: positive CMV antigenemia	1—Clinical judgment. 2—The diagnosis of CMV antigenemia was defined by a positive CMV pp65 antigenemia assay result	16.8	50[α]	28[α]
2006	von Muller et al. [53]	Prospective observational single center	Anesthesiological intensive care unit. Non-immunocompromized CMV IgG-seropositive patients with septic shock with ICU stay for at least 7 days	23	Serology CMV antigenemia Blood. CMV reactive T helper 1 lymphocytes Positive cases: positive CMV antigenemia	Twice during 1st week then weekly until discharge Positive cases: positive antigenemia	30.4	57*	38*
2008	Ziemann et al. [2]	Retrospective, single center	Mixed ICU Patients treated for at least 14 days in ICU	99	CMV DNA PCR Blood. Positive cases: at least two positive samples	Based on the decision of the treating team	35[Σ]	28.6[α]	10.9[α]
2008	Limaye et al. [1]	Prospective, multicenter	Mixed ICU, positive anti-CMV IgG	120	PCR Blood Positive cases: positive blood CMV PCR	Thrice weekly until death or discharge	33	CMV disease was significantly associated with death or continued hospitalization after 30 days	

Table 2 continued

Year of publication	Study	Study design	Patient population	Patients no.	Method and specimen	Frequency of monitoring	Incidence (%)	Mortality (%)	
								CMV positive[a]	CMV negative[b]
2009	Chiche et al. [26]	Prospective, single center	MICU Ventilated patients for at least 2 days	242	CMV serology and antigenemia. CMV culture on BAL if VAP suspected, antigenemia on the day of BAL. Other organ Virologic studies based on clinical suspicion. Positive cases: positive antigenemia or BAL CMV culture	Within 48 h of ICU admission and once weekly until discharge	16.1	54*	37*
2010	Chilet et al [54]	Prospective observational Single center	Anesthesiological ICU Single center CMV-seropositive, ICU stay longer than 5 days	53	CMV PCR Tracheal aspirate and plasma Plasma tumor necrosis factor alpha	Once a week	39.7	61*	46*
2010	Smith et al. [55]	Prospective single center	Tertiary ICU Mechanically ventilated patients	174	Respiratory secretions CMV PCR Thrice weekly		19	NA	
2011	Iahangard	Prospective	ICU CMV-seropositive patients	132	CMV IgG serology PCR in blood	Weekly	34	The overall mortality rate associated with active CMV infection was 1.93 times higher than that without CMV infection	
2011	Bordes et a . [56]	Prospective Single center	Severe burn unit Burn surface area more than 15%	29	CMV DNA Blood	First sample on admission then one to twice weekly until discharge	55	33*	20*
2011	Uegaki	Retrospective Single center	ICU	67	CMV antigenemia	After 7 days of admission if intensivists suspected CMV	52	NA	

Table 2 continued

Year of publication	Study	Study design	Patient population	Patients no.	Method and specimen	Frequency of monitoring	Incidence (%)	Mortality (%)	
								CMV positive[a]	CMV negative[b]
2011	Heininger et al. [38]	Prospective, observational, single center	Severe sepsis, positive anti-CMV IgG	86	Viral culture from tracheal secretions. Qualitative CMV DNA PCR from leukocytes, plasma, tracheal secretions Quantitative CMV DNA PCR from positive plasma and tracheal secretions HSV DNA PCR from tracheal secretions Positive cases: positive PCR from any source	Once weekly until discharge from hospital or death	40.7	37.1*	35.3*
2012	De Vlieger et al. [57]	Prospective, MICU and SICU, single center (Van Den Berge study)	Admitted for at least 3 days in ICU Mechanically ventilated in SICU MICU regardless of mechanical ventilation	1504	CMV IgG serology	Within first 2 days of admission	64	19.2*	17.1*
2012	Chiche et al. [10]	Prospective Single center	MICU CMV-seropositive patients	82	CMV serology CMV antigenemia Lymphocyte subset Interferon-γ	Within 48 h of admission then once weekly until discharge	27	40*	13.3*
2012	Coisel et al. [37]	Prospective single center	MICU Mechanically ventilated suspected of having pneumonia 10% were previously immunocompromized	93	1—Serology (IgM and IgG) for cytomegalovirus (CMV) and herpes simplex (HSV) using (ELISA) Blood PCR was not routinely done 2—CMV antigen detection in blood 3—CMV and HSV DNA PCR on BAL Positive cases: positive CMV PCR in BAL or positive antigenemia or positive IgM	Within 12 h of pneumonia diagnosis	24	55[α]	20[α]
2013	Clari et al. [9]	Prospective single center	SICU Mechanically ventilated patients CMV seropositive	31	CMV serology at baseline CMV-specific interferon-γ-producing CD8, CD4 T lymphocytes CMV PCR in blood and tracheal aspirate	2–8 samples per patient were analyzed for T lymphocytes subset and CMV PCR	54.8	47*	35*

Table 2 continued

Year of publication	Study	Study design	Patient population	Patients no.	Method and specimen	Frequency of monitoring	Incidence (%)	Mortality (%)	
								CMV positive[a]	CMV negative[b]
2014	Ishioka et al. [58]	Prospective Single center	Cardiac ICU Post-surgery	100	CMV PP65 antigenemia Serum	On admission, day 7 and day 14	4	0*	1*
2014	Osman	Prospective Single center	Respiratory and geriatric ICU	51	CMV PCR Blood	NA	68.6	74.3[α]	31.3[α]
2014	Walton et al. [59]	Prospective Single center	MICU and SICU Critically ill septic and non-septic patients versus healthy volunteers	560	CMV IgG CMV PCR Blood	Daily Starting within 24–72 h of admission	24.2	Significant increase in 90 days mortality in CMV-positive patients compared to CMV-negative ones	
2015	Ong et al. [40]	Multicenter prospective cohort	Mixed ICU (tertiary care referral centers) ARDS patients on mechanical ventilation for at least 4 days	271	CMV IgG if positive CMV PCR in blood	Weekly for maximum 30 days	27	46[α]	28[α]
2015	Frantzeskaki et al. [12]	Prospective, observational two centers	Mixed ICU, mechanically ventilated, seropositive anti-CMV IgG	80	CMV DNA PCR Blood	At admission, then weekly until day 28 or discharge from ICU or death	13.75	18*	22*
2015	Ong et al. [60]	Multicenter prospective cohort	Mixed ICU (tertiary care referral centers) ARDS patients on mechanical ventilation for at least 4 days	209	CMV IgG between days 5 and 14 of admission If positive CMV DNA PCR in plasma	CMV DNA PCR on day 14 or ICU discharge date (whichever first) then weekly	26	28*,[δ]	16*

Positive serology: positive anti-CMV IgG or IgM

ELISA enzyme-linked immunosorbent assay, *PCR* polymerase chain reaction, *CMV* cytomegalovirus, *ARDS* acute respiratory distress syndrome, *BAL* bronchoalveolar lavage, *MICU* medical intensive care unit, *SICU* surgical intensive care unit, *SAPS* simplified acute physiology score, *ICU* intensive care unit, *ELISA* enzyme-linked immunosorbent assay

[a] CMV positive based on study methodology

[b] CMV negative based on study methodology

* Nonsignificant difference in mortality

[α] Statistically significant difference in mortality between groups

[δ] 24% in seropositive without reactivation

[Σ] Considered infected if at least two positive results

In general, CMV affects multiple organs at varying rates and severity. ICU-acquired pneumonia, especially VAP, appears to be a common CMV-associated disease that draw attention of ICU physicians and researchers.

Diagnosis

Critically ill patients have dynamic immune system that affects the CMV detection window. The fact that immune suppression is not expected usually on presentation to intensive care, coupled with the ability of infected individuals to control the disease and eventually clear the virus at some point, affects the accuracy of diagnostic methods for CMV, all of that in addition to the differential sensitivities and clinical utilities of the techniques used to detect CMV (Table 3). In one major study assessing the rate of CMV disease in ICU patients, 50% of viremia was detected within the first 12 days of admission, but CMV infection was not detected earlier than the first 3 days [1].

Testing for CMV for the diagnosis of CMV disease should be based on predictors of CMV disease in addition to signs and other laboratory investigations directing toward viral origin of the current clinical status as indicators of liver and gastrointestinal involvement [41].

Serology

The most commonly used tests to measure CMV-specific IgM or IgG levels are the enzyme-linked immune assays and anticomplement immunofluorescence assays. The presence of IgM antibodies indicates an acute CMV infection and can last for 4–6 months [42]. Because IgG seropositivity is long lasting, the measurement of IgG antibodies is not a reliable method to diagnose CMV infection. Critically ill patients may develop immune paralysis (anergy) that limits their ability to mount immune responses; therefore, it is important to note that negative serology does not exclude CMV infection. The main utility of serology testing at present is to screen for the potential of latent CMV reactivation [42].

PCR

Due to its high sensitivity and rapid turnaround time, PCR is considered the gold standard method of diagnosing CMV infection [8]. Both qualitative and quantitative (viral load) PCR assays are available. However, quantitative tests are preferred as it quantifies viral load, which has prognostic importance [1]. Whole blood testing is more sensitive than plasma testing because it enables the detection of cell-free and intracellular viruses [43].

CMV antigen assays

Antigen assays using immunofluorescent antibodies are quick and easy to perform and can be used to detect the CMV pp65 antigen in leukocytes [4]. In one study that compared PCR to antigen detection to diagnose CMV infection in critically ill patients, the antigen detection method was unable to identify 5 of the 11 CMV-positive patients detected by PCR. In addition, the diagnostic time of the PCR method was ahead than that of the antigen detection method [29]. However, meta-analyses performed by Osawa and Kalil revealed that the sensitivities and specificities of antigen detection methods are comparable to those of PCR detection methods [8, 44]. The only potential limitation of antigen assays is their low sensitivity in patients with leukopenia [5].

Viral culture

Culture-based assays are not clinically used due to their low sensitivity and delay in receiving the results [8]. In a meta-analysis by Osawa and Singh [8], detection rate of CMV infection among studies using culture was 0–20% of CMV infections, whereas it was 0–32% using PCR and antigen assays. In a meta-analysis performed by Kalil and Florescu [34], the PCR/antigen detection methods achieved a CMV detection rate of 20%, whereas that the culture method was only 12%.

Histopathology

Histopathology is the most specific method for diagnosing CMV, especially by detecting organ-specific

Table 3 Diagnostic methods of CMV, advantages, and disadvantages

Diagnostic method	Advantages	Disadvantages
Anti-CMV immunoglobulins	Might be used for screening for latent CMV infection	Low sensitivity and specificity for active infection
CMV PCR assays	High sensitivity and specificity and considered gold standard, quick easy to perform, gives information of viral load, can be used for wide variety of samples	Better to be performed on whole blood, qualitative might be so sensitive and detect "innocent viral shedding" quantitative might be superior
CMV antigen assays	Quick and easy to perform, has comparable sensitivity and specificity to PCR	Might be inferior to PCR in case of leukopenia
Viral culture	Highly specific, can be performed on wide variety of samples	Time-consuming, low sensitivity
Histopathology	Highly specific, confirm CMV disease and pathogenicity and invasiveness	Invasive, low sensitivity, liable to sampling error, needs skilled pathologist and so operator dependent

manifestations related to CMV. However, this method is invasive and has a limited sensitivity that depends on the sampling site and pathologist's skills.

We suggest using CMV PCR or CMV antigen detection assays to diagnose CMV disease not earlier than 3 days and up to 2 weeks after the onset of critical illness, especially when the pretest probability of the disease is high [1, 8].

Prognosis

Studies addressing association of CMV disease and outcome in critically ill patients revealed inconsistent results.

A systematic review by Osawa and Singh [8] concluded that CMV disease in critically ill patients was associated with hepatic, respiratory, and renal dysfunctions; prolonged ICU stay, prolonged mechanical ventilation, increased incidence of bacterial and fungal infections, and increased mortality.

In a landmark prospective cohort study by Limaye et al. [1] of 120 CMV-seropositive critically ill patients, he found significant association between CMV disease and 30-day mortality and increased ICU length of stay. Notably high levels of viremia were associated with increased mortality and morbidity rates, as well as prolonged lengths of stay in the hospital, the latter of which increased with each log increase in the number of CMV copies (>1000 copies/ml up to 28 days of hospital length of stay). In addition, he observed higher rate of hospitalization beyond 30 days in CMV-infected patients indicating a long-term effect of CMV disease that persists beyond ICU discharge and even after clearance of the viremia. Of note, the study could not identify a relationship between the severity of critical illness (APACHE) and the risk of CMV disease, probably refuting the idea that CMV disease might be a marker of the underlying disease severity.

Regarding specific ICU population, a recent observational prospective study that included 86 CMV-seropositive septic patients found an association between CMV disease and longer ICU stay, prolonged mechanical ventilation, and impaired pulmonary gas exchange [38]. Coisel examined critically ill patients with ventilator-associated pneumonia and found a significant increase in ICU and 60-day mortality (50% CMV group vs. 20% in control group), longer ICU stay, and less ventilator-free days in patient with CMV disease [37].

On the other hand, a prospective observational study of 80 mechanically ventilated patients that were seropositive for CMV found no association between CMV disease and 28-day mortality, ICU mortality, ICU length of stay, or duration of mechanical ventilation, although the SOFA score was significantly higher in CMV-infected group [12]. Similar findings were also reported in a study that used CMV pp65 antigenemia as evidence of CMV disease [28].

These inconsistent findings are probably related to differences of studied populations, retrospective nature of several studies, differences in diagnostic tests, the unmeasured confounders; therefore, it is difficult to establish proved causality based on the existing studies, necessitating future studies with strict methodology in relation to blinding, studied population, testing timing, and method of testing preferably with tissue studies to clarify the causal relation between CMV disease and ICU mortality and morbidity.

In conclusion, although the current literature is inconsistent, there is strong evidence suggesting an association between CMV disease and higher morbidity and mortality in the ICU.

Treatment and prevention

The central controversy of CMV disease in critically ill patients is whether to treat or not and whether treatment makes a difference to the patient's outcomes or not.

Treatment of CMV disease as any other disease should be based on a benefit/risk ratio, taking into consideration all other factors associated with the diagnostic process and treatment such as invasiveness of the diagnostic method, side effects of anti-CMV medications which might be serious especially in critical ill patients, and risk of emergence of CMV resistance to the medications [45]. There is an agreement regarding treatment of established CMV disease and prophylactic treatment for certain populations of immunocompromized patients as is the case in organ transplant recipients, for whom the guidelines are well established [7, 44].

Similarly, the curative treatment of clinically confirmed CMV disease (detection of significant CMV viral load by PCR or antigen detection based on diagnostic method threshold, in addition to clinical condition attributed to CMV and ruling out other potential causes) in immunocompetent critically ill patients has been recommended, and support for such approach comes from studies like the one by Eddleston et al. [46] that examined the outcome of previously reported 34 cases of severe CMV disease in immunocompetent patients. It was found that multiorgan involvement was associated with poor outcome compared with isolated central nervous system involvement. Among patients with multiorgan involvement, 5 of 6 patients who received treatment of either ganciclovir or foscarnet recovered, while only 4 of 18 patients who did not receive either one of the abovementioned drugs survived. The outcome noticed in this review pointed toward a potential benefit of antiviral treatment in this group of patients.

Table 4 Anti-CMV medications and common associated side effects

Agent	Mechanism of action	Common side effects
Ganciclovir	Competitively inhibits the binding of deoxyguanosine triphosphate to DNA polymerase resulting in inhibition of viral DNA synthesis	Thrombocytopenia, leukopenia, increased creatinine, fever, vomiting, diarrhea
Valganciclovir	Converted to ganciclovir in the body, much higher bioavailability of ganciclovir compared to oral ganciclovir	As ganciclovir
Foscarnet	Non-competitive inhibitor of many viral RNA and DNA polymerases	Electrolyte abnormalities, fever, vomiting, diarrhea, anemia, granulocytopenia, renal insufficiency, cardiotoxicity, central nervous system toxicity, hepatic toxicity
Cidofovir	Suppresses CMV replication by selective inhibition of viral DNA synthesis	Fever, alopecia, rash, ocular, renal, and gastrointestinal toxicity, cough, dyspnea

However, the benefit of preemptive treatment of subclinical detected viral replication with no proven direct organ pathology attributed to CMV, and the prophylactic treatment in immunocompetent patients deemed to be at risk of developing CMV disease is much less clear [45]. It is plausible to assume that the best strategy to handle CMV disease in the ICU is to prevent reactivation in seropositive patients as these are at high risk of developing the disease. At present randomized clinical trials examining the safety and efficacy of preventative strategies in critically ill patients are still going on.

Challenges for CMV preemptive and prophylactic treatment includes discouraging safety profiles of anti-CMV medications on the kidney and bone marrow especially in critically ill patients who already have organ dysfunction that puts them at extra risk of further dysfunctions and secondary infections (Table 4).

The other challenge is the detection of CMV, the current used methods, namely CMV PCR and CMV antigenemia, are highly accurate regarding sensitivity and specificity, but the challenge is that detection of CMV is highly sensitive to the timing and frequency of testing which is related to the window of emergence of CMV infection within the first 2 weeks of critical illness but not earlier than 3 days [8, 44]; secondly, it is unclear whether some cases represent innocent viral DNA or antigen shedding not necessarily related to tissue invasiveness and thus does not require therapy, which stress against random screening for CMV [13].

Papazian recommended in his recent review that treatment for evident CMV replication (blood or BAL significant viral load or antigen titer) is not indicated unless it is associated with lung infiltrates and at least two factors (prolonged mechanical ventilation, absence of bacterial agent, leukopenia, hemophagocytosis, high liver enzymes, hyperbilirubinemia, fever, or diarrhea) which if found points for CMV being a pathogen invading multiple organs and not only a bystander or innocent viral shedding [41].

So far no definite criterion is available to guide which critically ill patients should be screened for CMV disease. According to available literature certain populations as septic, burns, trauma, ICU-acquired pneumonia especially mechanically ventilated patients have been found at high risk of developing CMV disease across multiple studies [26, 41, 47]. Many authors recommended in these populations especially in case of prolonged mechanical ventilation with evidence of pneumonia, unexplained liver derangement or fever or unexplained digestive tract pathology, to screen for CMV disease and in case of CMV detection using PCR or antigenemia detection methods; then, treatment should be taken as benefit/risk ratio [37, 41, 48] (Table 4).

Regarding preemptive treatment, immunological assessment of IFN-γ produced by CMV-specific CD8+ T cells and NK cell function as mentioned in virulence section might be a strong trigger to start preemptive treatment for detected CMV, because there is evidence that impaired CMV-specific CD8+ T cells IFN-γ production prior to CMV reactivation predicts poor outcome, which favors treatment. This has not been applied clinically so far but might be promising in the future for challenging cases [10].

CMV might acquire resistance to the limited number of medications that are currently available; hence, their prophylactic use should be confined to confirmed cases or preemptive treatment until clear risk assessment tools for prophylactic therapy are developed in high-risk groups in the ICU [48].

Conclusion

There are many uncertainties about CMV disease in the critically ill patients. First, while identification of the virus is common in critically ill patients, the actual rate of CMV as a disease in critically ill patients is unclear. Second, the importance of CMV detection in critically ill patients remains questionable, especially in the absence of histologic evidence of infection. On the other hand, the existing evidence is strong regarding the association between CMV detection and increased mortality and morbidity rates in ICU settings.

Still there are no high-quality data to guide the decision regarding when to treat detected CMV in ICU patients if there is no definite clinical confirmation of CMV disease (preemptive treatment), and there is no risk assessment tool to guide prophylactic therapy in ICU setting.

There is a need for well-conducted studies to develop risk assessment tool of CMV disease in critically ill patients, to estimate the real burden of CMV disease, and to examine the effect of prophylactic and preemptive treatment on morbidity and mortality. Potential answers to these questions will hopefully be answered by currently ongoing trials related to CMV in critical care. "Cytomegalovirus Control in Critical Care trial" (NCT01503918) is addressing the safety and success rate regarding preventing reactivation of latent cytomegalovirus infection in critically ill patients when treated with one of two different antiviral regimens: "Valaciclovir/Aciclovir or not." "Study of Ganciclovir/Valganciclovir for Prevention of Cytomegalovirus Reactivation in Acute Injury of the Lung and Respiratory Failure" (NCT01335932) is addressing whether administration of ganciclovir in CMV-seropositive patients reduces serum IL-6 levels in immunocompetent adults with severe sepsis or trauma-associated respiratory failure based on the hypothesis that pulmonary and systemic CMV reactivation amplifies both lung and systemic inflammation mediated through specific cytokines. "Preemptive Treatment of Herpesviridae trial" (NCT02152358) is addressing whether preemptive treatment by ganciclovir (for positive CMV viremia) or aciclovir (for positive HSV oropharyngeal PCR) is able to increase the number of ventilator-free days at day 60 in ICU patients with prolonged mechanical ventilation having evident viral replication.

Authors' contributions

AA carried out the literature review of the studies addressing CMV prevalence and participated in drafting the manuscript. FA participated in reviewing the literature of clinical manifestations, risk factors and treatment and prevention sections and participated in drafting the manuscript. SS participated in reviewing literature addressing CMV diagnosis. YA and WA participated in drafting the manuscript. All authors read and approved the final manuscript.

Author details

[1] Critical Care and Infection Control Department, Dr. Sulaiman Al Habib Medical Group, Riyadh, Saudi Arabia. [2] AlFaisal University, Riyadh, Saudi Arabia. [3] Intensive Care Department, King Khalid University Hospital, King Saud University Medical City, King Saud University, Riyadh, Saudi Arabia. [4] Department of Medicine, McMaster University, Hamilton, Canada. [5] Department of Internal Medicine, Dr. Sulaiman Al Habib Medical Group, Riyadh, Saudi Arabia. [6] Intensive Care Department, King Abdullah International Medical Research Center, King Saud Bin Abdulaziz University for Health Sciences, Riyadh, Saudi Arabia.

Competing interests

The authors declare that they have no competing interests.

Funding

The authors declare that they have not received any funding from any source.

References

1. Limaye AP, Kirby KA, Rubenfeld GD, Leisenring WM, Bulger EM, Neff MJ, et al. Cytomegalovirus reactivation in critically ill immunocompetent patients. JAMA. 2008;300(4):413–22.
2. Ziemann M, Sedemund-Adib B, Reiland P, Schmucker P, Hennig H. Increased mortality in long-term intensive care patients with active cytomegalovirus infection. Crit Care Med. 2008;36(12):3145–50.
3. Sinclair J. Human cytomegalovirus: latency and reactivation in the myeloid lineage. J Clin Virol. 2008;41(3):180–5.
4. Ljungman P, Griffiths P, Paya C. Definitions of cytomegalovirus infection and disease in transplant recipients. Clin Infect Dis. 2002;34(8):1094–7.
5. Kotton CN, Kumar D, Caliendo AM, Asberg A, Chou S, Danziger-Isakov L, et al. Updated international consensus guidelines on the management of cytomegalovirus in solid-organ transplantation. Transplantation. 2013;96(4):333–60.
6. Andrews PA, Emery VC, Newstead C. Summary of the British Transplantation Society guidelines for the prevention and management of CMV disease after solid organ transplantation. Transplantation. 2011;92(11):1181–7.
7. Tomblyn M, Chiller T, Einsele H, Gress R, Sepkowitz K, Storek J, et al. Guidelines for preventing infectious complications among hematopoietic cell transplant recipients: a global perspective. Preface. Bone Marrow Transplant. 2009;44(8):453–5.
8. Osawa R, Singh N. Cytomegalovirus infection in critically ill patients: a systematic review. Crit Care. 2009;13(3):R68.
9. Clari MA, Aguilar G, Benet I, Belda J, Gimenez E, Bravo D, et al. Evaluation of cytomegalovirus (CMV)-specific T-cell immunity for the assessment of the risk of active CMV infection in non-immunosuppressed surgical and trauma intensive care unit patients. J Med Virol. 2013;85(10):1802–10.
10. Chiche L, Forel JM, Thomas G, Farnarier C, Cognet C, Guervilly C, et al. Interferon-gamma production by natural killer cells and cytomegalovirus in critically ill patients. Crit Care Med. 2012;40(12):3162–9.
11. Venet F, Davin F, Guignant C, Larue A, Cazalis MA, Darbon R, et al. Early assessment of leukocyte alterations at diagnosis of septic shock. Shock. 2010;34(4):358–63.
12. Frantzeskaki FG, Karampi ES, Kottaridi C, Alepaki M, Routsi C, Tzanela M, et al. Cytomegalovirus reactivation in a general, nonimmunosuppressed intensive care unit population: incidence, risk factors, associations with organ dysfunction, and inflammatory biomarkers. J Crit Care. 2015;30(2):276–81.
13. Cook CH, Trgovcich J. Cytomegalovirus reactivation in critically ill immunocompetent hosts: a decade of progress and remaining challenges. Antivir Res. 2011;90(3):151–9.
14. Hummel M, Abecassis MM. A model for reactivation of CMV from latency. J Clin Virol. 2002;25(Suppl. 2):S123–36.
15. Guedes MI, Risdahl JM, Wiseman B, Molitor TW. Reactivation of porcine cytomegalovirus through allogeneic stimulation. J Clin Microbiol. 2004;42(4):1756–8.
16. Emery VC. Progress in understanding cytomegalovirus drug resistance. J Clin Virol. 2001;21(3):223–8.
17. Shuster EA, Beneke JS, Tegtmeier GE, Pearson GR, Gleaves CA, Wold AD, et al. Monoclonal antibody for rapid laboratory detection of cytomegalovirus infections: characterization and diagnostic application. Mayo Clin Proc. 1985;60(9):577–85.
18. Penfold ME, Dairaghi DJ, Duke GM, Saederup N, Mocarski ES, Kemble GW, et al. Cytomegalovirus encodes a potent alpha chemokine. Proc Natl Acad Sci USA. 1999;96(17):9839–44.
19. Roberts ET, Haan MN, Dowd JB, Aiello AE. Cytomegalovirus antibody levels, inflammation, and mortality among elderly Latinos over 9 years of follow-up. Am J Epidemiol. 2010;172(4):363–71.
20. Sullivan V, Talarico CL, Stanat SC, Davis M, Coen DM, Biron KK. A protein kinase homologue controls phosphorylation of ganciclovir in human cytomegalovirus-infected cells. Nature. 1992;359(6390):85.
21. Beersma MF, Bijlmakers MJ, Ploegh HL. Human cytomegalovirus down-regulates HLA class I expression by reducing the stability of class I H chains. J Immunol. 1993;151(9):4455–64.

22. Littler E, Stuart AD, Chee MS. Human cytomegalovirus UL97 open reading frame encodes a protein that phosphorylates the antiviral nucleoside analogue ganciclovir. Nature. 1992;358(6382):160–2.
23. Cook CH, Yenchar JK, Kraner TO, Davies EA, Ferguson RM. Occult herpes family viruses may increase mortality in critically ill surgical patients. Am J Surg. 1998;176(4):357–60.
24. Heininger A, Jahn G, Engel C, Notheisen T, Unertl K, Hamprecht K. Human cytomegalovirus infections in nonimmunosuppressed critically ill patients. Crit Care Med. 2001;29(3):541–7.
25. Prosch S, Wendt CE, Reinke P, Priemer C, Oppert M, Kruger DH, et al. A novel link between stress and human cytomegalovirus (HCMV) infection: sympathetic hyperactivity stimulates HCMV activation. Virology. 2000;272(2):357–65.
26. Chiche L, Forel JM, Roch A, Guervilly C, Pauly V, Allardet-Servent J, et al. Active cytomegalovirus infection is common in mechanically ventilated medical intensive care unit patients. Crit Care Med. 2009;37(6):1850–7.
27. Cook CH, Martin LC, Yenchar JK, Lahm MC, McGuinness B, Davies EA, et al. Occult herpes family viral infections are endemic in critically ill surgical patients. Crit Care Med. 2003;31(7):1923–9.
28. Jaber S, Chanques G, Borry J, Souche B, Verdier R, Perrigault PF, et al. Cytomegalovirus infection in critically ill patients: associated factors and consequences. Chest. 2005;127(1):233–41.
29. Kutza AS, Muhl E, Hackstein H, Kirchner H, Bein G. High incidence of active cytomegalovirus infection among septic patients. Clin Infect Dis. 1998;26(5):1076–82.
30. von Muller L, Klemm A, Weiss M, Schneider M, Suger-Wiedeck H, Durmus N, et al. Active cytomegalovirus infection in patients with septic shock. Emerg Infect Dis. 2006;12(10):1517–22.
31. Domart Y, Trouillet JL, Fagon JY, Chastre J, Brun-Vezinet F, Gibert C. Incidence and morbidity of cytomegaloviral infection in patients with mediastinitis following cardiac surgery. Chest. 1990;97(1):18–22.
32. Soderberg-Naucler C, Fish KN, Nelson JA. Reactivation of latent human cytomegalovirus by allogeneic stimulation of blood cells from healthy donors. Cell. 1997;91(1):119–26.
33. Bowden RA, Sayers M, Flournoy N, Newton B, Banaji M, Thomas ED, et al. Cytomegalovirus immune globulin and seronegative blood products to prevent primary cytomegalovirus infection after marrow transplantation. N Engl J Med. 1986;314(16):1006–10.
34. Kalil AC, Florescu DF. Prevalence and mortality associated with cytomegalovirus infection in nonimmunosuppressed patients in the intensive care unit. Crit Care Med. 2009;37(8):2350–8.
35. Rafailidis PI, Mourtzoukou EG, Varbobitis IC, Falagas ME. Severe cytomegalovirus infection in apparently immunocompetent patients: a systematic review. Virol J. 2008;5:47.
36. Papazian L, Doddoli C, Chetaille B, Gernez Y, Thirion X, Roch A, et al. A contributive result of open-lung biopsy improves survival in acute respiratory distress syndrome patients. Crit Care Med. 2007;35(3):755–62.
37. Coisel Y, Bousbia S, Forel JM, Hraiech S, Lascola B, Roch A, et al. Cytomegalovirus and herpes simplex virus effect on the prognosis of mechanically ventilated patients suspected to have ventilator-associated pneumonia. PLoS One. 2012;7(12):e51340.
38. Heininger A, Haeberle H, Fischer I, Beck R, Riessen R, Rohde F, et al. Cytomegalovirus reactivation and associated outcome of critically ill patients with severe sepsis. Crit Care. 2011;15(2):R77.
39. Papazian L, Fraisse A, Garbe L, Zandotti C, Thomas P, Saux P, et al. Cytomegalovirus. An unexpected cause of ventilator-associated pneumonia. Anesthesiology. 1996;84(2):280–7.
40. Ong DS, Spitoni C, Klein Klouwenberg PM, Verduyn Lunel FM, Frencken JF, Schultz MJ, et al. Cytomegalovirus reactivation and mortality in patients with acute respiratory distress syndrome. Intensive Care Med. 2016;42(3):333–41.
41. Papazian L, Hraiech S, Lehingue S, Roch A, Chiche L, Wiramus S, et al. Cytomegalovirus reactivation in ICU patients. Intensive Care Med. 2016;42(1):28–37.
42. Chou S. Newer methods for diagnosis of cytomegalovirus infection. Rev Infect Dis. 1990;12(Suppl. 7):S727–36.
43. Lisboa LF, Asberg A, Kumar D, Pang X, Hartmann A, Preiksaitis JK, et al. The clinical utility of whole blood versus plasma cytomegalovirus viral load assays for monitoring therapeutic response. Transplantation. 2011;91(2):231–6.
44. Kalil AC, Levitsky J, Lyden E, Stoner J, Freifeld AG. Meta-analysis: the efficacy of strategies to prevent organ disease by cytomegalovirus in solid organ transplant recipients. Ann Intern Med. 2005;143(12):870–80.
45. Chanques G, Jaber S. Treating HSV and CMV reactivations in critically ill patients who are not immunocompromised: con. Intensive Care Med. 2014;40(12):1950–3.
46. Eddleston M, Peacock S, Juniper M, Warrell DA. Severe cytomegalovirus infection in immunocompetent patients. Clin Infect Dis. 1997;24(1):52–6.
47. Kalil AC, Florescu DF. Is cytomegalovirus reactivation increasing the mortality of patients with severe sepsis? Crit Care. 2011;15(2):138.
48. Forel JM, Martin-Loeches I, Luyt CE. Treating HSV and CMV reactivations in critically ill patients who are not immunocompromised: pro. Intensive Care Med. 2014;40(12):1945–9.
49. Florescu DF, Kalil AC. Cytomegalovirus infections in non-immunocompromised and immunocompromised patients in the intensive care unit. Infect Disord Drug Targets. 2011;11(4):354–64.
50. Docke WD, Prosch S, Fietze E, Kimel V, Zuckermann H, Klug C, et al. Cytomegalovirus reactivation and tumour necrosis factor. Lancet. 1994;343(8892):268–9.
51. Stephan F, Meharzi D, Ricci S, Fajac A, Clergue F, Bernaudin JF. Evaluation by polymerase chain reaction of cytomegalovirus reactivation in intensive care patients under mechanical ventilation. Intensive Care Med. 1996;22(11):1244–9.
52. Razonable RR, Fanning C, Brown RA, Espy MJ, Rivero A, Wilson J, et al. Selective reactivation of human herpesvirus 6 variant A occurs in critically ill immunocompetent hosts. J Infect Dis. 2002;185(1):110–3.
53. von Muller L, Klemm A, Durmus N, Weiss M, Suger-Wiedeck H, Schneider M, et al. Cellular immunity and active human cytomegalovirus infection in patients with septic shock. J Infect Dis. 2007;196(9):1288–95.
54. Chilet M, Aguilar G, Benet I, Belda J, Tormo N, Carbonell JA, et al. Virological and immunological features of active cytomegalovirus infection in nonimmunosuppressed patients in a surgical and trauma intensive care unit. J Med Virol. 2010;82(8):1384–91.
55. Smith CA, Conroy LT, Pollock M, Ruddy J, Binning A, McCruden EA. Detection of herpes viruses in respiratory secretions of patients undergoing artificial ventilation. J Med Virol. 2010;82(8):1406–9.
56. Bordes J, Maslin J, Prunet B, d'Aranda E, Lacroix G, Goutorbe P, et al. Cytomegalovirus infection in severe burn patients monitoring by real-time polymerase chain reaction: a prospective study. Burns. 2011;37(3):434–9.
57. De Vlieger G, Meersseman W, Lagrou K, Wouters P, Wilmer A, Peetermans WE, et al. Cytomegalovirus serostatus and outcome in nonimmunocompromised critically ill patients. Crit Care Med. 2012;40(1):36–42.
58. Ishioka H, Sanui M, Tsutsumi Y, Yanase F, Shiotsuka J. Low prevalence of active cytomegalovirus infection in a cardiovascular intensive care unit. J Intensive Care. 2014;2(1):12.
59. Walton AH, Muenzer JT, Rasche D, Boomer JS, Sato B, Brownstein BH, et al. Reactivation of multiple viruses in patients with sepsis. PLoS One. 2014;9(2):e98819.
60. Ong DS, Klein Klouwenberg PM, Verduyn Lunel FM, Spitoni C, Frencken JF, Dekker HA, et al. Cytomegalovirus seroprevalence as a risk factor for poor outcome in acute respiratory distress syndrome. Crit Care Med. 2015;43(2):394–400.

Permissions

All chapters in this book were first published in AIC, by Springer; hereby published with permission under the Creative Commons Attribution License or equivalent. Every chapter published in this book has been scrutinized by our experts. Their significance has been extensively debated. The topics covered herein carry significant findings which will fuel the growth of the discipline. They may even be implemented as practical applications or may be referred to as a beginning point for another development.

The contributors of this book come from diverse backgrounds, making this book a truly international effort. This book will bring forth new frontiers with its revolutionizing research information and detailed analysis of the nascent developments around the world.

We would like to thank all the contributing authors for lending their expertise to make the book truly unique. They have played a crucial role in the development of this book. Without their invaluable contributions this book wouldn't have been possible. They have made vital efforts to compile up to date information on the varied aspects of this subject to make this book a valuable addition to the collection of many professionals and students.

This book was conceptualized with the vision of imparting up-to-date information and advanced data in this field. To ensure the same, a matchless editorial board was set up. Every individual on the board went through rigorous rounds of assessment to prove their worth. After which they invested a large part of their time researching and compiling the most relevant data for our readers.

The editorial board has been involved in producing this book since its inception. They have spent rigorous hours researching and exploring the diverse topics which have resulted in the successful publishing of this book. They have passed on their knowledge of decades through this book. To expedite this challenging task, the publisher supported the team at every step. A small team of assistant editors was also appointed to further simplify the editing procedure and attain best results for the readers.

Apart from the editorial board, the designing team has also invested a significant amount of their time in understanding the subject and creating the most relevant covers. They scrutinized every image to scout for the most suitable representation of the subject and create an appropriate cover for the book.

The publishing team has been an ardent support to the editorial, designing and production team. Their endless efforts to recruit the best for this project, has resulted in the accomplishment of this book. They are a veteran in the field of academics and their pool of knowledge is as vast as their experience in printing. Their expertise and guidance has proved useful at every step. Their uncompromising quality standards have made this book an exceptional effort. Their encouragement from time to time has been an inspiration for everyone.

The publisher and the editorial board hope that this book will prove to be a valuable piece of knowledge for researchers, students, practitioners and scholars across the globe.

List of Contributors

Roosmarijn T. M. van Hooijdonk, Jan M. Binnekade and Janneke Horn
Department of Intensive Care Medicine, Academic Medical Center, University of Amsterdam, Meibergdreef 9, 1105 AZ Amsterdam, The Netherlands

Lieuwe D. J. Bos, Nicole P. Juffermans and Marcus J. Schultz
Department of Intensive Care Medicine, Academic Medical Center, University of Amsterdam, Meibergdreef 9, 1105 AZ Amsterdam, The Netherlands
Laboratory of Experimental Intensive Care and Anesthesiology (L·E·I·C·A), Academic Medical Center, University of Amsterdam, Amsterdam, The Netherlands

Ameen Abu-Hanna
Department of Medical Informatics, Academic Medical Center, University of Amsterdam, Amsterdam, The Netherlands

Kerstin Weidner
Department of Psychotherapy and Psychosomatic Medicine, Medizinische Fakultät Carl Gustav Carus, Technische Universität Dresden, Dresden, Germany

Gloria-Beatrice Wintermann
Department of Psychotherapy and Psychosomatic Medicine, Medizinische Fakultät Carl Gustav Carus, Technische Universität Dresden, Dresden, Germany
Center for Sepsis Control and Care, Jena University Hospital, Friedrich-Schiller University, Jena, Germany
Institute of Psychosocial Medicine and Psychotherapy, Jena University Hospital, Friedrich-Schiller University, Stoystr. 3,07743 Jena, Germany

Bernhard Strauß and Jenny Rosendah
Institute of Psychosocial Medicine and Psychotherapy, Jena University Hospital, Friedrich Schiller University, Stoystr. 3,07743 Jena, Germany

Katja Petrowski
Department of Workplace Health Promotion, German Sport University Cologne, Cologne, Germany

Yoanna Skrobik
Soins Intensifs, Hôpital Maisonneuve Rosemont, Montréal, QC H1T 2M4, Canada

Gerald Chanques
Intensive Care and Anaesthesiology Department (DAR), Saint Eloi Hospital, Montpellier University Hospital, 80, Avenue Augustin Fliche, Montpellier cedex 5 34295, France

Guillaume Grillet
Service des Maladies Infectieuses et Réanimation Médicale, CHU Rennes, 2 rue Henri Le Guilloux, 35033 Rennes, France

Pierre Bouju, Julien Letheulle and Pierre Fillatre
Service des Maladies Infectieuses et Réanimation Médicale, CHU Rennes, 2 rue Henri Le Guilloux, 35033 Rennes, France
Faculté de Médecine, Biosit, Université Rennes 1, 35043 Rennes, France

Angélique Goepp and Nicolas Barbarot
Réanimation polyvalente, CH Saint-Brieuc, 22000 Saint-Brieuc, France

Fabrice Uhel, Jean-Marc Tadié, Yves Le Tulzo and Arnaud Gacouin
Service des Maladies Infectieuses et Réanimation Médicale, CHU Rennes, 2 rue Henri Le Guilloux, 35033 Rennes, France
Faculté de Médecine, Biosit, Université Rennes 1, 35043 Rennes, France
Inserm-CIC-1414, Université Rennes I, IFRI 40, 35033 Rennes, France

Emeline Dubief and Tanissia Boukertouta
Service de Réanimation Médico-Chirurgicale, Hôpital Louis Mourier, AP-HP, 178 rue des Renouillers, 92700 Colombes, France

Stéphane Gaudry
Service de Réanimation Médico-Chirurgicale, Hôpital Louis Mourier, AP-HP, 178 rue des Renouillers, 92700 Colombes, France
ECEVE, UMRS 1123, Sorbonne Paris Cité, Univ Paris Diderot, Paris, France
ECEVE, U1123, CIC 1421, INSERM, Paris, France

Jonathan Messika, Jean-Damien Ricard and Didier Dreyfuss
Service de Réanimation Médico-Chirurgicale, Hôpital Louis Mourier, AP-HP, 178 rue des Renouillers, 92700 Colombes, France
IAME, UMR 1137, INSERM, 75018 Paris, France
IAME, UMR 1137, Sorbonne Paris Cité, Univ Paris Diderot, 75018 Paris, France

Sylvie Guillo
ECEVE, UMRS 1123, Sorbonne Paris Cité, Univ Paris Diderot, Paris, France
ECEVE, U1123, CIC 1421, INSERM, Paris, France
Département de Biostatistiques, Santé Publique et Informatique Médicale, CIC 1421, Hôpital Pitié Salpétrière, AP-HP, Paris, France
Unité de Recherche Clinique Paris Nord, Hôpital Bichat, AP-HP, Paris, France

Florence Tubach
ECEVE, UMRS 1123, Sorbonne Paris Cité, Univ Paris Diderot, Paris, France
ECEVE, U1123, CIC 1421, INSERM, Paris, France
Département de Biostatistiques, Santé Publique et Informatique Médicale, CIC 1421, Hôpital Pitié Salpétrière, AP-HP, Paris, France
Unité de Recherche Clinique Paris Nord, Hôpital Bichat, AP-HP, Paris, France
Université Pierre et Marie Curie, Sorbonne Universités, Paris, France

Blandine Pasquet
Département de Biostatistiques, Santé Publique et Informatique Médicale, CIC 1421, Hôpital Pitié Salpétrière, AP-HP, Paris, France
Unité de Recherche Clinique Paris Nord, Hôpital Bichat, AP-HP, Paris, France

Jaume Montanya
Centro de Investigación Biomédica En Red en Enfermedades Respiratorias (CIBERES), Instituto de Salud Carlos III, Madrid, Spain

Josefina Lopez-Aguilar and Rudys Magrans
Centro de Investigación Biomédica En Red en Enfermedades Respiratorias (CIBERES), Instituto de Salud Carlos III, Madrid, Spain
Institut d'Investigacióí Innovació Parc Taulí (I3PT), Fundació Parc Taulí, Sabadell, Spain

Joan Carles Oliva
Institut d'Investigacióí Innovació Parc Taulí (I3PT), Fundació Parc Taulí, Sabadell, Spain

Marc Turon
Centro de Investigación Biomédica En Red en Enfermedades Respiratorias (CIBERES), Instituto de Salud Carlos III, Madrid, Spain
Institut d'Investigacióí Innovació Parc Taulí (I3PT), Fundació Parc Taulí, Sabadell, Spain
Department of Clinical and Health Psychology, Universitat Autònoma de Barcelona, International Excellence Campus, Bellaterra, Spain

Lluís Blanch
Centro de Investigación Biomédica En Red en Enfermedades Respiratorias (CIBERES), Instituto de Salud Carlos III, Madrid, Spain
Institut d'Investigacióí Innovació Parc Taulí (I3PT), Fundació Parc Taulí, Sabadell, Spain
Critical Care Department, Parc Taulí Hospital Universitari, Institut d'Investigació i Innovació Parc Taulí (I3PT), Universitat Autònoma de Barcelona, Sabadell, Spain

Sol Fernandez-Gonzalo
Institut d'Investigacióí Innovació Parc Taulí (I3PT), Fundació Parc Taulí, Sabadell, Spain
Centro de Investigación Biomédica En Red en Salud Mental (CIBERSAM), Instituto de Salud Carlos III, Madrid, Spain

Mercè Jodar
Department of Clinical and Health Psychology, Universitat Autònoma de Barcelona, International Excellence Campus, Bellaterra, Spain
Centro de Investigación Biomédica En Red en Salud Mental (CIBERSAM), Instituto de Salud Carlos III, Madrid, Spain
Neurology Department, Parc Taulí Hospital Universitari, Institut d'Investigació i Innovació Parc Taulí (I3PT), Universitat Autònoma de Barcelona, Sabadell, Spain

Candelaria de Haro and Victor Gomez-Simon
Critical Care Department, Parc Taulí Hospital Universitari, Institut d'Investigació i Innovació Parc Taulí (I3PT), Universitat Autònoma de Barcelona, Sabadell, Spain

Gemma Gomà
Institut d'Investigacióí Innovació Parc Taulí (I3PT), Fundació Parc Taulí, Sabadell, Spain
Critical Care Department, Parc Taulí Hospital Universitari, Institut d'Investigació i Innovació Parc Taulí (I3PT), Universitat Autònoma de Barcelona, Sabadell, Spain

David Hernando and Raquel Bailón
BSICOS Group, I3A, Universidad de Zaragoza&CIBER-BBN, Saragossa, Spain

Melcior Martinez-Perez
Centro de Investigación Biomédica En Red en Enfermedades Respiratorias (CIBERES), Instituto de Salud Carlos III, Madrid, Spain
Critical Care Department, Parc Taulí Hospital Universitari, Institut d'Investigació i Innovació Parc Taulí (I3PT), Universitat Autònoma de Barcelona, Sabadell, Spain

Dong-kai Li, Xiao-ting Wang and Da-wei Liu
Department of Critical Care Medicine, Peking Union Medical College Hospital, Peking Union Medical College, Chinese Academy of Medical Science, 1 Shuaifuyuan, Dongcheng District, Beijing 100730, China

S. R. Hamada, A. Harrois, S. Figueiredo and J. Duranteau
Department of Anaesthesia and Critical Care, AP-HP, Hôpital Bicêtre, Hôpitaux Universitaires Paris Sud, University Paris-Sud, 78 rue du Général Leclerc, 94275 Le Kremlin Bicêtre, France

C. Espina
Department of Anaesthesia and Critical Care, AP-HP, Hôpital Cochin, Hôpitaux Universitaires Paris Centre, University Paris Descartes, 27 Rue du Faubourg Saint-Jacques, 75014 Paris, France

T. Guedj and R. Buaron
Department of Radiology, Hôpital Bicêtre, Hôpitaux Universitaires Paris Sud, University Paris-Sud, 78 rue du Général Leclerc, 94275 Le Kremlin Bicêtre, France

Laura Van Coile
Faculty of Medicine and Health Sciences, Ghent University, Ghent, Belgium

Alexander Decruyenaere
Faculty of Medicine and Health Sciences, Ghent University, Ghent, Belgium
Department of Internal Medicine, Ghent University Hospital, Ghent, Belgium

Astrid Van den broecke, Kirsten Colpaert, Dominique Benoit and Johan Decruyenaere
Faculty of Medicine and Health Sciences, Ghent University, Ghent, Belgium
Department of Intensive Care Medicine, Ghent University Hospital, De Pintelaan 185, 9000 Ghent, Belgium

Hans Van Vlierberghe
Faculty of Medicine and Health Sciences, Ghent University, Ghent, Belgium
Department of Hepatology and Gastro-Enterology, Ghent University Hospital, Ghent, Belgium

Dana Y. Fuhrman
Children's Hospital of Pittsburgh, 4401 Penn Avenue, Children's Hospital Drive, Faculty Pavilion Suite 2000, Pittsburgh, PA 15224, USA

Sandra Kane-Gill
School of Pharmacy, University of Pittsburgh, 638 Salk Hall, 3501 Terrace Street, Pittsburgh, PA 15261, USA

Stuart L. Goldstein
Center for Acute Care Nephrology, Cincinnati Children's Hospital Medical Center, 3333 Burnet Avenue, Cincinnati, OH 45229, USA

Priyanka Priyanka and John A. Kellum
The Center for Critical Care Nephrology, 3347 Forbes Avenue, Ste 220, Pittsburgh, PA 15213, USA

François Vincent
Medical-Surgical Intensive Care Unit, Le Raincy-Montfermeil General Hospital, 10, rue du Général Leclerc, 93370 Montfermeil, France

Marcio Soares
D'Or Institute for Research and Education, Rio de Janeiro, Brazil
Programa de Pós-Graduação em Oncologia, Instituto Nacional de Câncer, Rio de Janeiro, Brazil

Djamel Mokart
Anesthesiology and Intensive Care Unit, Paoli Calmette Institute, Marseille, France

Virginie Lemiale and Michaël Darmon
Medical Intensive Care Unit, Saint-Louis University Hospital, AP-HP, Paris, France

Fabrice Bruneel
Medical-Surgical Intensive Care Unit, Mignot Hospital, Le Chesnay, France

Marouane Boubaya
Clinical Research Unit, Avicenne University Hospital, AP-HP, Bobigny, France

Frédéric Gonzalez and Yves Cohen
Medical-Surgical Intensive Care Unit, Avicenne University Hospital, AP-HP, Bobigny, France

Elie Azoulay
ECSTRA Team, Biostatistics and Clinical Epidemiology, UMR 1153 (Center of Epidemiology and Biostatistics, Sorbonne Paris Cité, CRESS), INSERM, Paris Diderot Sorbonne University, Paris, France

Richard Brunner, Christian Zauner, Michael Trauner and Bruno Schneeweiss
Division of Gastroenterology and Hepatology, Department of Internal Medicine III, Medical University of Vienna, Vienna, Austria

Andreas Drolz, Thomas Horvatits, Kevin Roedl, Karoline Rutter and Valentin Fuhrmann
Division of Gastroenterology and Hepatology, Department of Internal Medicine III, Medical University of Vienna, Vienna, Austria
Department of Intensive Care Medicine, University Medical Center, Hamburg-Eppendorf, Martinistraße 52, 20246 Hamburg, Germany

Peter Schellongowski
Division of Oncology and Infectious Diseases, Department of Internal Medicine I, Medical University of Vienna, Vienna, Austria

Gottfried Heinz
Division of Cardiology, Department of Internal Medicine II, Medical University of Vienna, Vienna, Austria

Georg-Christian Funk
Department of Respiratory and Critical Care Medicine, and Ludwig Boltzmann Institute for COPD, Otto-Wagner Hospital, Vienna, Austria

Karim Jaffal
Critical Care Center, CHU Lille, 59000 Lille, France

Julien Poissy, Anahita Rouze, Sébastien Preau and Saad Nseir
Critical Care Center, CHU Lille, 59000 Lille, France
U995-LIRIC-Lille Inflammation Research International Center, Univ. Lille, 59000 Lille, France
Inserm, U995, 59000 Lille, France

Boualem Sendid and Marjorie Cornu
U995-LIRIC-Lille Inflammation Research International Center, Univ. Lille, 59000 Lille, France
Inserm, U995, 59000 Lille, France
Laboratory of Mycology and Parasitology, CHU Lille, 59000 Lille, France

Claudia Scorcella, Elisa Damiani, Roberta Domizi, Silvia Pierantozzi, Stefania Tondi, Andrea Carsetti, Silvia Ciucani, Valentina Monaldi, Mara Rogani, Benedetto Marini, Erica Adrario, Rocco Romano and Abele Donati
Anaesthesia and Intensive Care, Department of Biomedical Sciences and Public Health, Università Politecnica delle Marche, via Tronto 10/a, 60126 Ancona, Italy

Can Ince
Department of Translational Physiology, Academic Medical Centre, University of Amsterdam, Meibergdreef 9, 1105 AZ Amsterdam, The Netherlands

E. Christiaan Boerma
Department of Intensive Care, Medical Centre Leeuwarden, Henri Dunantweg 2, 8934 AD Leeuwarden, The Netherlands

Ulrich Mayr, Leonie Fahrenkrog-Petersen, Gonzalo Batres-Baires, Alexander Herner, Sebastian Rasch, Roland M. Schmid, Wolfgang Huber and Tobias Lahmer
Klinik und Poliklinik für Innere Medizin II, Klinikum rechts der Isar, Technische Universität München, Ismaninger Strasse 22, 81675 Munich, Germany

Xiukai Chen
Pittsburgh Heart, Lung, Blood and Vascular Medicine Institute, University of Pittsburgh, 200 Lothrop Street, BST E1240, Pittsburgh, PA 15261, USA

Xiaoting Wang and Dawei Liu
Department of Critical Care Medicine, Peking Union Medical College Hospital, Peking Union Medical College, Chinese Academy of Medical Sciences, 1 Shuaifuyuan, Dongcheng District, Beijing 100073, China

Patrick M. Honore
Department of Intensive Care, Centre Hospitalier Universitaire Brugmann, Brugmann University Hospital, 4 Place Van Gehuchtenplein, 1020 Brussels, Belgium

Herbert D. Spapen
Department of Intensive Care, University Hospital, Vrije Universiteit Brussel (VUB), 101, Laarbeeklaan, Jette 1090 Brussels, Belgium

Christian Niederwanger, Andreas Entenmann and Agnes Balog
Department of Pediatrics, Pediatrics I, Medical University of Innsbruck, Anichstrasse 35, 6020 Innsbruck, Austria

Mirjam Bachler
Institute for Sports Medicine, Alpine Medicine and Health Tourism, UMIT - University for Health Sciences, Medical Informatics and Technology, Eduard Wallnöfer Zentrum 1, 6060 Hall in Tirol, Austria

Tobias Hell
Department of Mathematics, Faculty of Mathematics, Computer Science and Physics, University of Innsbruck, Technikerstraße 13, 6020 Innsbruck, Austria

Caroline Linhart
Department of Medical Statistics, Informatics and Health Economics, Medical University of Innsbruck, Anichstrasse 35, 6020 Innsbruck, Austria

Katharina Auer
Department of General and Surgical Critical Care Medicine, Medical University of Innsbruck, Anichstrasse 35, 6020 Innsbruck, Austria

Petra Innerhofer
Department of Anaesthesiology and Critical Care Medicine, Medical University of Innsbruck, Anichstrasse 35, 6020 Innsbruck, Austria

Bertrand Guidet
Assistance Publique - Hôpitaux de Paris (AP-HP), Service de Réanimation Médicale, Hôpital Saint-Antoine, 184 rue du Faubourg Saint-Antoine, 75012 Paris, France
Sorbonne Universités, Université Pierre et Marie Curie - Paris 06, Paris, France
INSERM, UMR_S 1136, Institute Pierre Louis d'Épidémiologie et de Santé Publique, 75013 Paris, France

Helene Vallet
INSERM, UMR_S 1136, Institute Pierre Louis d'Épidémiologie et de Santé Publique, 75013 Paris, France
Assistance Publique - Hôpitaux de Paris (AP-HP), Service de gériatrie, Hôpital Pitié salpêtrière, 75013 Paris, France

Jacques Boddaert
Sorbonne Universités, Université Pierre et Marie Curie - Paris 06, Paris, France
Assistance Publique - Hôpitaux de Paris (AP-HP), Service de gériatrie, Hôpital Pitié salpêtrière, 75013 Paris, France

Dylan W. de Lange
Department of Intensive Care, University Medical Center Utrecht, University Utrecht, Utrecht, The Netherlands

Alessandro Morandi
Department of Rehabilitation Hospital Ancelle di Cremona, Cremona, Italy
Geriatric Research Group, Brescia, Italy

Guillaume Leblanc
Division of Critical Care Medicine, Department of Anesthesiology and Critical Care Medicine, Université Laval, Québec City, QC, Canada
Centre de recherche du CHU de Québec – Université Laval, Population Health and Optimal Health Practices Research Unit (Trauma – Emergency – Critical Care Medicine), Université Laval, Québec City, QC, Canada

Antonio Artigas
Department of Intensive Care Medecine, CIBER Enfermedades Respiratorias, Corporacion Sanitaria Universitaria Parc Tauli, Autonomous University of Barcelona, Sabadell, Spain

Hans Flaatten
Department of Anaesthesia and Intensive Care, Haukeland University Hospital, Bergen, Norway
Department of Clinical Medicine, University of Bergen, Bergen, Norway

Flora Cipriani, Laurent Camous, Pierre Sentenac, Martin Dres, Nadia Anguel, Christian Richard and Jean-Louis Teboul
Service de réanimation médicale, Hôpital de Bicêtre, Hôpitaux universitaires Paris-Sud, 78, rue du Général Leclerc, 94270 Le Kremlin-Bicêtre, France
Faculté de médecine Paris-Sud, Inserm UMR S_999, Univ Paris-Sud, 63, rue Gabriel Péri, 94270 Le Kremlin-Bicêtre, France

Evguenia Krastinova
Faculté de médecine Paris-Sud, Inserm UMR S_999, Univ Paris-Sud, 63, rue Gabriel Péri, 94270 Le Kremlin-Bicêtre, France
Service de santé publique, Hôpital de Bicêtre, Hôpitaux universitaires Paris-Sud, 78, rue du Général Leclerc, 94270 Le Kremlin-Bicêtre, France

Xavier Monnet
Service de réanimation médicale, Hôpital de Bicêtre, Hôpitaux universitaires Paris-Sud, 78, rue du Général Leclerc, 94270 Le Kremlin-Bicêtre, France
Faculté de médecine Paris-Sud, Inserm UMR S_999, Univ Paris-Sud, 63, rue Gabriel Péri, 94270 Le Kremlin-Bicêtre, France
Service de réanimation médicale, Centre Hospitalier Universitaire de Bicêtre, 78, rue du Général Leclerc, 94270 Le Kremlin-Bicêtre, France

Emilie Greau, Jean-Baptiste Lascarrou, Nathalie Maquigneau, Yolaine Alcourt, Anne Coutolleau, Cécile Rousseau and Vanessa Erragne
Medical-Surgical Intensive Care Unit, District Hospital Center, La Roche-sur-Yon, France

Aurélie Le Thuaut
Clinical Research Unit, District Hospital Center, La Roche-sur-Yon, France
Délégation à la Recherche Clinique et à l'Innovation, CHU Hôtel Dieu, 44093 Nantes Cedex, France

Jean Reignier
Medical-Surgical Intensive Care Unit, District Hospital Center, La Roche-sur-Yon, France
UPRES EA-3826, Clinical and Experimental Therapies for Infections, University of Nantes, Nantes, France
Medical Intensive Care Unit, Nantes University Hospital, Nantes, France

Roosmarijn TM van Hooijdonk and Tineke Winters
Department of Intensive Care, Academic Medical Center, University of Amsterdam, Room, Meibergdreef 9, 1105 AZ, Amsterdam, the Netherlands

Johan C Fischer and Edmée C van Dongen-Lases
Department of Clinical Chemistry, Academic Medical Center, University of Amsterdam, Amsterdam, the Netherlands

James S Krinsley
Division of Critical Care, Stamford Hospital, Columbia University College of Physicians and Surgeons, Stamford, CT, USA

Jean-Charles Preiser
Department of Intensive Care, Erasme University Hospital, Brussels, Belgium

Marcus J Schultz
Department of Intensive Care, Academic Medical Center, University of Amsterdam, Room, Meibergdreef 9, 1105 AZ, Amsterdam, the Netherlands
Laboratory of Experimental Intensive Care and Anesthesiology (LEICA), Academic Medical Center, University of Amsterdam, Amsterdam, the Netherlands

Awad Al-Omari
Critical Care and Infection Control Department, Dr. Sulaiman Al Habib Medical Group, Riyadh, Saudi Arabia
AlFaisal University, Riyadh, Saudi Arabia

Fadi Aljamaan
Intensive Care Department, King Khalid University Hospital, King Saud University Medical City, King Saud University, Riyadh, Saudi Arabia

Waleed Alhazzani
Department of Medicine, McMaster University, Hamilton, Canada

Samer Salih
Department of Internal Medicine, Dr. Sulaiman Al Habib Medical Group, Riyadh, Saudi Arabia

Yaseen Arabi
Intensive Care Department, King Abdullah International Medical Research Center, King Saud Bin Abdulaziz University for Health Sciences, Riyadh, Saudi Arabia

Index

www.ingramcontent.com/pod-product-compliance
Lightning Source LLC
LaVergne TN
LVHW080716210926
848485LV00003B/472
* 9 7 8 1 6 3 9 2 7 1 0 1 6 *